W9-DDG-172

Color
Atlas of
Pediatric
Dermatology

Color Atlas of
Pediatric Dermatology

Third Edition

Samuel Weinberg, M.D., F.A.A.P., F.A.C.P.
Clinical Professor of Dermatology
New York University Medical Center
New York, New York

Neil S. Prose, M.D., F.A.A.P.
Associate Professor of Medicine
(Dermatology) and Pediatrics
Duke University Medical Center
Durham, North Carolina

Leonard Kristal, M.D., F.A.A.P.
Clinical Assistant Professor of Dermatology and Pediatrics
State University of New York at Stony Brook
Chief, Pediatric Dermatology
Schneider Children's Hospital
Long Island Jewish Medical Center
New Hyde Park, New York

McGraw-Hill
HEALTH PROFESSIONS DIVISION

New York   St. Louis   San Francisco   Auckland   Bogotá   Caracas   Lisbon   London
Madrid   Mexico City   Milan   Montreal   New Delhi   San Juan
Singapore   Sydney   Tokyo   Toronto

McGraw-Hill

*A Division of The **McGraw·Hill** Companies*

Color Atlas of Pediatric Dermatology

4567891011 QPKQPK 098765432

ISBN 0-07-069249-1

This book was set in Times Roman by York Graphic Services, Inc.
The editors were Martin Wonsiewicz and Lester A. Sheinis.
The production supervisor was Richard C. Ruzycka.
The cover designer was Marsha Cohen/Parallelogram.
The indexer was Alexandra Nickerson.
Quebecor Printing/Kingsport was printer and binder.
This book is printed on acid-free paper.

Library of Congress Cataloging-in-Publication Data

Weinberg, Samuel, date.
    Color atlas of pediatric dermatology / Samuel Weinberg, Neil S.
Prose, Leonard Kristal.—3d ed.
        p.   cm.
    Includes bibliographical references and index.
    ISBN 0-07-069249-1
    1. Pediatric dermatology—Atlases.   I. Prose, Neil S.
II. Shapiro, Lewis.   III. Title.
    [DNLM: 1. Skin Diseases—in infancy & childhood—atlases.   WS 17
W423c 1997]
RJ511.W44   1997
618.92′5′00222—dc21
DNLM/DLC
for Library of Congress   97-42667
                                                                            CIP

To the late Dr. Maurice J. Costello, mentor, friend, and inspiration; and to Pearl, for all her patience in helping this book to fruition.

S.W.

To my mother, Jessie Rubin.

N.P.

To Sam Weinberg and Paul Honig, two great teachers and colleagues; and to Manda, my parents, and my children, for their unending love and support.

L.K.

Credits for Photographs

Arturo Aballi
A. Bernard Ackerman
J. O'D. Alexander
William G. Ballinger
Charles S. Baraf
Robert Baron
Alexander G. Bearn
Jerrold M. Becker
Bernard W. Berger
Eugene L. Bodian
Martin H. Brownstein
Philip Charney
Platon J. Collipp
Maurice J. Costello
Vincent Derbes
Anthony N. Domonkos
Lawrence Eichenfeld
Leon Eisenbud
Nancy B. Esterly
Robert P. Feinstein
Ilona J. Frieden

Alexander A. Fisher
Robert W. Goltz
Ralph W. Grover
Paul Honig
Jonathan Horwitz
Sidney Hurwitz
Kathleen L. Hussey
Josef E. Jelinek
S. Wayne Klein
Irwin H. Krasna
Jose Kriner
Saul Krugman
Teresita A. Laude
Lawrence Leiblich
Chester M. Lessenden, Jr.
Luther B. Lowe
John McSorley
Seth J. Orlow
Lamar S. Osment
John R. T. Reeves
Perry Robins

Victor Torres Rodriguez
Avron Ross
James P. Rotchford
Wiley M. Sams
Arthur Sawitsky
Lawrence A. Schachner
Keith M. Schneider
Edward Shapiro
Meyer H. Slatkin
Roy Stephens
Conrad Stritzler
Ronald Stritzler
Joel A. Teisch
Louis Tobin
Donald Waldorf
William A. Welton
Zelma Wessely
Constance Y. Wong
Alex W. Young, Jr.
Erwin Zimmerman

Department of Dermatology, College of Physicians and Surgeons, Columbia University

New York University School of Medicine (Skin and Cancer Unit) permitted use of photographs for the following figures: 16, 62, 73, 78, 96, 183, 185, 224, 233, 234, 235, 238, 240, 243, 247, 284, 321, 322, 323, 330, 332, 337, 338, 354, 357, 358, 367, 370, 376, 388, 395, 396, 403, 405, 432, 449, 464, 466, 469, 472, 480, 483, 528, 562, 607, 626, 645, 694, 715, 741, 770, 803, 815, 832, 834, 841, 853, 855

The following figures have been used with permission:

Figure 34: I. J. Frieden, N. S. Prose, V. Fletcher, and M. L. Turner, "Granulomatous Perioral Dermatitis in Children." Copyright © 1989, American Medical Association. *Archives of Dermatology* 125:369–373, 1989. **Figures 473** and **474:** Ilona J. Frieden and Nancy B. Esterly, "Selected Granulomatoses in Infants and Children." Copyright © 1988 by Lippincott/Harper & Row, *Clinics in Dermatology,* Vol. 3, No. 1, Jan.–Mar., 1988, p. 22. **Figures 584, 591,** and **592:** *Journal of the American Academy of Dermatology.* **Figure 586:** *Pediatric Dermatology* 4:67–74, 1987. **Figures 587** and **590:** *Advances in Dermatology.*

Contents

Section 9   Papulosquamous, Lichenoid, and Perforating Disorders   Page 87

Section 10   Nutritional and Metabolic Disorders   Page 105

Section 27   Miscellaneous Anomalies   Page 255

Preface

Twenty-three years have passed since the publication of the first edition of this color atlas. Eight years ago a second edition was published to represent the explosion of knowledge in the field of pediatric dermatology.

Since the second edition many exciting advances have taken place that have influenced pediatric dermatology. The greater sophistication of molecular genetic techniques has enabled us to identify specific genetic defects in many genodermatoses, such as neurofibromatosis type 1 and nonbullous ichthyosiform erythroderma. New viruses have been identified to be the causes of previously unexplained exanthems, such as human parvovirus B19, which causes erythema infectiosum, and human herpes viruses 6 and 7, which cause roseola infantum. New disease entities such as palmoplantar eccrine hidradenitis and unilateral laterothoracic exanthem continue to be identified and described.

The text of the third edition of the atlas bears the indelible imprint of the late Dr. Morris Leider, a coauthor of the first edition. His warmth, wit, dermatologic knowledge, and dedication to the precise and imaginative use of the English language can be appreciated in the several passages that have been left intact. The connoisseur of his unique writing style will immediately recognize his continued literacy influence in the humorous discussions of insect "bites" and branchial-cleft cysts.

The format of this atlas allows for only a brief discussion of the etiology and clinical appearance of each disease entity. We have also tried to include some very basic therapeutic suggestions. We ask the reader to bear in mind that this volume is not a textbook and that it should be used in conjunction with one of the several comprehensive references on pediatric dermatology. It is our hope that this atlas will be of practical use to all health practitioners who are involved in the care of children.

*Color
Atlas of*
Pediatric
Dermatology

1

Benign Neonatal Dermatoses

Figure 1

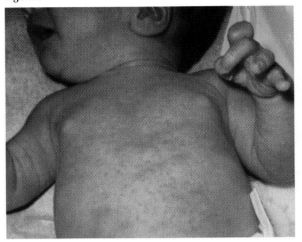

Figure 2

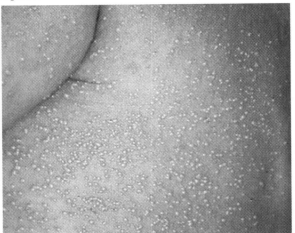

Erythema toxicum neonatorum This very common and completely benign condition usually arises in the first 2 days of life. It is seen in about half of healthy newborns and occurs less frequently in preterm infants. The lesions are erythematous macules, within which papules and pustules may develop. The trunk is the most common site, but all other body surfaces, except for the palms and soles, may be involved. The eruption in Fig. 1 began 2 hours after delivery and involved the face and trunk. The eruption in Fig. 2 was unusual in that it was so widespread and vesiculopustular. Occasionally, this unimportant eruption must be differentiated from more serious infectious processes, such as neonatal herpes simplex. Tzanck smear of a pustule of erythema toxicum neonatorum will reveal numerous eosinophils but no multinucleated giant cells or bacteria. Occasionally, peripheral eosinophilia is also present. The cause of this condition is not known, and it resolves spontaneously within 10 days. No treatment is required.

Figure 3

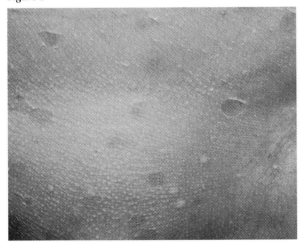

Figure 4

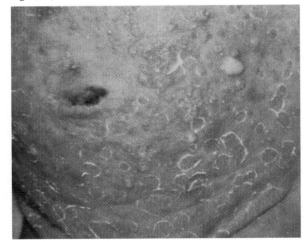

Transient neonatal pustular melanosis This is a benign neonatal dermatosis that is most common among African-American infants. The original lesion is a vesiculopustule, which may be present at birth. This small blister quickly ruptures and leaves a typical collarette of superficial scale. Both intact pustules and collarettes are seen in the newborn in Fig. 3. Figure 4 shows the brownish pigmented macules that develop at the site of each resolving pustule. These macules may be sparse or numerous and resolve without residua over a period of several weeks to several months. In some infants, the pustule and collarette stages seem to occur in utero, and the sole cutaneous manifestations are the typical macules. Lesions of transient neonatal pustular melanosis favor the forehead, neck, chin, and lower back but may be very widespread and may involve the palms and soles. Scraping the base of an unroofed pustule reveals polymorphonuclear leukocytes but no bacteria, pseudohyphae, or multinucleated giant cells. A biopsy of a pustule, which is rarely necessary, shows an intraepidermal collection of polymorphonuclear leukocytes.

2

Milia, Miliaria, and Pustular and Acneiform Disorders

Figure 5

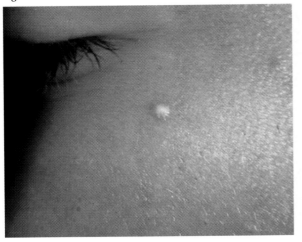

Figure 6

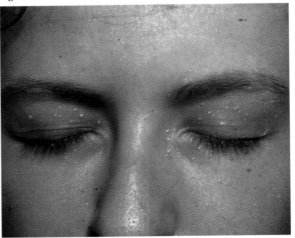

Milia   A milium is a white papule, 1–2 mm in size, composed of laminated, keratinous material and situated as a solid cyst in a pilosebaceous follicle. Milia are fairly common on the brow, glabella, and nose in newborn infants and in such infants tend to disappear quickly and spontaneously. There may be few or many, and they may develop later in infancy, in childhood, and in adolescence. In older children and adolescents, they tend to persist, may precede acne or be associated with incipient acne,

and commonly develop on or about the eyelids. Milia may be ablated, if desirable, by delicate incision and expression of their keratinous content. Lesions so treated do not recur, but if new lesions appear, they have to be treated in the same way. The operation is trivial and uncomplicated. There are no preventive measures. When acne is associated, it is the more serious and difficult condition to manage.

Figure 7

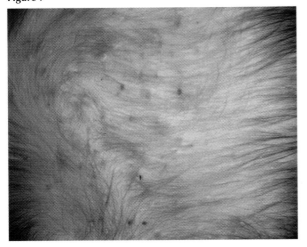

Figure 8

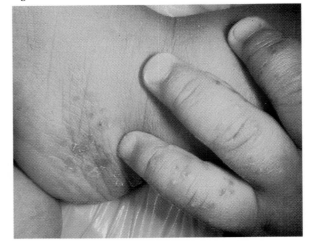

Eosinophilic pustular folliculitis of infancy   Children with this rare disorder develop repeated crops of pruritic yellow or white pustules, which vary in size from 1 to 3 mm. Most lesions are located on the scalp and distal extremities. Tzanck smear reveals numerous eosinophils, and there may also be a peripheral eosinohilia. Eosinophilic pustular folliculitis is associated with no systemic symptoms and eventually resolves spontaneously. Therapy with topical steroids is somewhat beneficial.

Infantile acropustulosis   This cutaneous disorder is characterized by recurrent episodes of intensely pruritic pustules and papulovesicles on the hands and feet. Lesions are most common on the palms and soles but may be seen on the dorsal surfaces as well. Lesions may also occur on the ankles, forearms, and, rarely, the face, scalp, and upper trunk. The age at onset is typically between 2 and 10 months.

Figure 9

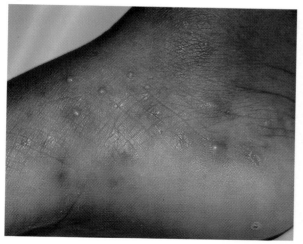

Figure 10

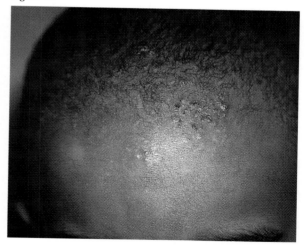

Infantile acropustulosis Individual episodes last for 7 to 10 days and may recur as often as every 2 weeks at the beginning of the disease and tend to become less frequent and severe over time. The disease resolves spontaneously by 2 to 3 years of age. Stained smears of an individual lesion will reveal numerous neutrophils, although eosinophils may be present early in the course of the disorder.

Infantile acropustulosis This photograph shows involvement of the forehead in a patient with infantile acropustulosis. The individual lesions in this condition resolve with scale and post-inflammatory hyperpigmentation. Infantile acropustulosis may be seen after scabies infestation in infants ("postscabies syndrome").

Figure 11

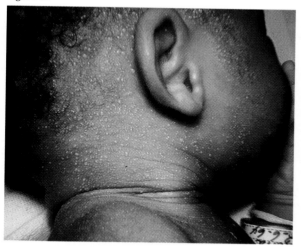

Figure 12

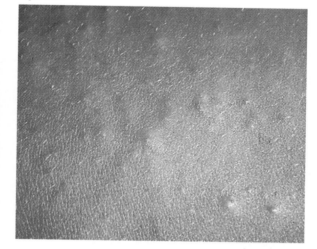

Miliaria crystallina The lesions in this condition are small, clear, thin-roofed vesicles that develop when the sweat duct is obstructed within the stratum corneum. They occur after sunburn or in response to excessive sweating in high environmental heat and humidity. Fever may also be a cause. The scalp, face, trunk, and intertriginous areas are sites of lesions. Itching is not a symptom. The vesicles resolve rapidly with the elimination of the causative environmental factor.

Miliaria rubra (prickly heat) This is the most common form of miliaria. It occurs when there is plugging of the eccrine ducts within the malpighian layer and release of sweat into the adjacent skin. Miliaria rubra is characterized by discrete erythematous papules and papulovesicles. The forehead, upper trunk, and intertriginous areas are commonly affected. Unlike miliaria crystallina, miliaria rubra is characterized by spasmodic pricking sensations. A decrease in environmental heat and humidity is the only treatment required.

Figure 13

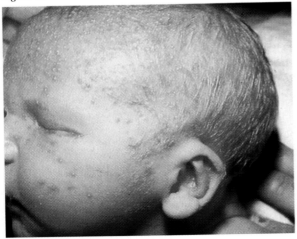

Figure 14

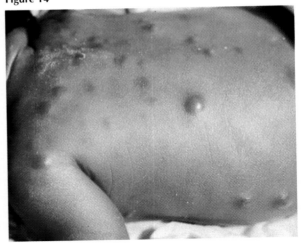

Miliaria pustulosa   Progression from miliaria rubra to miliaria pustulosa is related to duration of sweat-duct occlusion, the amount of sweat retention, and the degree of inflammation around the ducts. In affected patients one sees the typical erythematous papules of miliaria rubra and, in addition, lesions that are frankly pustular. Although this condition may resemble a bacterial pyoderma, it responds well to the appropriate adjustment in environmental heat and humidity.

Multiple sweat-gland abscesses (miliaria profunda)   The forms of miliaria described above are limited to the portion of the sweat apparatus within the epidermis. Occasionally, obstruction of deeper portions of the sweat glands (the dermal ducts and coils) results in spillage of sweat into the dermis, inflammation, and secondary infection. The resultant abscesses are firm and are slow to resolve by spontaneous rupture and discharge to the surface.

Figure 15

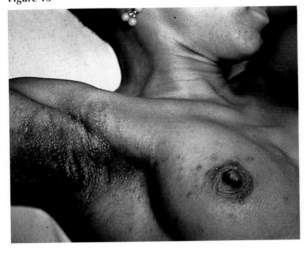

Figure 16

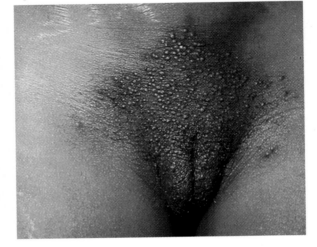

Fox-Fordyce disease (apocrine miliaria)   This chronic and intensely pruritic papular eruption is localized to the axillae, areolae, and pubic areas. It occurs almost exclusively in young women, frequently with onset during adolescence. The follicular papules result from the obstruction of the intraepidermal sweat duct, with release of apocrine sweat into the surrounding skin. Figure 15 shows the process in an axilla; Fig. 16 shows it in the pubic area. The etiology of Fox-Fordyce disease is unknown, and treatment is difficult. Topical and intralesional corticosteroids, estrogen therapy, and antimicrobial therapy are sometimes helpful.

Figure 17

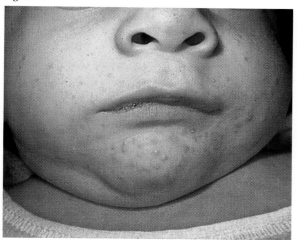

Figure 18

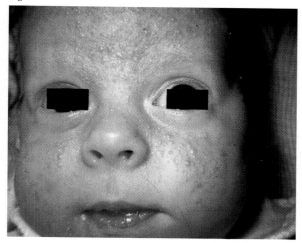

Neonatal and infantile acne   Mild comedonal acne is fairly common in the newborn. The typical eruption consists of closed comedones. Open comedones, inflammatory papules and pustules, and small cysts may also occur. Neonatal acne is attributed to the stimulation of sebaceous glands by androgens from both mother and infant. The lesions of neonatal acne usually resolve during the first few months of life. Acne, in varying degrees of severity, may also appear in infants after the neonatal period. This form of infantile acne may persist for 1 or 2 years and may rarely eventuate in scarring. Children with early onset of acne and a strong family history are particularly at risk for a severe course of the disease during puberty. Most cases of neonatal and infantile acne do not require treatment. If necessary, a mild benzoyl peroxide solution may be used.

Figure 19

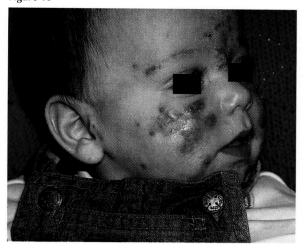

Infantile cystic acne   Comedones generally predominate in infantile acne, although more inflammatory papules and pustules may be seen. Rarely, an infant may develop cystic nodules, as seen in this photograph, that occasionally heal with scarring. Infants with severe acne should be evaluated for sexual precocity or abnormal virilization.

Figure 20

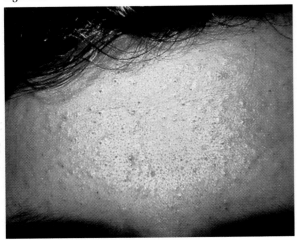

Figure 21

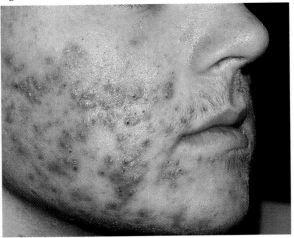

Acne vulgaris   The common varieties of acne generally begin to develop in late childhood or early adolescence. The earliest lesions are open or closed comedones, and these may progress to inflammatory papules, pustules, and cysts. Figure 20 shows the comedo stage, and Fig. 21, the beginning of progression to inflammatory papules and pustules. Acne during adolescence is caused by the effect of androgenic hormones on the pilosebaceous unit. The increased activity of the sebaceous gland pro-

vides a substrate for *Propionibacterium acnes,* whose lipolytic enzymes convert triglycerides in sebum to free fatty acids. This primary irritant causes the formation of comedones. Abnormal keratinization in the pilosebaceous follicle also plays a role in the development of acne. Topical therapies are aimed at decreasing skin colonization by *P. acnes* (topical antibiotics) and at normalizing keratinization within the follicle (tretinoin).

Figure 22

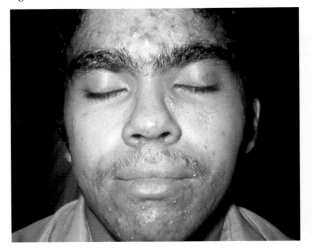

Figure 23

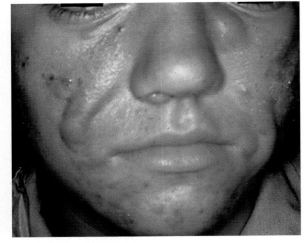

Cystic acne   Many cases of acne progress from open and closed comedones (blackheads and whiteheads) to inflammatory forms that are marked by papules, pustules, and cysts. Figure 22 shows a combination of these. Severe cystic acne is more difficult to control or cure and causes scarring. Topical therapy with combinations of antibiotics and tretinoin is of value. In addition, systemic antibiotics, such as tetracycline and erythromycin, are useful because of their antibacterial and anti-inflammatory properties. The intralesional injection of corticosteroids may also be helpful.

Acne conglobata   In conglobate acne, the most severe form of acne, cysts tend to be large, irregular, and intercommunicating and tend to result in severe scarring. Severe cystic acne can sometimes be controlled with topical therapy and systemic antibiotics. The patient who does not respond to these measures may be a candidate for 13-*cis*-retinoic acid. Side effects of this therapy range from dry lips and skin to elevation of cholesterol and triglycerides. In addition, all female patients must be advised that 13-*cis*-retinoic acid is a potent teratogen and that pregnancy must be avoided.

Figure 24

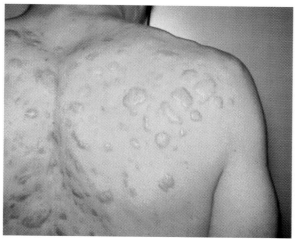

Keloids following acne Hypertrophic scars and keloids following resolution of inflammatory lesions of acne are an uncommon but particularly distressing complication. The chest and upper back are sites of predilection. Keloids occur less commonly on the face. The tendency toward keloid formation is more common in African-American adolescents and is sometimes familial. Successful control of the acne itself, through topical or systemic therapy, will minimize the extent of future scarring. The use of intralesional corticosteroids is the most effective treatment of keloids once they have formed.

Figure 25

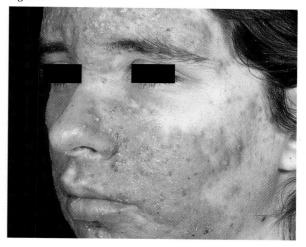

Pyoderma faciale This condition is an uncommon acneiform eruption that begins abruptly in young women, usually in their early twenties. With a background of facial erythema, these patients develop purulent nodules on the forehead, cheeks, and chin that coalesce and form draining sinuses. The cause is unknown.

Figure 26

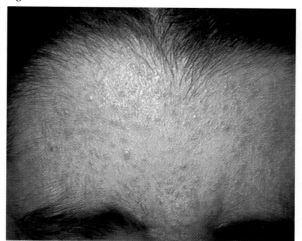

Acne and precocious puberty from a pinealoma In this 4-year-old child, persistent acne, precocious puberty, and frequent headache were the presenting signs and symptoms of a pinealoma. Occasionally, acne in a preadolescent may be an indication of an endocrine abnormality in which either androgen or glucocorticoids are present in excess. For example, a typical eruption of monomorphic follicular papules, usually concentrated on the back and chest, is seen in Cushing's disease. The same type of acne occurs in some children undergoing systemic steroid therapy for any reason.

Figure 27

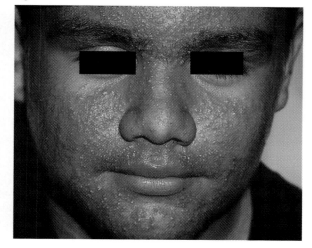

Steroid acne (dexamethasone) This form of acne may be caused by systemic or topical corticosteroids, as is seen in this photograph of a patient receiving systemic dexamethasone. The eruption is monomorphous, characterized by the presence of small erythematous papules or pustules primarily seen on the upper trunk, arms, neck, and, less commonly, the face.

Figure 28

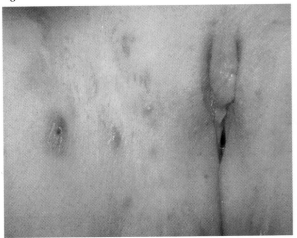

Figure 29

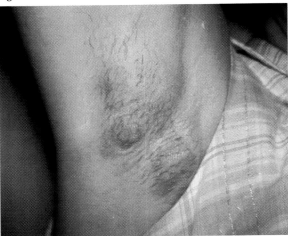

Hidradenitis suppurativa This condition is a chronic, recurrent inflammatory process of unknown etiology that involves the apocrine sweat glands. The favored locations are the axillae, groin, and buttocks. The disease begins just before or during puberty and persists, with remissions and exacerbations, for years. It is more common in women and is sometimes associated with acne conglobata and dissecting cellulitis of the scalp. Worsening of the disease may be seen during summer months or at the time of menstruation. Hidradenitis suppurativa is ag-

gravated by obesity. Apocrine gland occlusion in the involved axilla or groin leads to the formation of pustules, nodules, abscesses, and sinus tracts. The disease process is complicated by chronic overgrowth with *Staphylococcus aureus* and a wide variety of anaerobes and gram-negative bacteria. The process pictured in Fig. 28 is situated in the anogenital region and is not particularly severe. The patient in Fig. 29 has more severe disease in the axilla.

Figure 30

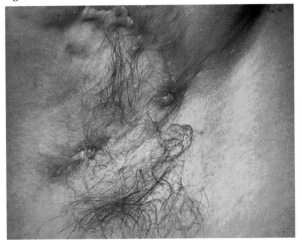

Hidradenitis suppurativa In this photograph, the condition has partially, and temporarily, abated. Corded hypertrophic and keloidal scarring has developed. The treatment of hidradenitis suppurativa is often difficult. Topical and systemic antibiotics are most commonly used; the choice of an agent should be guided by repeated culture and sensitivity testing of the organisms in the purulent exudate. Intralesional steroids, incision and drainage of abscesses, and even surgical excision of the involved area are sometimes indicated.

Figure 31

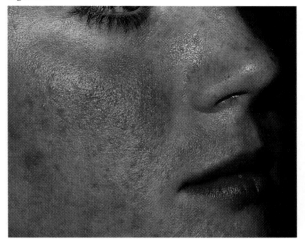

Rosacea   This is an inflammatory condition of the midface characterized by the presence of erythema, papules, pustules, telangiectasias, and, in the later stages, hyperplasia of the sebaceous glands of the nose. The absence of comedones helps to distinguish this condition from acne vulgaris, although the two conditions may coexist. Although usually seen in middle age, this condition may start in late adolescence.

Figure 32

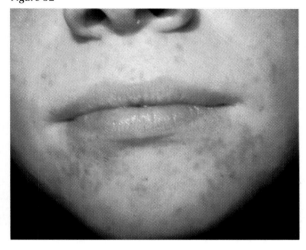

Periorificial granulomatous dermatitis   This condition is a chronic eruption of fine papules and pustules located on the skin around the mouth and nose, and sometimes around the eyes. The condition may initially present with perinasal scaling, which then progresses to involve the perioral area. The etiology of this condition is not completely understood.

Figure 33

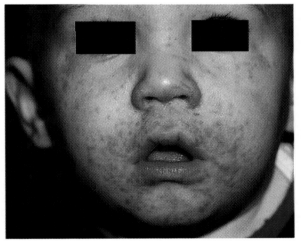

Periorificial granulomatous dermatitis   This condition usually begins in early childhood, with males and females equally affected. Periorificial granulomatous dermatitis is different from the type of perioral dermatitis that occurs in young women as a result of the frequent use of topical steroids in the affected areas.

Figure 34

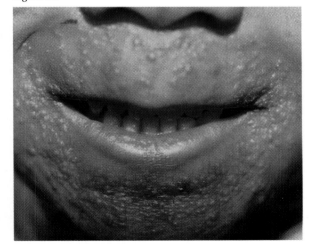

Periorificial granulomatous dermatitis   Topical steroids may perpetuate this condition in childhood. In most instances, perioral granulomatous dermatitis responds to oral tetracycline (in children over the age of 9 years) or erythromycin or to the application of topical metronidazole. Histopathologically, the lesions have a granulomatous infiltrate, and the condition may be confused with sarcoid.

Figure 35

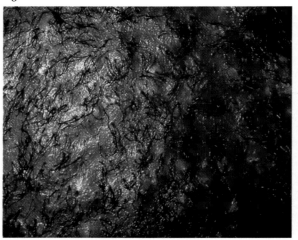

Figure 36

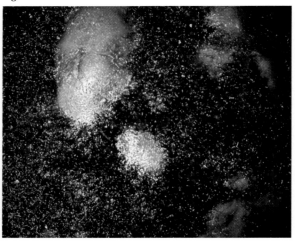

Folliculitis et perifolliculitis capitis abscedens et suffodiens
This imposing title translates as an inflammation in and around hair follicles of the scalp that flows (pus) and channels under or through (tissue). A less imposing title is dissecting cellulitis of the scalp. This chronic condition resembles, and sometimes accompanies, acne conglobata and hidradenitis suppurativa (the follicular occlusion triad). Like them, it is marked by inflammation, purulence, intercommunicating abscesses, cysts and si-nuses, and scarring. This disease appears to be somewhat more common among African-Americans, and onset may occur during adolescence. A number of therapies are routinely used. These include topical and systemic antibiotics, incision and drainage of abscesses, and intralesional steroids. There are usually many remissions and exacerbations, and the process often eventuates in a scarring alopecia.

3

Bacterial Infections

Figure 37

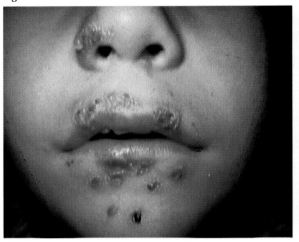

Figure 38

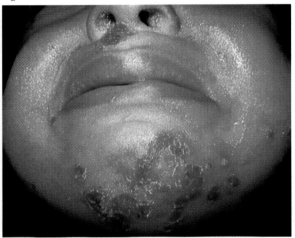

Impetigo contagiosa (vulgaris) Impetigo is a primary superficial infection of the skin. It is more prevalent in humid climates and occurs most commonly in the summer months. Trauma to the skin, such as a small abrasion or insect bite, sometimes provides the site of entry for the infective bacteria. The lesions evolve from discrete small vesicles into pustules. The fluid content of the primary lesions dries into a thick yellowish crust (Fig. 37), and removal of the crust may reveal bright-red and shiny erosions (Fig. 38). The causative streptococcus

has been associated with epidemics of impetigo-induced acute glomerulonephritis. Because the "honey-crusted" lesions of impetigo are frequently caused by a combination of *Staphylococcus aureus* and *Streptococcus pyogenes,* systemic antibiotic therapy should be effective against both organisms. The use of topical mupirocin ointment appears to be an effective treatment and may replace the need for systemic therapy in some patients with localized lesions.

Figure 39

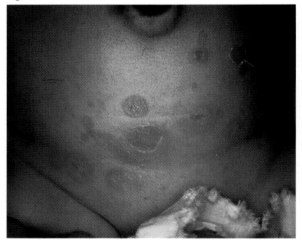

Figure 40

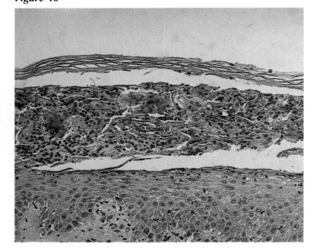

Bullous impetigo This form of impetigo consists of flaccid blisters that quickly rupture and evolve into superficial round or oval erosions with a varnished surface and minimal crust. Blisters are caused by the local effect of staphylococcal toxin. Pictured here are lesions in varying stages of evolution. Bullous impetigo is associated with a pure culture of *Staphylococcus aureus.* Oral treatment with dicloxacillin, erythromycin, or a cephalosporin is an effective mode of therapy.

Histopathology of impetigo contagiosa In the common form of impetigo, whether caused by a pathogenic staphylococcus or streptococcus or both together, a subcorneal vesicle or bulla is produced as the initial or primary lesion. Neutrophils migrate through the living cellular portion of the epidermis (the stratum malpighii) and accumulate between it and the overlying dead, cornified portion (the stratum corneum). In this photomicrograph one sees intact and degenerating leukocytes together with epithelial debris in a pustule.

Figure 41

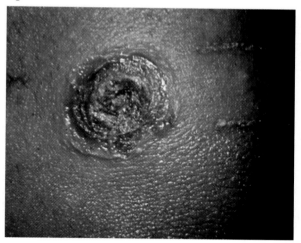

Figure 42

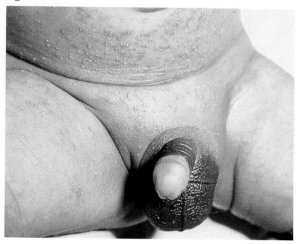

Ecthyma   Impetigo vulgaris is the most superficial of pyoder-mas; ecthyma is the next grade in depth. If impetigo is infec-tion by streptococci and/or staphylococci superficially in the epidermis, ecthyma is infection by the same organisms through the entire thickness of the epidermis (0.1 mm) to the upper reaches of the dermis (perhaps to a depth of 0.5 mm). The le-sion of ecthyma then becomes not a bulla but a firm crust on a superficial ulcer, surrounded by erythema.

Staphylococcal pustulosis   This condition is one that is seen usually at 3–5 days of age, more commonly in males. It is char-acterized by discrete pustules with a slight erythematous base located in the diaper area, in the periumbilical area, on the lat-eral aspect of the chest, and on the neck. The condition may be seen in an epidemic setting. The diagnosis is made by doing a Gram's stain and culture of a pustule. Treatment is with a sys-temic β-lactamase–resistant antibiotic.

Figure 43

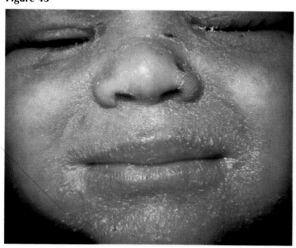

Figure 44

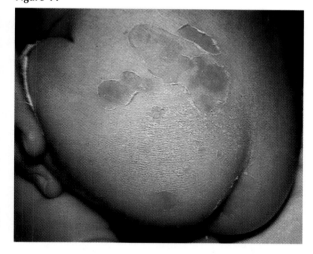

Staphylococcal scalded skin syndrome   This eruption oc-curs most commonly in children under the age of 5 years. It is characterized by a generalized tender, macular erythema, which is most prominent on the skin around the mouth and nose and in intertriginous areas. Within 1 or 2 days, the rash begins to peel. Typically, the large superficial flaccid bullae ("scalded skin") are quickly unroofed, revealing areas of slightly erythe-matous and shiny skin. These areas crust and then heal. Chil-dren with this syndrome are often extremely irritable and febrile, but the overall prognosis is good. Figure 43 shows the typical

crusting and fissuring around the lips and nose, and Fig. 44 illustrates superficial blistering on the buttock. The scalded skin syndrome is caused by an epidermolytic toxin that may be produced by several strains of *Staphylococcus aureus*. These causative organisms may be present in the nose, throat, con-junctiva, or an infected wound. Staphylococcal scalded skin syn-drome resolves without scarring within a period of two weeks. Treatment consists of appropriate supportive care and penicil-linase-resistant antibiotics.

Figure 45

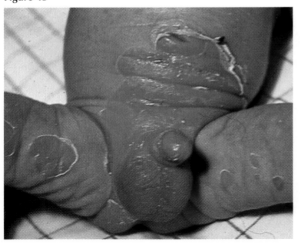

Staphylococcal scalded skin syndrome   The staphylococcal toxin exfoliatin may sometimes produce extensive areas of desquamation. Infants with this degree of involvement must be managed carefully with respect to fluid and electrolyte levels and must also receive topical therapy to minimize the risk of cutaneous infection by other organisms. Scalded skin syndrome must be differentiated from scarlet fever, Kawasaki's disease, toxic shock syndrome, and drug-induced toxic epidermal necrolysis.

Figure 46

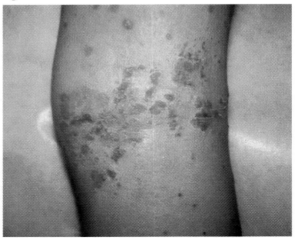

Impetiginization   This is the term for superficial pyoderma imposed upon preexisting dermatosis. Eruptions that are pruritic are particularly susceptible to secondary infection. Scratching disrupts the integrity of the epidermal barrier to infection and implants bacteria into the area of denuded skin. The most common organisms are *Streptococcus pyogenes* and *Staphylococcus aureus*. Pictured here is a case of impetiginized atopic dermatitis. The development of such "honey-crusted" lesions in a child with eczema suggests the need for antibiotic therapy.

Figure 47

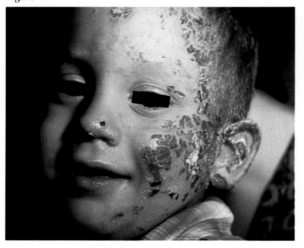

Pyoderma complicating a thermal burn   Secondary infection is a feared complication of thermal burns. Depending on the extent and depth of a burn and on the infecting microorganism, pyodermatous complication may vary from trivial to life-threatening. *Pseudomonas aeruginosa* and mixed infections are the most difficult to overcome. In the patient pictured here, the burn was limited to the face, and the infecting organism was susceptible to antibiotics. The consequence was scarring, mostly from the burn.

Figure 48

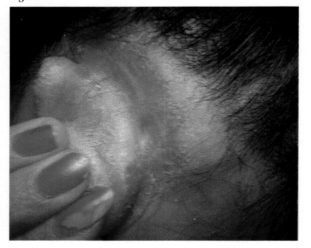

Infectious eczematoid dermatitis   This term should be reserved for that superficial inflammatory condition of the skin caused by pus overrunning from a nearby source. It is common from the nostril down on the upper lip from chronic nasal discharge, on the pinna of the ear from the meatus outward where there has been a run of pus from otitis externa, and around draining sinuses from a process, as in mastoiditis or osteomyelitis.

Figure 49

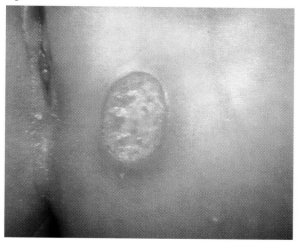

Figure 50

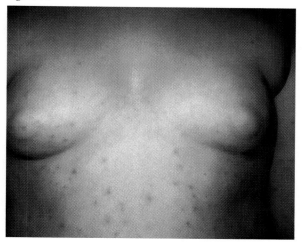

Chancriform pyoderma   It sometimes happens that infection with a banal organism like a staphylococcus, or more often with organisms like *Pseudomonas aeruginosa* or a species of the genus *Proteus* and combinations thereof, results in chancriform ulcers. Such conditions are more difficult to cure than the usual run of pyodermatous ulcers. In addition to effective systemic antibiotics, wet dressings, adequate drainage, and topical antiseptics may be required.

Hot tub folliculitis   This condition is seen after immersion in a hot tub in which gram-negative organisms, predominantly *Pseudomonas* species, proliferate as a result of improper maintenance. Patients develop numerous discrete erythematous papules and pustules on the upper trunk, groin, buttocks, and thighs. Lesions may be tender. The eruption is self-limited, although topical gentamicin and/or diluted white vinegar soaks may hasten resolution. Hot tubs must be properly cleaned and maintained.

Figure 51

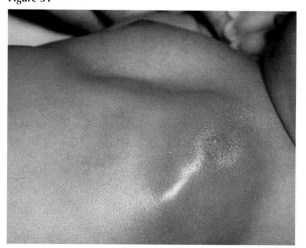

Figure 52

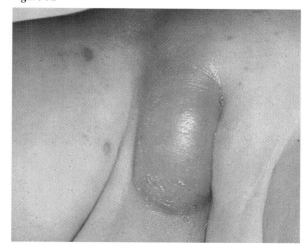

Furuncle   A furuncle is a skin abscess or boil. Lesions of this type are usually caused by a coagulase-positive *Staphylococcus aureus*. The organism invades through either an area of damaged skin, a hair follicle, or a sebaceous gland. As bacteria multiply, a deep cavity containing polymorphonuclear leukocytes and bacteria is formed. Here pictured, in Fig. 51, is a furuncle on the chest and in Fig. 52, on the labia. Abscesses can form anywhere on the body but are most common on the extremities, neck, buttocks, and axillae.

A carbuncle is a multiloculated abscess that forms when two or more neighboring furuncles become confluent. Many individuals with recurrent furuncles are found to be harboring the causative strain of *S. aureus* in the nares. Rarely, recurrent furunculosis is a sign of an underlying immune deficiency. In the earliest stages, intermittent warm compresses and systemic antibiotics may abort or mature lesions quickly. When lesions have pointed, incision and drainage is the treatment of choice.

Figure 53

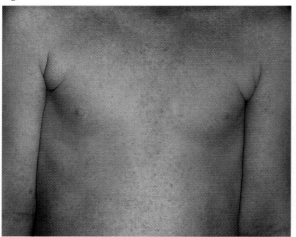

Scarlet fever   Scarlet fever is a generalized exanthem of childhood, with the highest incidence between the ages of 2 and 10 years. The cause is infection of the oropharynx by group A β-hemolytic streptococcus. The rash results from an erythrogenic toxin produced by this bacteria. The disease begins after a short incubation period of 2–4 days with a pharyngitis, fever, and malaise. The skin then begins to show a diffuse punctate erythema, which has a fine "sandpaper" texture.

Figure 54

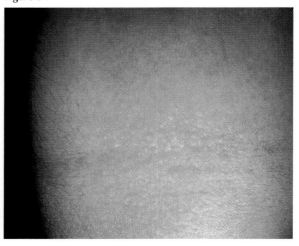

Scarlet fever   The face may become flushed but does not become as erythematous as the body. Characteristically, there is pallor around the mouth and the tip of the nose. Erythema is deepest in skin folds, especially the antecubital fossae and the axillary lines, where petechiae in linear arrangement may develop, known as Pastia's lines, as seen in this photograph. Tender cervical adenopathy is usual.

Figure 55

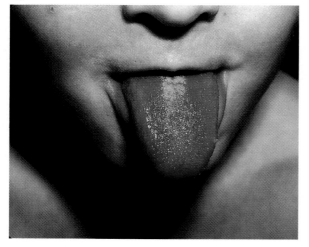

Scarlet fever   A red pharynx, purulent tonsillitis, and palatal petechiae may be present. The tongue develops a thin white coating with erythema and mild swelling of the papillae ("strawberry tongue"), as seen in this figure.

Figure 56

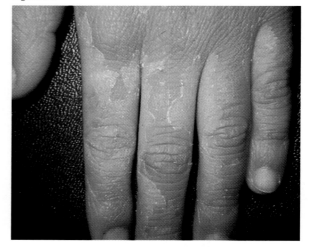

Scarlet fever   Desquamation of the hands, feet, elbows, and knees occurs during healing. Occasionally, peeling in these locations may be the sole cutaneous manifestation of a mild, resolving streptococcal infection.

Figure 57

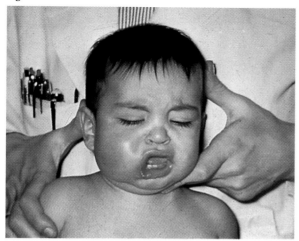

Figure 58

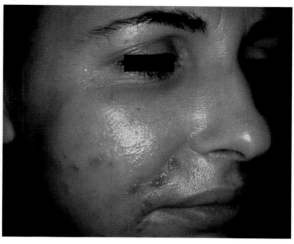

Facial cellulitis Cellulitis of the face may present in young children with a pink-to-purple edematous and warm discoloration of the cheek. In these cases, etiology is often *Hemophilus influenzae* or *Streptococcus pneumoniae*. There is usually high fever and toxicity, and often a preceding history of an otitis media. Complications of this form of infection include meningitis and sepsis. Rapid antibiotic therapy is mandatory, and the choice of antibiotic can be revised on the basis of blood and tissue aspirate cultures.

Erysipelas This is a rare form of superficial cellulitis caused by group A β-hemolytic streptococci. Erysipelas frequently occurs on the face, and presents as a tense, warm, tender, erythematous plaque with a well-demarcated border. The patient may be severely ill, with fever and local lymphadenopathy. Parenteral penicillin is often required in the initial, acute phase.

Figure 59

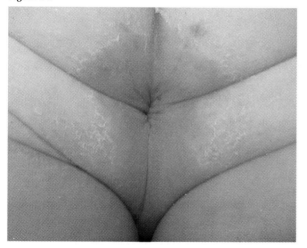

Figure 60

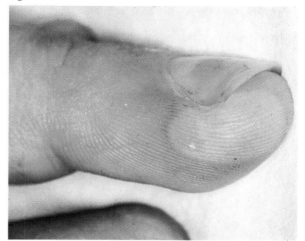

Perianal streptococcal disease Group A β-hemolytic streptococcus is sometimes the cause of perianal inflammation in a child. This localized infection is accompanied by painful defecation or pruritus. Examination of the area reveals a bright-red erythema surrounding the rectum and oozing from the infected area of skin. Diagnosis may be confirmed by perianal swab and culture, and treatment consists of oral penicillin.

Blistering distal dactylitis This is a distinctive cutaneous infection that is caused by group A β-hemolytic streptococcus. The clinical appearance, as illustrated here, is a superficial blister over the anterior fat pad of the distal phalanx. One or more fingers may be involved. The blister fluid is culture-positive for the causative bacteria, and treatment consists of incision and drainage along with the appropriate antibiotic by mouth.

Figure 61

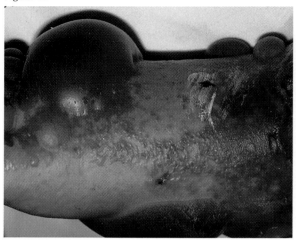

Figure 62

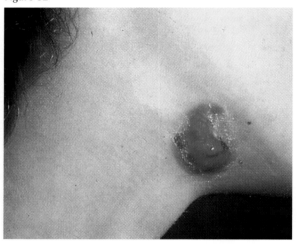

Invasive group A streptococcal disease   Group A β-hemo-lytic streptococcus may, though rarely, cause severe invasive disease with clinical findings such as pneumonia, septicemia, necrotizing fasciitis, and a toxic shock–like illness. A small pro-portion of patients with varicella also may develop secondary infection with streptococcus, leading to severe invasive disease.

Actinomycosis   This is a chronic granulomatous disease of worldwide distribution caused by gram-positive obligate para-sites that are most closely related to bacteria. Illustrated here is the most common, cervicofacial form of the disease. Deep to this superficial neck mass is a focus of actinomycosis. The pu-rulent discharge from the underlying sinus contains yellowish particles, the so-called sulfur granules. These granules are colonies of the causative agent, which is usually *Actinomyces israelii*. Diagnosis is made by culture of the organism on anaer-obic media, and the treatment of choice is penicillin.

Figure 63

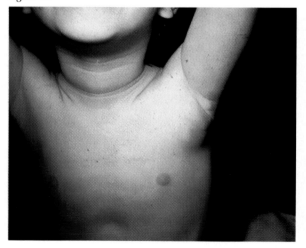

Figure 64

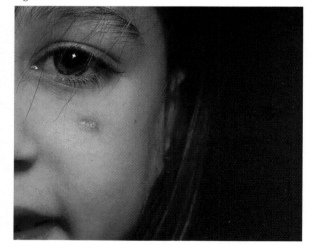

Cat-scratch disease   This disease is characterized by the ap-pearance of a papule or pustule at the site of a scratch from a cat. Within several weeks, enlarged regional lymph nodes (Fig. 63) develop and become tender and fluctuant. Cat-scratch dis-ease is accompanied by fever and malaise in about one-third of

cases. Localized adenopathy may last from several weeks to months and then resolves spontaneously. Central nervous sys-tem involvement is a very rare but sometimes serious compli-cation. The disease is caused by *Bartonella henselae*.

Figure 65

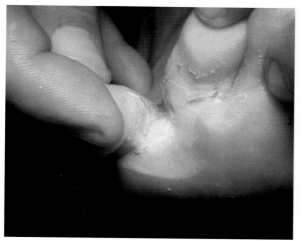

Figure 66

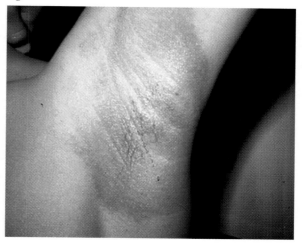

Erythrasma This is a fairly common condition that is occasionally seen during childhood and increases in frequency with age. Lesions occur in the axillae, groin, and toe webs. The causative organism is a diphtheroid, *Corynebacterium minutissimum.* Involvement in the axilla, as seen in Fig. 65, appears as a well-demarcated brown-to-red plaque. Maceration and scaling between the toes (Fig. 66) is another clinical presentation.

A characteristic of the lesion is that it fluoresces coral-red under the Wood's light (3650 Å), because the causative organism produces porphyrins in the stratum corneum. Erythrasma is exceedingly superficial but can become extensive. A 10-day course of oral erythromycin, 250 mg four times a day, is the treatment of choice.

Figure 67

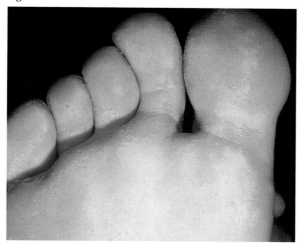

Pitted keratolysis This condition is characterized by numerous shallow, discrete pits on the plantar surface of the feet, usually in the weight-bearing areas. Although the condition is asymptomatic, there is usually hyperhidrosis, and the feet may be malodorous. Painful erosions may occur. The condition is caused by *Micrococcus* species.

Spirochetal, Protozoal, and Mycobacterial Diseases

Figure 68

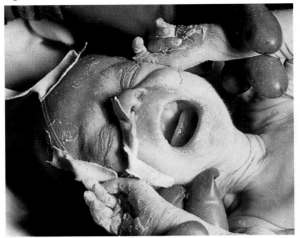

Figure 69

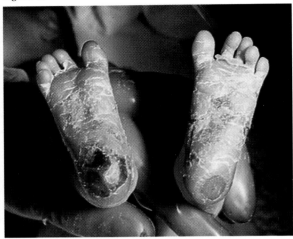

Congenital syphilis In utero infection by the spirochete *Treponema pallidum* can occur after the sixteenth week of gestation. Intrauterine disease, especially during early pregnancy, may result in spontaneous abortion or in a severely affected infant. Severe disease that is present at birth presents with hepatosplenomegaly, ascites, meningoencephalitis, and severe anemia. Osteochondritis is the most characteristic bone change. The cutaneous findings in severe congenital syphilis include bullae, pustules, macules, and papules. Fissuring and peeling of

the skin are also characteristic. The palms, soles, and periorificial skin are sites of predilection. Syphilitic rhinitis, with a copious and bloody nasal discharge, is an associated finding. If infection occurs late in pregnancy, signs and symptoms may be delayed for several weeks. In these cases, diagnosis is usually made on the basis of a positive syphilis serology in mother and infant. If the disease is allowed to progress, rhinitis, cutaneous macules, and mucous patches may be the presenting signs.

Figure 70

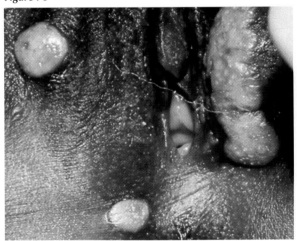

Figure 71

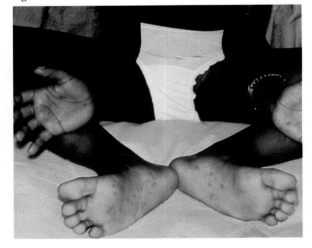

Acquired syphilis Unlike congenital syphilis, acquired syphilis in infants, children, and adolescents follows the classic course of syphilis in adults. Such an infection in a child should be assumed to be the result of sexual abuse. The first event in the development of syphilis is a dark-field positive chancre at the portal of entry of the treponeme. Shortly thereafter, serologic tests for syphilis become positive.

Acquired syphilis Secondary syphilis usually develops 6–8 weeks after the appearance of the chancre. Malaise, low-grade fever, myalgias, and lymphadenopathy are accompanied by a wide variety of cutaneous manifestations. The lesions illustrated in Fig. 70 are condylomata lata on the genitalia. Note the moist papules and plaques. Figure 71 shows the most consistent form of skin disease in secondary syphilis.

Figure 72

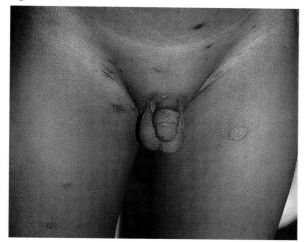

Figure 73

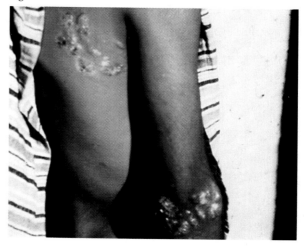

Acquired syphilis (cont.)   This condition consists of copper-colored papulosquamous lesions, most commonly on the palms and soles. Sometimes the eruption resembles pityriasis rosea, as seen in Fig. 72. Other cutaneous manifestations of secondary syphilis include papular lesions, pustules, nodules, plaques, and mucous patches.

Yaws   This is a nonvenereal treponematosis that is caused by *Treponema pertenue.* It is endemic in areas of Central and South America, Africa, and southeast Asia. The disease is acquired by physical contact, and the majority of cases occur during childhood. An ulceration occurs at the site of the primary inoculation. Secondary lesions are cutaneous nodules or moist or hyperkeratotic plaques; they appear within several weeks and resolve spontaneously. Recurrence of the latent disease, with gummata of the skin and bones, may occur many years later.

Figure 74

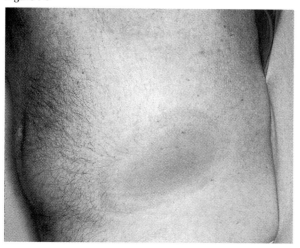

Figure 75

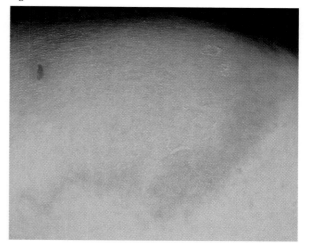

Erythema migrans (Lyme disease)   Lyme disease is caused by the spirochete *Borrelia burgdorferi* and is transmitted by the pinhead-sized Ixodid ticks. The illness is endemic in large areas of the continental United States. The early cutaneous manifestation, termed *erythema migrans,* is pictured here. It consists of an expanding annular lesion around the original tick bite. Satellite areas of involvement may also be present. Pruritus or burning may be present at the site of the lesion, and the rash may be accompanied by fever, malaise, and regional lymphadenopathy. The systemic manifestations of Lyme disease include neurologic dysfunction (e.g., Bell's palsy), cardiac conduction abnormalities, and arthritis. Early antibiotic therapy for the typical skin lesion will often prevent the development of the more serious and long-lasting systemic illness. Serologic testing is of some value in diagnosis, but results may be negative early on, especially in the absence of neurologic or joint symptoms.

Figure 76

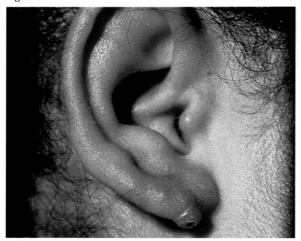

Figure 77

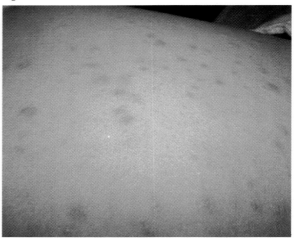

Lepromatous leprosy Leprosy, or Hansen's disease, is a chronic multisystem disease that is caused by *Mycobacterium leprae,* an acid-fast bacillus. The highest incidence of the disease is in areas of South America, Africa, and Asia. It is not rare in children. The clinical manifestations of this illness depend on the host response to infection. At one end of the spectrum is lepromatous leprosy (LL), which represents a diminished host response to the leprosy bacillus. Cutaneous lesions in this form of the disease vary. Macular lesions are symmetri-

cally distributed hypopigmented and erythematous patches. When widespread involvement occurs, the lesions may be difficult to differentiate from normal skin. The lesions pictured here are more infiltrative. Nodular lesions of the earlobe, as illustrated in Fig. 76, are particularly common in lepromatous leprosy. Annular plaques and papules (Fig. 77) may also be present. Lepromatous leprosy is the form most likely to cause widespread nerve damage and ocular disease.

Figure 78

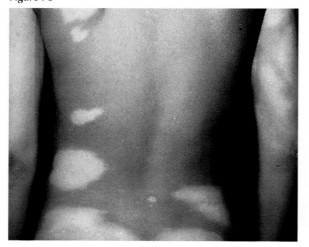

Figure 79

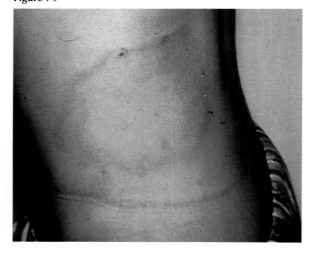

Tuberculoid leprosy Patients with tuberculoid leprosy (classification TT) are those who have the strongest immune response to chronic infection. The cutaneous lesions are typically sharply demarcated plaques with a firm raised border. Varying degrees of erythema, hypopigmentation, and anesthesia may be present. Note the large, sharply demarcated areas of decreased pigmentation in Fig. 78, and the raised border of the lesion in Fig. 79. In early disease, the loss of sensation and normal sweat-

ing in involved areas may be difficult to detect, and the lesions can easily be confused with vitiligo and pityriasis alba. Tuberculoid leprosy tends to remain a localized disease, and spontaneous resolution may occur. Nerve damage tends to be limited to one or two nerves. The treatment of all forms of leprosy is now complicated by the appearance of dapsone resistance. Combinations of rifampicin, clofazimine, and dapsone are now required in many cases.

Figure 80

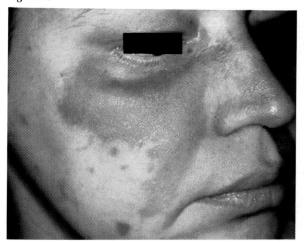

Figure 81

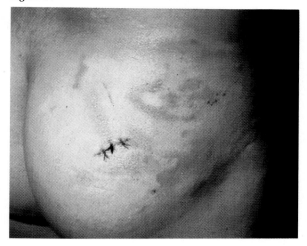

Dimorphous leprosy The terms *borderline* and *dimorphous* leprosy are used to refer to patients whose disease shows features of both the lepromatous and tuberculoid forms. Patients with dimorphous leprosy (classified as BL, BB, or BT) have varied skin lesions, including the plaques and annular lesions that are illustrated in Figs. 80 and 81. They often suffer widespread and rapidly progressive nerve damage. Knowledge of the proper treatment of leprosy must include an understanding of the acute

exacerbations that may accompany therapy. Treatment of non-lepromatous leprosy with antibiotics may induce erythema and edema of the skin lesions, accompanied by rapid damage to the peripheral nerves (type I reaction). Type II reaction, also termed erythema nodosum leprosum, is most common in patients who have lepromatous leprosy. It consists of painful dermal nodules accompanied by ocular disease, peripheral neuropathies, and a wide variety of constitutional symptoms.

Figure 82

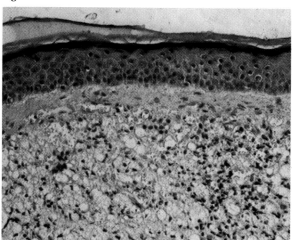

Figure 83

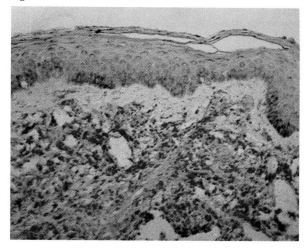

Histopathology of lepromatous leprosy Exposure to and contact with *Mycobacterium leprae, Mycobacterium tuberculosis,* and other microorganisms of the genus do not produce overt or detectable disease in all, or even in most, individuals. Only a few develop clinical disease. In the matter of leprosy, there are two polar types of overt disease, namely, lepromatous and tuberculoid leprosy. In the tuberculoid form, organisms are sparse, and the histologic response to them is granulomatous in a manner similar to that seen in sarcoidosis and some forms of

tuberculosis. In the lepromatous form, illustrated here, organisms are abundant, and the histologic response is characteristically in the form of sheets of histiocytes that are laden with lepra bacilli and that have foamy, vacuolated cytoplasm. Typically a zone of uninvolved connective tissue, well shown in the photomicrograph (Fig. 82), separates the epidermis from the disease process in the dermis. Lepra bacilli are readily revealed by any method of staining for acid-fast bacilli (Fig. 83).

Figure 84

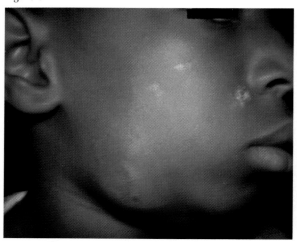

Primary complex of tuberculosis in the skin   A child who has an area of injury to the skin may develop a primary complex in that location when exposed to someone with active tuberculosis. After an incubation period of 1–3 weeks, a red papule develops and evolves into a nodule or plaque with ulceration. The tuberculous ulcer is accompanied by regional lymphadenopathy. This form of cutaneous tuberculosis is a self-limited disease, and slow healing with scar formation occurs. A stage in this process is shown here.

Figure 85

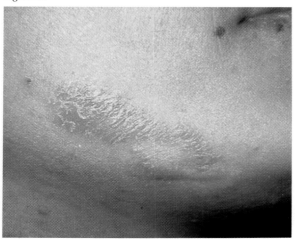

Lupus vulgaris   This is a progressive form of cutaneous tuberculosis that results from the hematogenous spread of *Mycobacterium tuberculosis*. It is seen in patients who are very sensitive to the organism. Favored locations are the central face, earlobes, and other parts of the head and neck. The lesions may be papules, nodules, or plaques, and the color is often described as "apple jelly." Older lesions, as pictured here, are brownish annular plaques; the area of central clearing represents an attempt at healing.

Figure 86

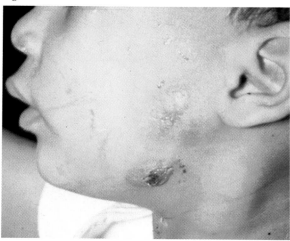

Tuberculosis cutis colliquativa (scrofuloderma)   This type of cutaneous tuberculosis results from the extension of infection from an underlying location to the skin. The original site of involvement may be a joint, bone, or visceral organ, but most commonly it is a lymph node. Illustrated here is a case of tuberculous cervical lymphadenitis, with the channeling of sinuses to the skin surface. This form of cutaneous infection by *M. tuberculosis* is particularly common in children.

Figure 87

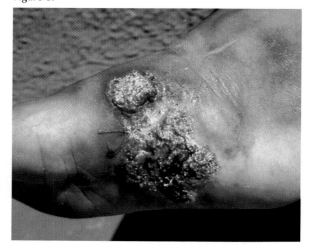

Tuberculosis cutis verrucosa   This form of cutaneous tuberculosis results from exogenous reinfection of an already tuberculin-sensitive individual. When the lesions are located on the hands or feet, they tend to develop a distinctly verrucous surface, beneath which is inflammation. This representation is characteristic. There is most likely a history of prior injury to the foot.

Figure 88

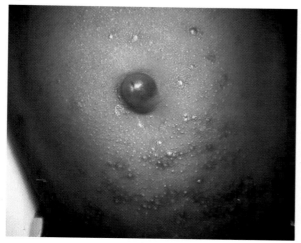

Figure 89

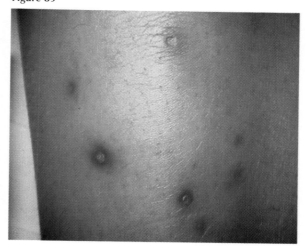

Lichen scrofulosorum This term describes a condition that consists of grouped lichenoid papules on the trunk. It occurs in children who have active tuberculosis in other locations. The individual lesions are flat-topped follicular papules and are either erythematous or flesh colored. The condition is asymptomatic and follows a benign course to spontaneous resolution.

Papulonecrotic tuberculid Clinically this condition is highly stereotypic. It consists of dusky red matchhead- to pea-sized, sterile papules that arise in symmetrical crops on the extensor aspects of the extremities, usually on the elbows and knees. Occasionally the buttocks are also involved. The condition is asymptomatic and heals spontaneously with varioliform scars.

Figure 90

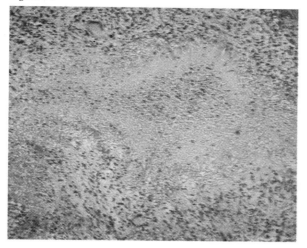

Figure 91

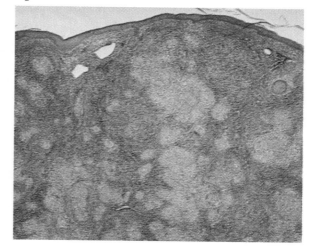

Histopathology of tuberculosis cutis Cutaneous tuberculosis may be divided into two categories, one in which the response is to living organisms present in tissue and another in which the response is to particulate or soluble products of organisms hematogenously disseminated from an occult focus of living organisms. The latter responses are commonly referred to as tuberculids. The histopathology of response to living organisms and their products depends on immunologic develop-

ments. When the skin becomes the portal of entry of tubercle bacilli, the early response is banal inflammation, and the later response is granulomatous with central necrosis (Fig. 90). Thereafter, responses to tubercle bacilli, endogenously disseminated or exogenously reacquired, are almost instantly granulomatous in the form of collections of epithelioid and giant cells seated in a sea of lymphocytes and with little or no necrosis (caseation). This is the typical picture of lupus vulgaris (Fig. 91).

Figure 92

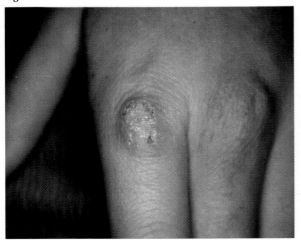

Figure 93

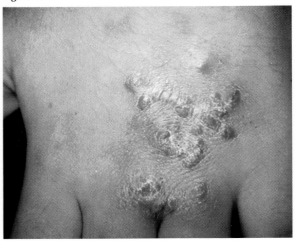

Infection with atypical mycobacteria   There are a number of cutaneous infections that are caused by mycobacteria other than *Mycobacterium tuberculosis* or *M. leprae*. Illustrated here is infection by *M. marinum*. This organism is known to contaminate fish tanks and swimming pools, and the cutaneous infection is sometimes termed *swimming pool granuloma*. In fact, the case in Fig. 92 was traced to a fish tank, and that in Fig. 93 to a swimming pool. The lesions usually appear at a point of

trauma, and the hands, feet, elbows, and knees are particularly common locations. After an incubation period of 2–6 weeks, the lesions evolve from small papules into single or grouped violaceous nodules. Satellite lesions may be present. Biopsy of a mature lesion reveals a caseating granuloma, and acid-fast organisms within histiocytes can sometimes be identified. Diagnosis can also be made by culture of biopsied material.

Figure 94

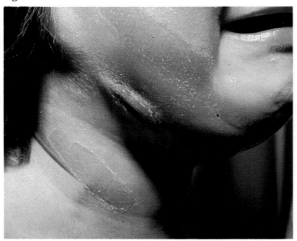

Figure 95

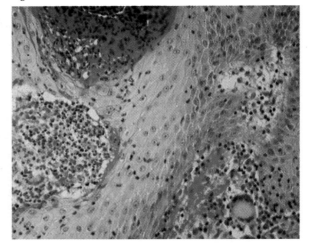

Infection with atypical mycobacteria   This illustration is another instance of a granulomatous process caused by a mycobacterium other than that of tuberculosis. In this case, the organism was *Mycobacterium intracellulare*. The lesion resembles that of tuberculosis cutis colliquativa. The causative organism was cultured from the discharge that issued from sinuses emerging from infected lymph nodes. The patient was positive in reaction to conventional tuberculin and to tuberculins derived from the so-called atypical mycobacteria.

Histopathology of infection with atypical mycobacteria   There are numerous mycobacteria that resemble *Mycobacterium tuberculosis* and have similar, though less virulent, pathogenicity. *M. marinum* is one such organism. The reaction that results depends again upon complex immunologic developments. The usual clinical picture is a verrucous process of which the histopathology, as shown here, is epidermal hyperplasia, intraepidermal abscess formation, and tuberculoid inflammatory process with giant cells in the dermis.

Figure 96

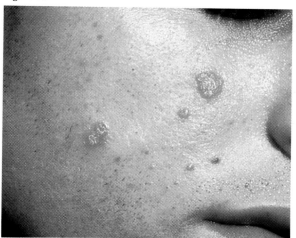

Figure 97

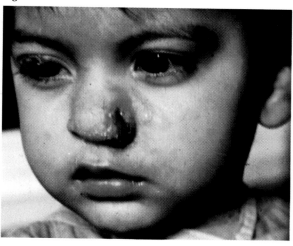

Leishmaniasis The cutaneous form of leishmaniasis is caused by a protozoan *(Leishmania tropica)* that is transmitted by the bite of a sandfly (of the genus *Phlebotomus*) in certain endemic regions (the Middle East, China, Africa, India, the former Soviet Union). The primary process in the skin starts as a macule of erythema, evolves into a papule (Fig. 96), and then develops into a granulomatous or ulcerous process (Fig. 97). The lesion takes up to 1 year to heal spontaneously in the form of a vac-

ciniform scar. *Systemic* or *visceral leishmaniasis* (kala-azar) is caused by the related protozoan *Leishmania donovani.* This form is characterized by fever, anemia, leukopenia, emaciation, and severe hepatosplenomegaly. The skin develops a grayish pigmentation, usually on the face. Finally, mucocutaneous leishmaniasis is caused by *Leishmania braziliensis,* is characterized by destructive mucosal lesions, and is endemic in some areas of Latin America.

Figure 98

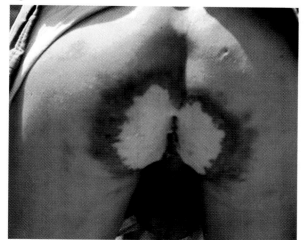

Amebiasis cutis *Entamoeba histolytica,* the cause of intestinal and cutaneous amebiasis, attains the skin from the intestinal infestation. Discharging from the ulcerous process in the lower part of the gut, viable amebas contaminate and may infect the perianal region especially. When the infection is seen in an active state, the process is a continually creeping, painful ulceration that has little tendency to heal spontaneously. When the infection is healed, the clinical appearance is a scar, as pictured.

Viral and Rickettsial Diseases

Figure 99

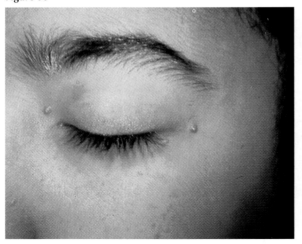

Figure 100

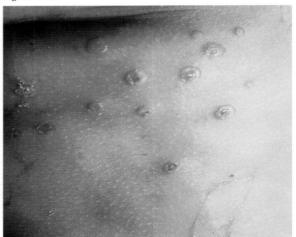

Molluscum contagiosum This condition is a benign viral infection that appears as crops of discrete, slightly umbilicated, flesh-colored or shiny papules. It is extremely common among children and may be seen in several children within a family. The lesions may become inflamed if traumatized or infected and sometimes become inflamed spontaneously as they resolve. Rarely is there only a solitary lesion; most commonly there are fewer than 20. However, the total number is sometimes in the hundreds. The lesions tend to be grouped, and the average size of a lesion is 2–3 mm in diameter and height. The trunk, face,

and genitalia are the most common sites of infection. Pruritus is an occasional symptom and may be the impetus for inoculating the viral infection from one area of the skin to another. Molluscum contagiosum is self-limited, but treatment is often required out of concern for appearance. Treatment should be individualized to the age and extent of involvement in each patient. Destruction of lesions with a sharp curette is the preferred mode in a cooperative child with limited disease. The child with numerous lesions poses a particular therapeutic challenge.

Figure 101

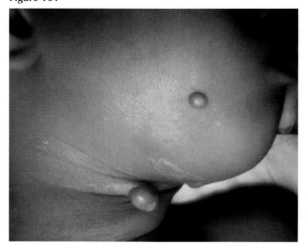

Figure 102

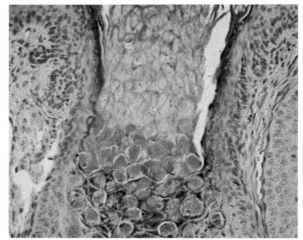

Molluscum contagiosum Occasionally, a lesion of molluscum contagiosum may grow to as large as 3 cm in diameter. Two such "giant mollusca" are pictured here. The diagnosis is usually suggested by the presence of more typical, smaller lesions on adjacent or distant skin surfaces. Treatment is again by surgical removal when possible. Local anesthesia would be a feasible and a kind thing to administer in such a case.

Histopathology of molluscum contagiosum Molluscum contagiosum is a viral disease that takes the form of small tumors in which the virus can be visualized within a characteristic histopathologic picture. In the upper layers of epidermal cells, viral inclusions are seen as collections known as *molluscum bodies* when they have developed to occupy the entire cytoplasmic space of those cells in the form of amphophilic or slightly basophilic structures. This phenomenon is most clearly seen in and about the stratum granulosum.

Figure 103

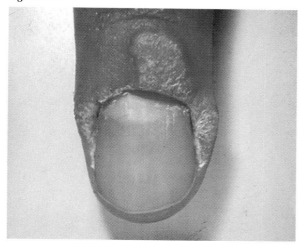

Figure 104

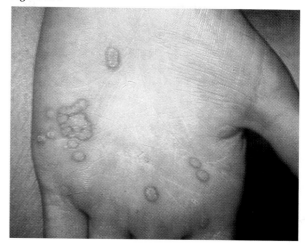

Verruca vulgaris The common wart is a benign growth caused by localized infection with one of the many types of human papillomavirus. These small DNA viruses are part of the papovavirus group. Warts are especially common among children and adolescents and may occur on any mucocutaneous surface. The hands are a particularly frequent location. The typical wart is a rough-surfaced nodule that may be either lighter or darker than the surrounding skin. Lesions involving the proximal and lateral nail folds are pictured in Fig. 103; Fig. 104 shows numerous verrucae on the palmar surface. Treatment must be individualized to the age and cooperative abilities of the patient, and to the size and location of the wart. For some lesions, the simplest and most effective approach is treatment by desiccation and curettage.

Figure 105

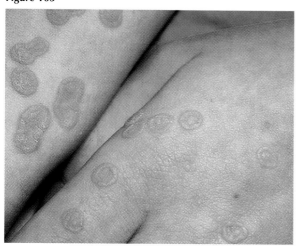

Figure 106

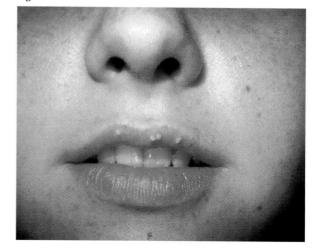

Ring verruca In other cases, cryotherapy or treatment with a salicylic acid preparation is preferable. The gentler forms of treatment are particularly good for periungual warts. In those areas, surgery may cause scarring of the nail matrix and nail dystrophy. Following the application of cantharidin or liquid nitrogen, blister formation may result. Upon resolution of the blister, a ring wart may develop, as seen in this figure.

Verruca filiformis The surfaces of common warts are influenced by their position on the body and by what goes on there. In general, they are rough of surface. On hands, the surfaces of warts are domed from wear and tear, so that troughs and crests are shallow; on soles, they are flat and smooth from the weight of the body; but where they are undisturbed, common warts tend to grow with fimbria or finger-like projections. They are then called *filiform* or *digitate* warts. The face and scalp are the most common sites where warts grow in this fashion.

Figure 107

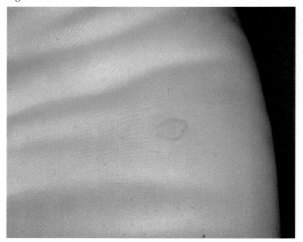

Figure 108

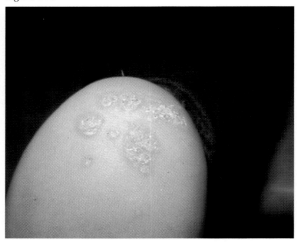

Verruca plantaris   Plantar warts appear as flat areas of firm hyperkeratosis on the soles of the feet. Lesions that occur at points of pressure may be associated with severe pain on walking. Figure 107 illustrates a solitary plantar wart. Note the obliteration of skin markings, which does not occur in a callus. The lesions in Fig. 108 are numerous and mosaic. Treatment of plantar warts requires perseverance on the part of both patient and

physician. Attempts at a rapid cure may result in scarring. One practical method involves the daily application of salicylic acid plasters or liquid salicylic acid preparations, along with repeated paring of the necrotic surface of the wart. The success of this routine may be hastened by gentle cryotherapy. Lesions that are small and in non–weight-bearing areas may be removed by curettage without electrocautery.

Figure 109

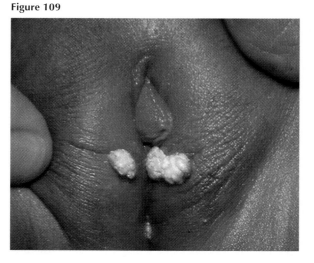

Figure 110

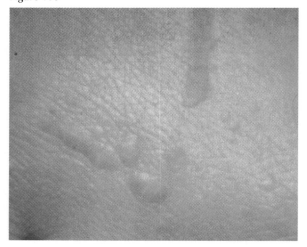

Condyloma acuminatum   Warts with this "cauliflower" appearance on the labia, penis, or around the rectum are termed *condylomata acuminata*. The presence of lesions of this type in a child should prompt the physician to consider the possibility of sexual abuse, although the true incidence of this association is not known. In some cases, condylomata acuminata may be the result of innocent contact with another infected individual, or perinatal transmission from a mother with cervical or vaginal lesions. Brief application of podophyllum resin is the preferred treatment.

Verruca plana   Plane, or flat, warts may be caused by several types of the human papillomavirus. They are common in children. The lesions are slightly raised, flesh-colored papules, usually 2–4 mm in diameter. The face and hands are the most frequent locations for these multiple small warts. The lesions may be discrete or confluent, and a linear array of flat warts may result from autoinoculation in a scratch. Gentle freezing or chemical destruction is the treatment of choice.

Figure 111

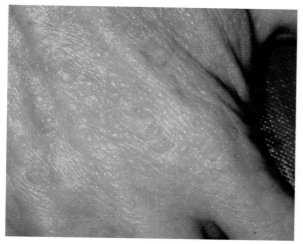

Figure 112

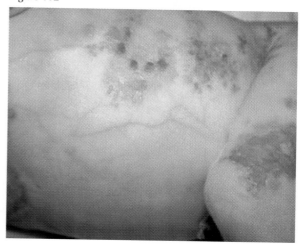

Epidermodysplasia verruciformis This rare familial disease usually has its onset during childhood. Patients develop numerous flat warts, initially involving the face and upper trunk. A number of human papillomavirus types have been implicated. As the lesions tend toward confluence, they may mimic the appearance of tinea versicolor. Most patients with epidermodysplasia verruciformis have depressed cell-mediated immunity. They are also at risk for squamous cell carcinomas, which generally arise on sun-exposed skin.

Neonatal herpes simplex Neonatal herpes simplex infection is acquired during passage through an infected birth canal. The cutaneous involvement may be as extensive as pictured here, or it may be subtle. The scalp is the most common site for the typical clustered vesicles. Because of the very high frequency of concurrent disseminated disease, cutaneous herpes simplex in the newborn must be considered a pediatric emergency. Early treatment with an intravenous antiviral agent offers the infant the best possibility of survival.

Figure 113

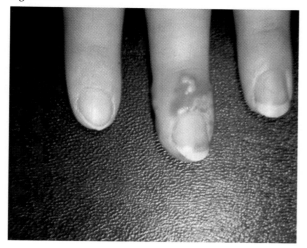

Figure 114

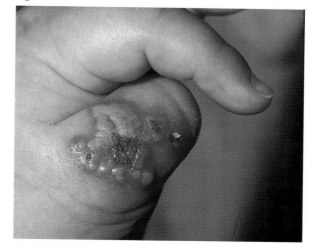

Herpetic whitlow Herpes simplex infection of the distal phalanx may occur in infants and young children. The first episode may accompany herpetic gingivostomatitis. Herpetic whitlow presents with pain or paresthesia and with erythema and vesiculation.

Herpes simplex The original infection is occasionally misdiagnosed as bacterial paronychia. Subsequent recurrences of lesions at the same site, which occur in about 20 percent of patients, will lead the practitioner to the correct diagnosis.

Figure 115

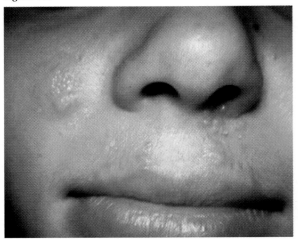

Figure 116

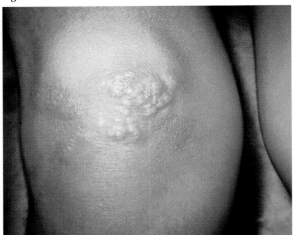

Herpes simplex, recurrent Following an episode of primary herpes simplex, the virus may remain dormant within a nerve ganglion. A number of triggering factors, including febrile illness, emotional or physical stress, excessive sun exposure, and trauma, may cause the virus to replicate and spread to the skin surface. The typical "fever blister" or "cold sore" is a recurrent herpes simplex infection on the lip or vermilion border. Geni-

tal herpes simplex infection, more often than not, is also characterized by periodic recurrence. Patients with recurrent disease will often experience prodromal pain or paresthesia in the involved area. Most episodes last from 7 to 10 days. Represented here are lesions on the face (Fig. 115) and on the knee (Fig. 116). The latter is a less common location, serving to illustrate that recurrent herpes simplex may occur on any area of the skin.

Figure 117

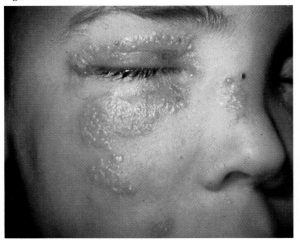

Figure 118

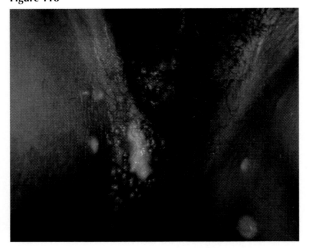

Herpes simplex, recurrent Here illustrated is a severe case of recurrent herpes simplex on the eyelids, cheek, and nose. Without a clear history of recurrence, herpes zoster would enter into the differential diagnosis. Repeated corneal ulceration, with scarring, may lead to visual impairment. Herpes simplex keratitis has become the major cause of infectious blindness in the United States.

Herpes progenitalis Herpes simplex infection in the genital region is a sexually transmitted disease. It is not uncommon in the sexually active adolescent, as pictured here. In the young child, genital herpes simplex should create a high index of suspicion for sexual abuse. This figure illustrates the multiple painful erosions that may occur in primary infection. Regional lymphadenopathy and fever may also be present. Recurrences of genital herpes are very common but are generally much milder in both extent and duration than the primary disease.

Figure 119

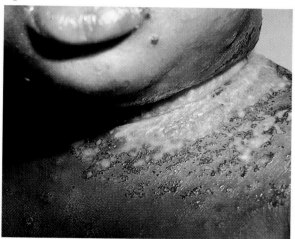

Figure 120

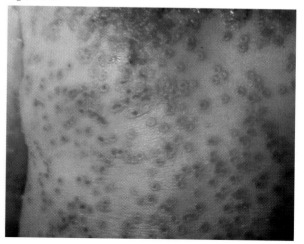

Eczema herpeticum (Kaposi's varicelliform eruption) Disseminated cutaneous herpes simplex infection is a serious complication of atopic dermatitis. It may also occasionally occur in individuals with other dermatologic disorders. Patients rapidly develop numerous umbilicated vesicles in the areas of eczematous involvement. Children with eczema herpeticum often become seriously ill with high fever. Bacterial superinfection and sepsis can be a complication, and the disease is occasionally fa-

tal. The patients pictured here developed involvement of the entire skin surface. The lesions in Fig. 119 are typical umbilicated vesicles; those in Fig. 120 are equally extensive and are beginning to crust. Skillful and attentive supportive treatment is required in order to maintain fluid and electrolyte balance and prevent superinfection. Treatment with intravenous acyclovir seems to hasten clinical improvement and is often recommended for children with extensive or rapidly increasing involvement.

Figure 121

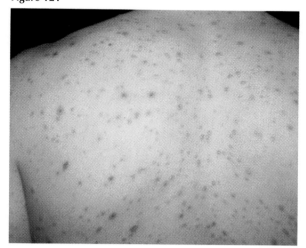

Figure 122

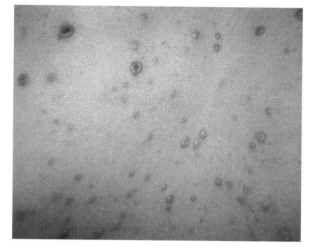

Varicella Chickenpox is caused by a virus of the herpes group. The disease is highly contagious and is spread by droplet or direct contact. The incubation period for chickenpox ranges from 11 to 21 days. Prodromal symptoms consist of low-grade fever, headache, anorexia, and malaise. On the following day, the characteristic rash begins to appear. The lesions evolve from erythematous macules to form small papules. Quickly, a clear vesicle arises on this erythematous base. The classic lesion of

chickenpox has been poetically described as a "dewdrop on a rose petal." Over the next several days, the vesicles rupture and then crust. The rash begins on the chest and back, and spreads centrifugally to involve the face, scalp, and extremities. New lesions of chickenpox arise in crops over a period of several days. Since crops of macules-papules-vesicles-crusts are successive and overlapping, one sees lesions at all stages of development in given locations. Itching is a symptom and may be severe.

Figure 123

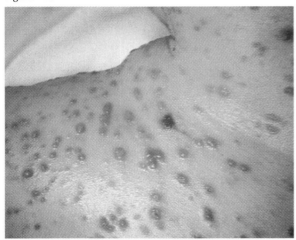

Figure 124

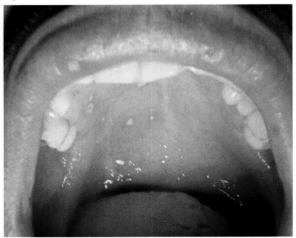

Varicella Lesions on the oral mucous membranes, which are common, are pictured in Fig. 123. They are most common on the palate and quickly evolve into small, superficial erosions. Fig. 124 depicts a case of chickenpox of unusual severity. The lesions tend to be large blisters and to become hemorrhagic. Cases of this type are more likely to occur in children with reticuloendothelial malignancies or immunologic defects, or in those under immunosuppressive or prolonged corticosteroid therapy. Complications of chickenpox in these children may include vari-

cella pneumonia, myocarditis, and hepatitis. There are also a number of complications of chickenpox in the child who was previously healthy. Secondary bacterial infection of the skin lesions is by far the most common. Other, less frequent, sequelae include thrombocytopenia, purpura fulminans, and postinfectious encephalitis. Finally, a significant number of cases of Reye's syndrome occur after chickenpox, and aspirin should therefore not be used as an antipyretic.

Figure 125

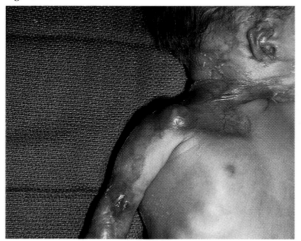

Figure 126

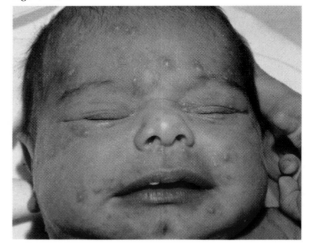

Congenital varicella syndrome On rare occasions, the infants of women who develop chickenpox during the first trimester of pregnancy are born with congenital defects. The congenital varicella syndrome is characterized by asymmetrical arm or leg lengths, ocular abnormalities, microcephaly, and intrauterine growth retardation. Cutaneous scarring in a dermatomal distribution is particularly characteristic of the constellation of birth defects caused by the varicella-zoster virus.

Neonatal varicella Maternal chickenpox in the several days before or after the birth of a child may lead to a significant health risk for the infant. The newborn who is exposed to varicella without the benefit of transplacental maternal antibody may go on to develop severe disseminated infection with pulmonary and hepatic involvement. This disease may sometimes be fatal. Pictured here is a newborn with numerous typical chickenpox lesions over the face. The hemorrhagic lesions that may be part of neonatal varicella are not present in this child.

Figure 127

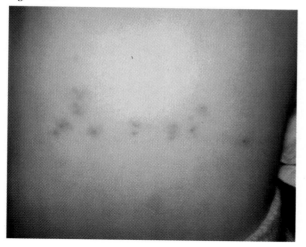

Figure 128

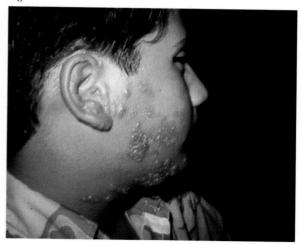

Herpes zoster Herpes zoster, or shingles, is an acute eruption characterized by vesicles and small bullae. Lesions are usually unilateral and confined to a single dermatome. The cause of herpes zoster is the varicella-zoster virus. After an initial episode of chickenpox, the virus lies dormant in the dorsal root or cranial nerve ganglia. Reactivation of the virus, usually years later, leads to the typical eruption. Herpes zoster is a relatively rare disease in children and is seen more frequently in those young people who had chickenpox at a very early age. Localized pain may precede the onset of the rash, but postherpetic neuralgia is unusual in childhood. Children with lesions around the eye or on the tip of the nose may have involvement of the nasociliary nerve and should be observed carefully for ocular involvement.

Figure 129

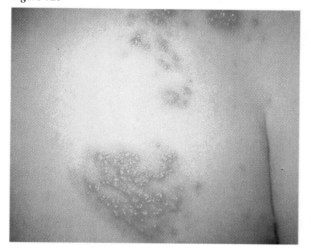

Figure 130

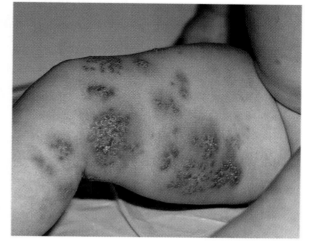

Generalized herpes zoster The child with herpes zoster may, in the normal course of the illness, develop several chickenpox-like lesions outside of the involved dermatome. However, rapid and widespread evolution of such lesions—generalized herpes zoster—is a problem of greater concern. Hematogenous spread of the viral infection in this fashion may be an indication of an underlying immune deficiency.

Herpes zoster, infantile Infants born to mothers who developed primary varicella infection during pregnancy may likewise have been infected during fetal life. These infants may develop herpes zoster without a clinical history of previous varicella. Associated with this may be a temporary paresis of the affected area.

Figure 131

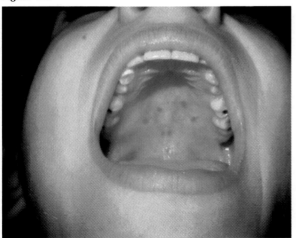

Figure 132

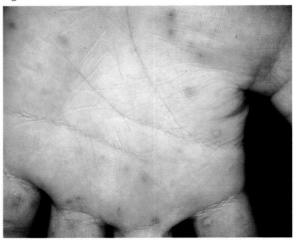

Hand-foot-mouth disease This common and benign viral disease of childhood is usually caused by the A16 strain of cox-sackievirus, although other strains of the same virus have been implicated. It most often occurs in late summer and early fall. The prodrome consists of low-grade fever and malaise. Shortly thereafter, vesicular lesions arise on the soft palate (Fig. 131), tongue, buccal mucosa, and uvula. The lips are usually spared. Occasionally, these lesions may be painful and cause some difficulty in eating. The cutaneous lesions develop 1 or 2 days after those in the mouth. They consist of asymptomatic round or oval vesiculopustules that evolve into superficial erosions. The edges of the palms and soles are a favored location (Fig. 132). The dorsae of the hands and feet may also be involved. There is sometimes an accompanying macular and papular eruption on the buttocks. The eruption lasts from 7 to 10 days, and no therapy is required. Although culture of the virus is possible, the diagnosis of hand-foot-mouth disease is usually made on clinical grounds.

Figure 133

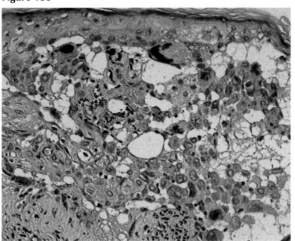

Histopathology of varicella and herpes zoster Chickenpox and shingles are caused by the same virus, one of the two in the herpes group that are pathogenic to man. Both viruses of the group produce intraepidermal blisters that are different from those caused by pox viruses. Distinctive features are enlargement of epithelial cells, margination of chromatin, frequent multinucleation, and sometimes nuclear atypia. In varicella and herpes zoster, inflammatory infiltrates are rare; the opposite is true in herpes simplex.

Figure 134

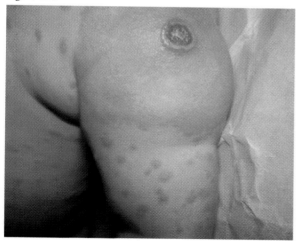

Figure 135

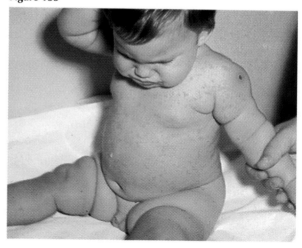

Complications of vaccinia The worldwide eradication of smallpox has eliminated the need for vaccination with the modified cowpox virus. Over the many years when this medical practice was necessary, a number of benign and some more serious dermatologic complications were observed. The sequelae of smallpox vaccination are as follows: 3–4 days after inoculation, there develops an area of erythema and edema at the in-

jection site (usually an arm or thigh); this rapidly evolves into edema, vesiculation, ulceration, crusting, and scar formation over a period of about 3 weeks. For most children, fever, malaise, and local discomfort are the major side effects. The complications of a severe local reaction (Fig. 134) and of a generalized eruption (Figs. 134, 135) are illustrated here.

Figure 136

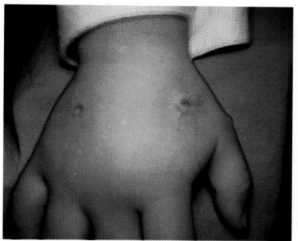

Figure 137

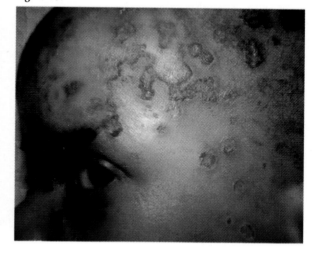

Complications of vaccinia Still another complication of premeditated induction of vaccinia was accidental autoinoculation on an undesirable site while the primary pock was in progress. Autoinoculation then resulted in a new lesion that began in 1 day (a reaction time) and rapidly repeated the whole process. The seriousness of such accidents were site specific: on the face, particularly around the eyes, blindness, and elsewhere on exposed skin, cosmetic defects, were serious consequences.

Eczema vaccinatum Disseminated vaccinia was the most dreaded complication of smallpox vaccination. Like eczema herpeticum, eczema vaccinatum occurred in children with underlying eczematous disorders. It was more serious because of the severity of the acute illness, the tendency toward scarring, and a higher incidence of mortality. The illustration suggests that the scarring from eczema vaccinatum can be disfiguring.

Figure 138

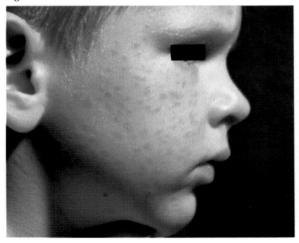

Figure 139

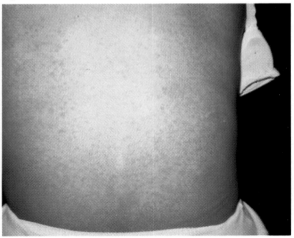

Echovirus disease   A wide variety of enteroviruses of the echovirus and coxsackievirus groups are responsible for similar systemic illnesses and cutaneous eruptions. These illnesses all occur most commonly in the late summer or early fall. In the case of echovirus, there is an incubation period of 3–7 days, followed by the sudden onset of fever and myalgia. Some combination of abdominal pain, vomiting, pharyngitis, and cervical adenopathy may also be present. Occasionally, nuchal rigidity may indicate the presence of aseptic meningitis. The eruption begins to develop on the face (Fig. 138), and within hours, generalization to the trunk (Fig. 139) and limbs occurs. The lesions, which are erythematous, papular, and rubelliform, persist for about 3–5 days and then recede. Occasionally, the virus can be recovered from throat, urine, or stool. There is no specific treatment, and little more than simple supportive therapy is required until spontaneous recovery takes place.

Figure 140

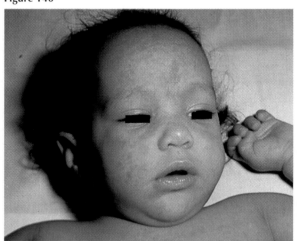

Figure 141

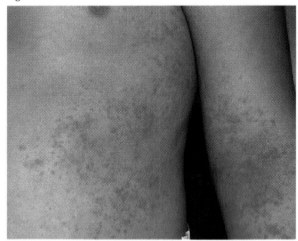

Exanthem subitum (roseola)   Roseola is a common childhood illness that is now known to be caused by human herpesvirus 6. Most cases occur during the first year of life. The disease is characterized by 3–5 days of high fever accompanied by minimal constitutional symptoms. Pharyngitis, periorbital edema, and cervical adenopathy may be present, and febrile convulsions sometimes occur. The disappearance of the fever is accompanied by the onset of rash. The typical eruption is macular and papular, and it is concentrated on the neck and trunk. The eruption clears in hours, or at most a day or two.

Unilateral laterothoracic exanthem   This condition of unknown etiology begins as an eruption first appearing in a periflexural area, the axillary fold being the most common. The eruption then spreads unilaterally in an asymmetric fashion, at times involving an entire side of the body. The eruption may then generalize to the rest of the body. The rash usually resolves in 2–6 weeks.

Figure 142

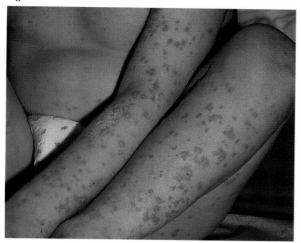

Figure 143

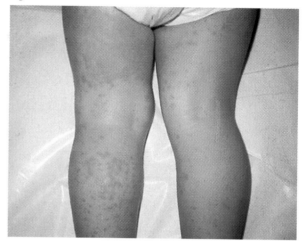

Papular acrodermatitis of childhood (Gianotti-Crosti syndrome) This condition is characterized by the eruption of firm erythematous papules on the extremities, cheeks, and buttocks. The papulonodular lesions may become confluent in some areas. This disease was originally seen in children with anicteric hepatitis B infection in Europe. Since that time, this syndrome

has been found to occur primarily in association with Epstein-Barr virus infection, although other causes include coxsackie, parainfluenza, poliovirus, vaccinia, β-hemolytic streptococcus, and bacille Calmette-Guérin (BCG). The disease is self-limiting, lasting 6–8 weeks.

Figure 144

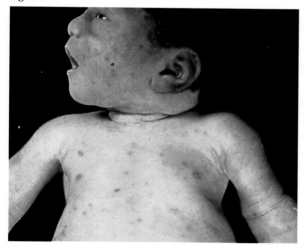

Figure 145

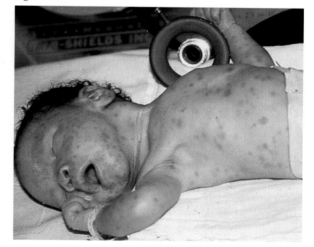

Cytomegalic inclusion disease Congenital infection with cytomegalovirus, a DNA virus of the herpes group, results in disease of varying severity. Whereas some neonates are completely asymptomatic, severely affected infants display intra-uterine growth retardation, microcephaly, and hepatosplenomegaly. The cutaneous manifestations, pictured here, are petechiae and purpura. The "blueberry muffin" spots are an indication of extramedullary hematopoiesis. Culture of the virus from urine is the most specific means of diagnosis.

Congenital rubella In utero infection by the rubella virus during the first 20 weeks of gestation may result in severe multi-system involvement and a variety of developmental defects. Illustrated here are the dark-blue-to-purple "blueberry muffin" lesions in the severely affected neonate. They are a sign of ex-tramedullary hematopoiesis. Thrombocytopenic purpura is an additional cutaneous manifestation. Congenital cataracts, deafness, and cardiac malformations form a classic triad in infants with the severe intrauterine infection.

Figure 146

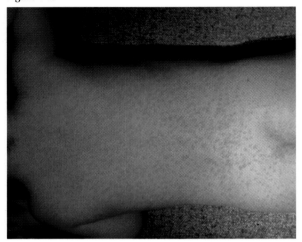

Figure 147

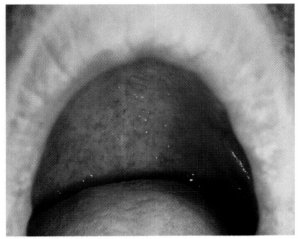

Rubella   This common viral disease affects both children and young adults. A mild prodrome consists of headache, coryza, and low-grade fever. The rash itself varies enormously in its course and duration. Most typically, it begins on the face and neck and spreads to the trunk and extremities, as pictured here, over 1–2 days. The lesions are small pink macules and maculopapules, which rapidly coalesce and then fade. The rash is so evanescent that it may begin to disappear on the face before developing on the trunk and extremities. Petechiae on the soft

palate, termed *Forchheimer's sign,* are present in some patients (Fig. 147). Systemic illness is generally mild. Enlargement of suboccipital and posterior auricular lymph nodes is a characteristic physical finding. The most serious aspect of rubella is the severe developmental defects that may result from intrauterine infection during the first trimester. Routine childhood immunization has resulted in fewer epidemics and therefore in a lower incidence of viral exposure to pregnant women.

Figure 148

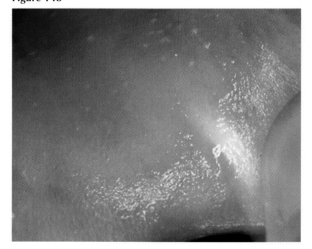

Figure 149

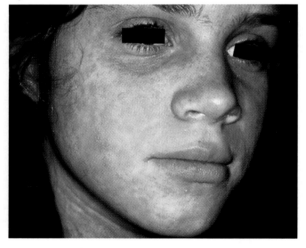

Measles   Rubeola, or measles, is a systemic illness caused by an RNA paramyxovirus. The incidence of this previously common childhood disease has decreased markedly since the advent of an effective vaccine, but measles has by no means been eradicated. After an incubation period of 1–2 weeks, the infected child develops fever, conjunctivitis, photophobia, and a distinctive brassy or barking cough. Frequently, the fever and constitutional symptoms are severe. A day or two after onset of these constitutional signs and symptoms, the enanthem (Kop-

lik's spots) appears as bright-red puncta with central blue-white flecks on the buccal mucosa opposite the second molars (Fig. 148). The characteristic rash is maculopapular and erythematous. It begins on the forehead and behind the ears and spreads to the face (Fig. 149), neck, trunk, and extremities. The rash disappears in the same sequence, sometimes leaving areas of fine desquamation. The duration of the entire illness is usually 5–7 days.

Figure 150

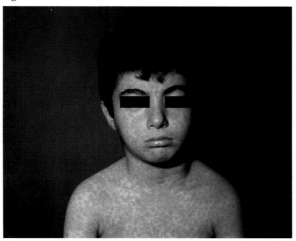

Figure 151

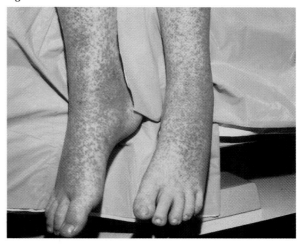

Measles (cont.) This picture shows the "measly" appearance of a child who clearly feels miserable. The disease is brief and self-limited for most children, and the treatment is entirely supportive. The incidence of complications is higher, however, than in the other childhood exanthems. Otitis media is the most common. Serious complications include bronchopneumonia and encephalitis, which may cause permanent neurologic damage. Subacute sclerosing panencephalitis is a late sequela of measles.

Atypical measles Children who received the "killed" measles vaccine, available during the mid-1960s, may have developed "atypical measles" upon exposure to the virus as young adults. This disease is characterized by high fever and severe respiratory symptoms. The accompanying rash is frequently compared to that of Rocky Mountain spotted fever (Figs. 154 and 155). The exanthem, which typically begins on the hands and feet, may be macular, vesicular, or purpuric. Children who receive the live attenuated measles vaccine, which is currently in use, are not susceptible to atypical measles.

Figure 152

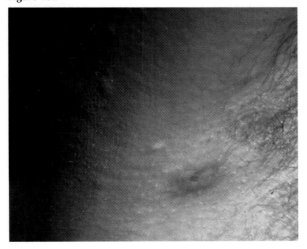

Figure 153

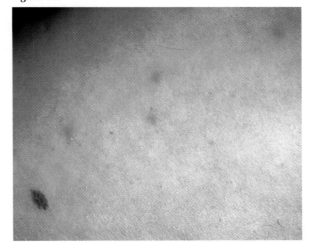

Rickettsialpox This self-limited febrile illness is caused by *Rickettsia akari*. It is transmitted to man by a mite that is an obligatory parasite of the common house mouse. One to two weeks after exposure, a nodule develops at the point of entry of a parasitized mite. The nodule becomes vesicular and then crusted with a black eschar (the pock, seen well developed on the neck in Fig. 152). Regional lymphadenopathy is usually present. Within sev-

eral days, the patient develops intermittent fever, photophobia, headache, myalgia, and lassitude. Two to three days later, a generalized exanthem, consisting of discrete macules that quickly become papular, appears (Fig. 153). Firm vesiculopustules arise atop the papules, and these subsequently form crusts. The eruption lasts 1–2 weeks. Unlike Rocky Mountain spotted fever, rickettsialpox shows a negative Weil-Felix reaction.

Figure 154

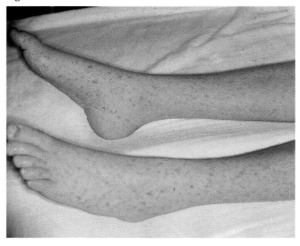

Figure 155

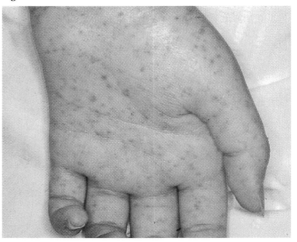

Rocky Mountain spotted fever   This disease is caused by *Rickettsia rickettsii* and is transmitted by a number of different ticks. Despite its geographical title, Rocky Mountain spotted fever is present in many locations throughout the United States and the entire Western Hemisphere. After infection by tick bite, there is an incubation period of 2–14 days. The abrupt onset of the disease includes severe headache, fever, chills, arthralgia, and myalgia. After 2–3 days of these constitutional symptoms, erythematous macules erupt on the wrists, hands, forearms, legs, and ankles, as seen in these figures. Lesions then spread to the palms and soles and the trunk. The macules originally blanch with pressure but soon become purpuric and even necrotic. The disease causes a severe vasculitis, and complications include disseminated intravascular coagulation, hemorrhage into the gastrointestinal and urinary tracts, and cardiovascular collapse. The Weil-Felix test is positive, but the disease must be treated immediately upon clinical suspicion. The high fatality rate is markedly reduced by prompt antibiotic therapy.

Figure 156

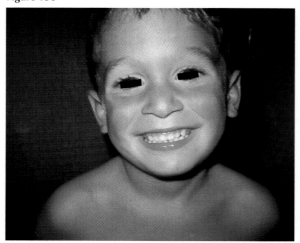

Figure 157

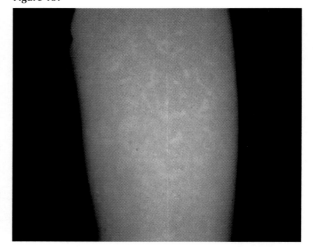

Erythema infectiosum (fifth disease)   Erythema infectiosum is a mild childhood disease that is now known to be caused by human parvovirus B19. This condition develops after a mean incubation period of 14 days. There are few if any prodromal symptoms. The rash evolves in three clinical stages. The first stage is characterized by the abrupt appearance of a bright-red malar blush. The appearance is so startling that it has been given the suggestive description of "slapped cheeks" (Fig. 156). During the second stage, the facial rash begins to fade, and a maculopapular, urticarial, or morbilliform exanthem develops on the extremities and trunk. Pruritus may be present. As portions of this rash fade over a period of several days, a reticular pattern emerges, mainly on the extremities, which gives the arms and legs a marbled appearance (Fig. 157). This reticular eruption, which is the third stage of the disease, may last only 1 week, or it may last continuously or by relapses for as long as 8 weeks. Exercise and variations in temperature may make the rash appear more or less prominent. No treatment is required.

Fungal Infections

Figure 158

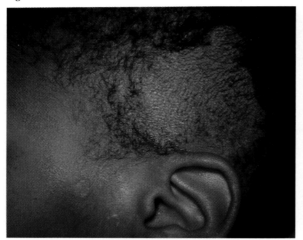

Figure 159

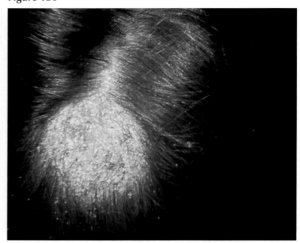

Tinea capitis Fungal infections of the scalp are extremely common in children. The diagnosis of tinea capitis should be entertained in any child in whom patches of incomplete alopecia, crusting, or scaling are found in the scalp. In previous decades, *Microsporum canis* and *M. audouinii* were the most common pathogenic fungi infecting the scalp. The latter frequently causes a discrete grayish patch of hair loss (Fig. 158). In most parts of the United States and in many other parts of the world, *Trichophyton tonsurans* is now the predominant organism causing tinea capitis. In the United States, this form of tinea capitis is seen almost exclusively in African-American children. In some children, this dermatophyte causes discrete and dramatic areas of hair loss studded by the stubs of broken hairs, the so-called black-dot ringworm (Fig. 159). In others, there are only small and unimpressive patches of "seborrheic" scale, with minimal hair loss, or groups of small pustules.

Figure 160

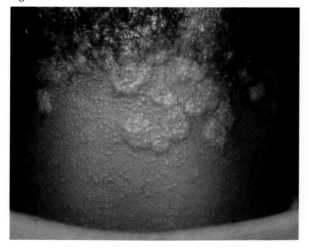

Figure 161

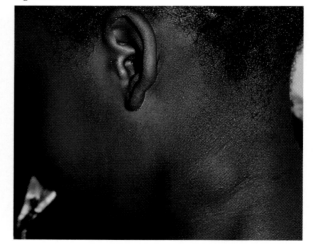

Tinea capitis Because *T. tonsurans* does not fluoresce, the Wood's light is no longer of use in most cases. However, diagnosis can be confirmed by the use of either potassium hydroxide preparation or fungal culture. Pictured here is an inflammatory response to infection with *T. tonsurans*. Children whose scalps are infected with this dermatophyte may also develop regional lymphadenopathy (Fig. 161) or a fine papular eruption that spreads from the face and neck to other skin surfaces (an id reaction). Attempts to treat tinea capitis with topical antifungal agents alone are doomed to failure. Oral griseofulvin is the most effective form of therapy. The use of selenium sulfide shampoo may be effective in preventing spread to classmates and siblings.

Figure 162

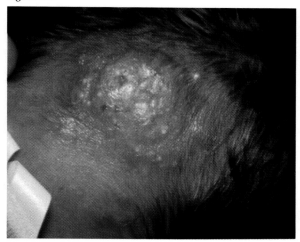

Figure 163

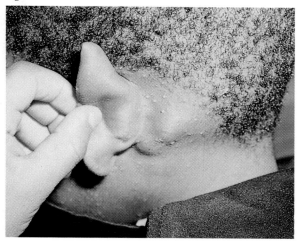

Kerion In some children, an exuberant inflammatory response to the infecting dermatophyte may occur. This boggy and tender mass is termed a *kerion,* a word that in Greek means a honeycomb, honey, or beeswax and is intended to describe the clinical appearance. Children with a kerion may also develop localized lymphadenopathy and fever. Misdiagnosis of a kerion as a bacterial infection of the scalp is an all too common pitfall. The proper treatment is oral griseofulvin. In some cases, a brief course of oral prednisone may minimize scarring.

Id reaction to tinea Before treatment or shortly after starting griseofulvin for tinea capitis, some patients develop a pruritic eruption that is a hypersensitivity reaction. These patients develop erythematous papules, papulovesicles, and sometimes oval plaques concentrated on the face, neck, trunk, and upper extremities. There is no need to discontinue the griseofulvin, for the eruption resolves in 1–2 weeks. Relief can be obtained with the application of low-potency topical corticosteroids. It is important to differentiate this from a true drug eruption.

Figure 164

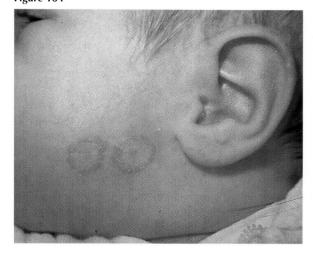

Figure 165

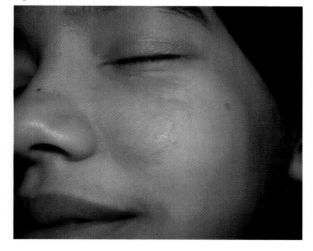

Tinea corporis (faciei) Superficial fungal infections of the skin are among the most common of all pediatric dermatoses. Infection at the sites pictured here may also be termed *tinea faciei.* Note the ring shape of the active periphery of the lesions in the infant in Fig. 164 and the more inflammatory process in the patient in Figs. 165 and 166.

Tinea corporis (faciei) *Trichophyton tonsurans, T. rubrum,* and *T. mentagrophytes* are common pathogens. Cutaneous infection with zoophilic species, such as *Microsporum canis,* usually results from close contact with a household pet. On the body, fungi lodge in the stratum corneum and do not invade lanugo hairs.

Figure 166

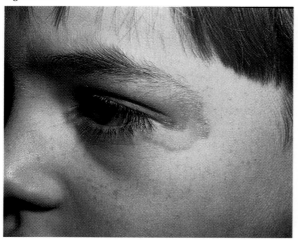

Tinea corporis (faciei) (cont.) Therefore, topically applied antifungal agents, such as the azole and allylamine agents, are effective therapy. Occasionally, a cutaneous fungal infection, particularly on the face, is misdiagnosed as atopic or contact dermatitis. The application of topical steroids to such a lesion will often cause dramatic worsening of the condition.

Figure 167

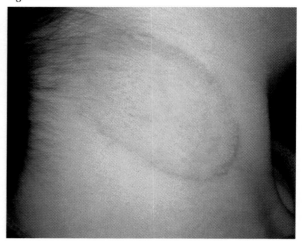

Tinea corporis The illustrations are of more superficial fungal infection of relatively hairless skin. The annular lesion in Fig. 167 resulted from infection with *Trichophyton tonsurans.* The numerous scaly rings in Fig. 168 are due to *Microsporum canis.* In the cases illustrated, clinical diagnosis of a superficial fungal infection is reasonably certain, and one may guess that the causative fungus is a microsporum or trichophyton.

Figure 168

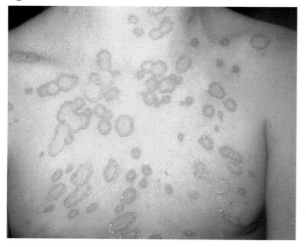

Tinea corporis Definitive diagnosis depends on mycologic culture of the scale from a lesion. In cases of candidiasis, favus, and tinea imbricata (see Fig. 182), the causative organism can frequently and confidently be guessed correctly. In general, one may say that *Microsporum canis, M. audouinii, Trichophyton tonsurans,* and *T. schoenleinii* can infect scalp and hairless skin, and *T. rubrum* and *Candida albicans,* hairless skin and nails.

Figure 169

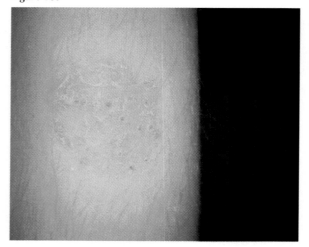

Tinea corporis Here illustrated is superficial fungal infection of glabrous skin caused by *Microsporum gypseum.* The clinical appearance is somewhat different from that of the condition caused by other dermatophytes in that, though a round lesion, it is not a ring of active periphery around a relatively healed center. Still, the superficiality, the scaling, and the low-grade inflammatory reaction are typical of a fungal infection; it can be proved by culture of the causative fungus.

Figure 170

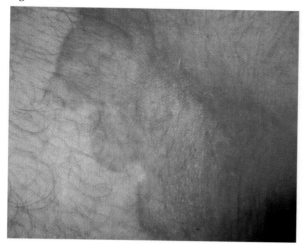

Tinea cruris   The groin is a common site of acute and then enduring superficial fungal infection. *Epidermophyton floccosum, Trichophyton rubrum,* and *Candida albicans* are the commonest infecting fungi. In infants, *C. albicans* is the usual pathogen; in older children and adults, all are common. Intertriginous spaces, such as groin, axillae, and digital webs, are particularly susceptible to fungal infection because the pH of these areas is less acid than elsewhere, temperature is higher, and humidity is greater.

Figure 171

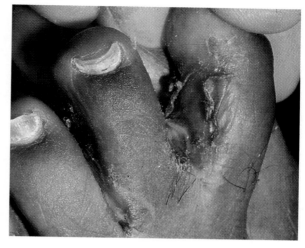

Tinea pedis   Superficial fungal infection of the feet is somewhat unique because of the location. Between the toes (most commonly the fourth and fifth), the condition appears as erythema, maceration, and scaling. This may in some cases become secondarily infected (Fig. 171). It is attended by itching or vague discomfort. On the sole and the lateral aspects of the feet, scattered pustules and vesicles with surrounding erythema and edema may occur. More commonly, there is persistent dry scale in a "moccasin" distribution with minimal inflammation.

Figure 172

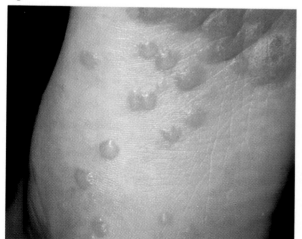

Tinea pedis   The fungi that are commonly found are *Epidermophyton floccosum, Trichophyton mentagrophytes, T. rubrum,* and *Candida albicans.* Fungal infections of the feet, although rare in infants and young children, must be considered when presented with erythema and scaling of the feet. More likely diagnoses with this presentation are juvenile plantar dermatosis and contact dermatitis.

Figure 173

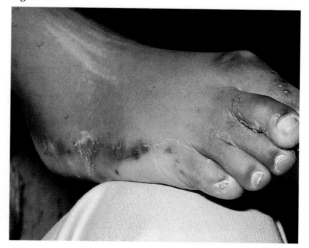

Tinea pedis   Sweating, friction, and debris promote fungal infection. During early adolescence, there is a marked increase in the incidence of tinea pedis. For most patients, the use of topical antifungal therapy, along with the wearing of sandals and light cotton socks, is adequate therapy.

Figure 174

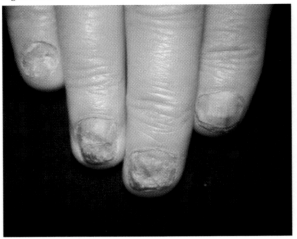

Figure 175

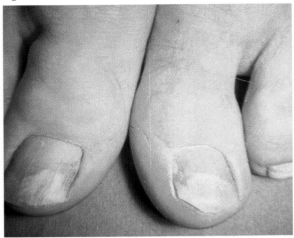

Onychomycosis Tinea unguium (fungal infection of the nails) is somewhat uncommon during childhood. After puberty, its frequency increases with age. Usually, onychomycosis is associated with tinea pedis. Fungal culture of the nails is sometimes difficult but extremely important in confirming the diagnosis. Onychomycosis is the most difficult of the superficial fungal infections to treat because the nail plate is not penetrated by topically applied agents. Newer systemic antifungal agents such as itraconazole and terbinafine appear promising in the treatment of onychomycosis. The illustrations show infection with dermatophytes. Note the distortion of nail plates in Fig. 174 and the onycholysis (separation of nail plates from nail beds) in Fig. 175. Infection by dermatophytes usually proceeds in a distal-to-proximal direction. Infection of nails by *Candida albicans* is different in that it is more acute (frequently purulent) and tends first to involve the lateral and proximal nail folds.

Figure 176

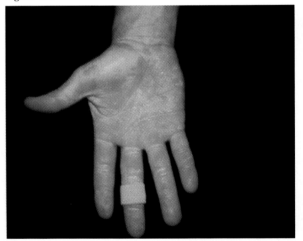

Figure 177

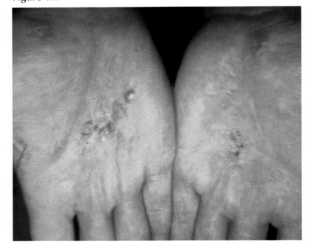

Tinea manuum Superficial fungal infection of the palms usually presents with erythema and whitish scale, predominantly in the palmar creases. It is almost always associated with tinea pedis. Generally tinea manuum involves one hand, but when both hands are involved, it is not symmetrical. The causative organism is usually *Trichophyton rubrum*. The condition may be treated with either topical imidazole creams or with oral griseofulvin. On the dorsa of the hands, the infecting fungi are more likely to be those that cause tinea corporis elsewhere.

Dermatophytids Fungal infections are sometimes accompanied by cutaneous eruptions that are the result of sensitization to the products of the fungi. Such cutaneous effects are called dermatophytids and are sterile of the fungi. Dermatophytids are papular and vesicular lesions, commonly on the hands. They usually stem from fungal infections of the foot that have become inflamed or irritated. The palmar blisters in this photograph are the result of such an event.

Figure 178

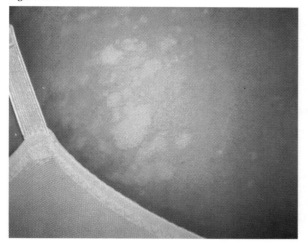

Figure 179

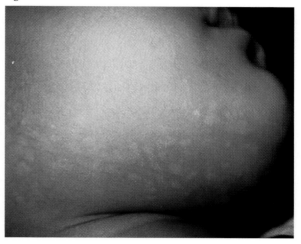

Tinea versicolor This title designates a superficial fungal infection *(tinea)* that changes color *(versicolor)*. The causative organism was originally called *Malassezia furfur* and is now called *Pityrosporum orbiculare*. Tinea versicolor typically causes numerous patchy scaling macules on the upper chest and back, proximal arms, and neck. Facial involvement may occur. The lesions may be hypopigmented, as illustrated here, or brown-orange, depending on the skin color of the patient and the degree of recent sun exposure. The organism is believed to prevent either the formation of melanin or the transfer of melanosomes into keratinocytes. The formation of azelaic acid is another suggested mechanism for the resultant hypopigmentation. Although tinea versicolor usually makes its appearance after puberty, it can develop in childhood and is occasionally seen in breast-fed infants. Tinea versicolor is usually asymptomatic but may itch slightly. The organism cannot be cultured, but diagnosis is aided by the orange or brown glow of lesional skin under a Wood's light, and by the "spaghetti and meatballs" appearance of clustered hyphae and spores on potassium hydroxide preparation.

Figure 180

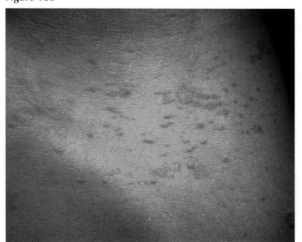

Figure 181

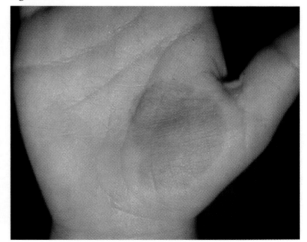

Tinea versicolor Illustrated here are small, scaly macules, which are in this case darker than the surrounding skin. There are several approaches to the treatment of tinea versicolor. Small areas of involvement can be eradicated by use of an imidazole cream. In patients with more extensive disease, the best approach is the use of a selenium sulfide or sodium thiosulfate lotion. Patients should be warned that treatment of tinea versicolor does not diminish the very high rate of recurrence and that the return to normal skin color may be delayed weeks to months after the completion of therapy.

Tinea nigra This is an infection of the stratum corneum, commonly on a palm, that is caused by the dematiaceous fungus *Exophiala (Cladosporium) werneckii.* It occurs most commonly in tropical regions. The clinical appearance is a tan-to-black discoloration with sharp borders that enlarge slowly. It can be mistaken for a melanocytic nevus, melanoma, or simple artifact. The correct diagnosis can be confirmed by potassium hydroxide examination or fungal culture. Treatment consists of a keratolytic lotion or topical imidazole cream.

Figure 182

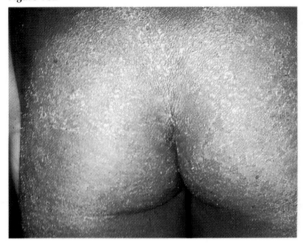

Tinea imbricata Tinea imbricata is a superficial fungal infection of the glabrous skin that is seen in a number of tropical countries. The causative organism is *Trichophyton concentricum*. Brown papules evolve into annular plaques. As the infection continues, many concentric ring lesions develop, which resemble the patterning of a tortoise shell. Griseofulvin is an effective therapy, but relapses occur.

Figure 183

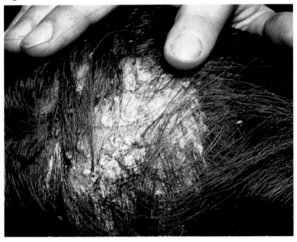

Favus This chronic form of tinea capitis is caused by *Trichophyton schoenleinii*. It occurs in parts of Europe, Africa, and South America as well as in some rural areas of the United States and Canada. Pictured here are the typical scaly patches seen in favus. The yellowish cup-like crusts, called *scutula,* are a distinctive part of this disease. The coalescent crusts form a plaque that emits a characteristic mousy odor. This form of fungal infection of the scalp may persist into adult life.

Figure 184

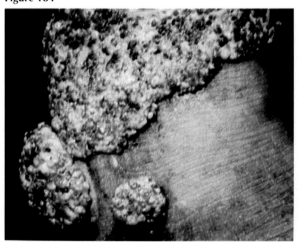

Chromoblastomycosis The parti-colored granulomatous process pictured here is of 12 years' duration. It started as a small nodule, developed slowly into a verrucous mass, and acquired satellite extensions. The condition, so reminiscent of a tuberculous process, is a deep fungal infection caused by species of *Phialophora, Fonsecaea,* and *Cladosporium,* which are indigenous to South America and other regions with warm climates. Lesions that are too large for surgical excision are treated with combinations of systemic flucytosine, amphotericin B, and ketoconazole.

Figure 185

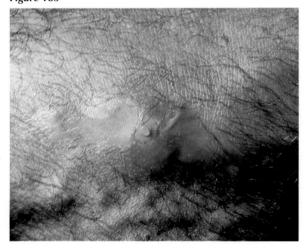

Coccidioidomycosis This disease, caused by the dimorphic fungus *Coccidioides immitis,* is endemic to the southwestern United States and parts of Central and South America. Most individuals in those areas develop the disease as an inconsequential upper-respiratory infection. However, severe disseminated disease can follow pulmonary infection and may involve the skin. In this case, the lesions are typically abscesses, nodules, or verrucous and inflammatory plaques. Primary infection of the skin, which is rare, is accompanied by regional lymphadenopathy. Amphotericin B is the customary treatment.

Figure 186

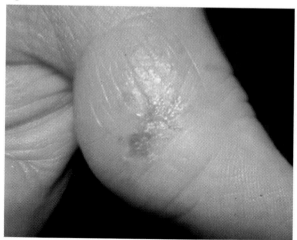

Figure 187

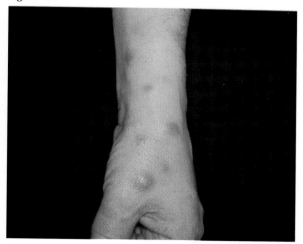

Sporotrichosis Cutaneous infection with *Sporothrix schenckii* is a disease with worldwide distribution. The majority of cases are seen in Central and South America, but outbreaks occur in the United States. The disease affects both children and adults and occurs when the causative fungus, in either contaminated soil or plant materials, contacts traumatized skin. The thorn of a rose bush may provide both the organism and a site of entry, and there have been outbreaks among children playing among bales of hay. Pictured here is the most common

form of sporotrichosis, the lymphocutaneous type. It causes an ulcerated lesion at the site of inoculation (Fig. 186) and a string of nodules or ulcerations along the lines of lymphatic drainage (Fig. 187). These tender secondary lesions may become chronic and extend into subcutaneous tissues. Very rarely, and especially in the immunocompromised host, disseminated or systemic sporotrichosis follows cutaneous infection. Diagnosis of sporotrichosis can be confirmed by culture of exudate or tissue from the skin lesions on Sabouraud's agar.

Figure 188

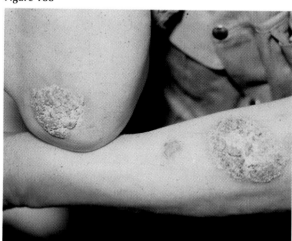

Figure 189

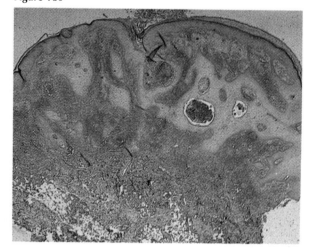

Sporotrichosis This figure illustrates a somewhat less common form of the disease, fixed cutaneous sporotrichosis. The patient fell on rocks while playing in the country and sustained abrasions on an arm and elbow. *Sporothrix schenckii* was cultured from the crusted plaques in both locations. In this clinical form, the deep fungal infection remains confined to one area of the skin and has no tendency toward lymphatic spread.

Histopathology of sporotrichosis Sporotrichosis is the most common deep fungal infection in which the skin is the portal of infection. The well-developed primary complex in the skin is clinically a chancriform or verrucous lesion that histologically shows epidermal hyperplasia and a dermal inflammatory infiltrate composed of neutrophils, mononuclear cells, and multinucleated giant cells, among which the infecting microorganism can sometimes be identified in the form of budding round bodies.

Figure 190

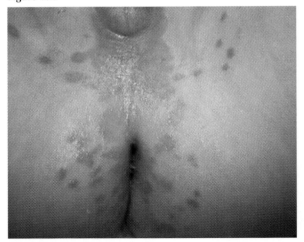

Figure 191

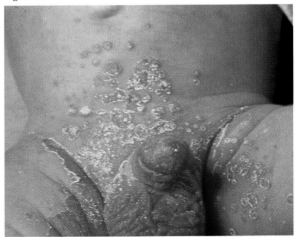

Candidiasis (moniliasis)   Cutaneous infection with *Candida albicans* tends to occur in areas that are chronically moist, warm, and macerated. For this reason, *Candida* is among the most common causes of diaper dermatitis. An early diaper rash in Fig. 190 illustrates some of the distinctive features of monilial infection. Note the confluent, glistening, beefy-red erythema, which begins in the perianal skin and spreads by local extension. There are numerous small satellite lesions. If untreated, this rash will go on to involve the gluteal folds, buttocks, and

inner thighs. More extensive involvement is seen in Fig. 191; note the peripheral scaling and again the satellite lesions. On occasion, these peripheral pustules and papules will involve the entire abdomen and back. Diagnosis of cutaneous candidiasis can be confirmed by potassium hydroxide preparation or by fungal culture. Treatment consists of the use of imidazole creams, such as ketoconazole, or nystatin. The several preparations that also contain a fluorinated topical steroid are not required for this condition and may lead to adverse local side effects.

Figure 192

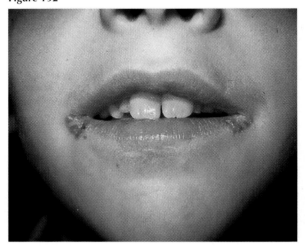

Figure 193

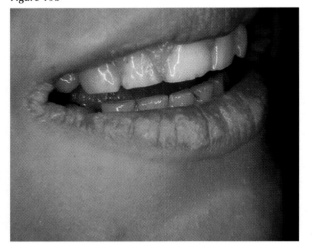

Candidiasis (moniliasis)   The angles of the mouth are also places where intertriginous conditions favor the overgrowth of ubiquitous *Candida albicans,* streptococci, staphylococci, and other ordinarily saprophytic but facultatively pathogenic microorganisms. The condition produced at the angles of the mouth (Fig. 192) is called *perlèche* or *angular stomatitis.* From such a beginning or even without it, the lips themselves may become involved in the manner pictured in Fig. 193. These con-

ditions are not to be confused with vitamin deficiencies, which are often overdiagnosed. Perlèche is more likely to be a mixed infection with *C. albicans* and bacteria. Therefore, treatment should be with a preparation that contains both an antimonilial agent like nystatin and a topical antibiotic. Candidal cheilitis is more difficult to treat and requires persistent application of a candicidal agent. Candidiasis in children with immunologic deficiency is particularly difficult to treat.

Figure 194

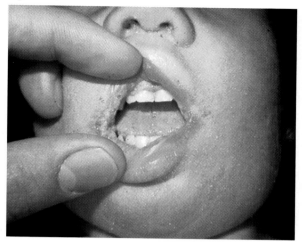

Figure 195

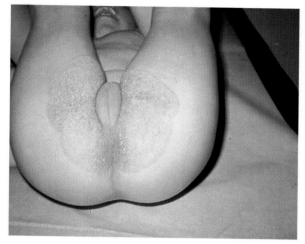

Chronic mucocutaneous candidiasis The immunologic inability to handle *Candida albicans* infection results in recurrent and severe infection of the mucous membranes, skin, and nails. Affected children have T-cell deficiencies due to a wide variety of underlying causes but manifest their mucocutaneous disease in similar fashion. Illustrated here are chronic perlèche and candidal cheilitis (Fig. 194) and a circumscribed, erythematous, and hyperkeratotic candidal rash in the diaper area (Fig. 195). Both areas of involvement in these patients have been resistant to con-

ventional antimonilial therapies. Chronic mucocutaneous candidiasis can also occur as an autosomal recessive syndrome, with no associated abnormalities. Early in their course, these children may be indistinguishable from those with profound immune deficiency disorders such as Swiss-type agammaglobulinemia, DiGeorge's syndrome, and Nezelof's syndrome. An identical clinical picture of unusual and persistent mucocutaneous monilial infection may be the presenting feature of infection with the human immunodeficiency virus.

Figure 196

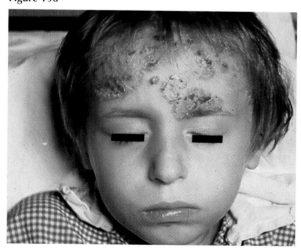

Figure 197

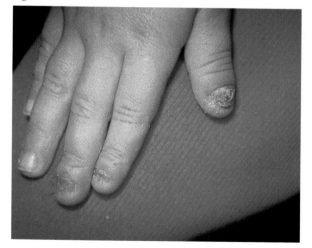

Chronic mucocutaneous candidiasis Chronic mucocutaneous candidiasis may in some patients lead to granuloma formation in the areas of infection. The face is a common site for the formation of these indurated and hyperkeratotic plaques. Note how the lesions on the forehead of the patient in Fig. 196 resemble some forms of tuberculosis cutis, sporotrichosis, and chromoblastomycosis, previously pictured and described. Figure 197 illustrates typical nail involvement in chronic mucocutaneous candidiasis. Patients develop swelling and tenderness

of the proximal and lateral nail folds. Eventually, the nails become brittle and discolored and may be destroyed by the process. Treatment with oral fluconazole is often effective. The use of intravenous amphotericin B and flucytosine should be reserved for unresponsive cases. Some patients with acrodermatitis enteropathica (zinc deficiency) and certain children with iron deficiency develop chronic mucocutaneous candidiasis. Dietary or parenteral replacement of the deficient mineral, as required, leads to resolution of the candidal infections.

Figure 198

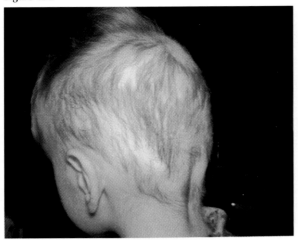

Figure 199

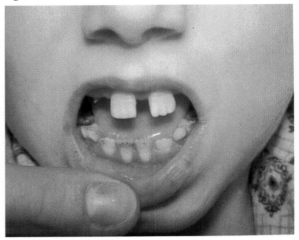

Chronic mucocutaneous candidiasis (cont.) In many patients, chronic mucocutaneous candidiasis is part of an autoimmune syndrome that has profound effects on the endocrine system. Hypoparathyroidism is the most common of these autoimmune syndromes and is present in more than 80 percent of the children with chronic mucocutaneous candidiasis. The sparse, brittle hair (Fig. 198) and the deforming effect of chronic hypocalcemia on tooth formation (Fig. 199) are both features of hypoparathyroidism. Other endocrine disorders that may be

associated with chronic mucocutaneous candidiasis include hypoadrenocorticism, gonadal insufficiency, and thyroid abnormalities. Alopecia areata and vitiligo may also occur in these patients. Children with the so-called candidiasis endocrinopathy syndrome have the same nail, skin, and mucous membrane involvement as do children with chronic mucocutaneous candidiasis from other causes. The onset of these manifestations usually occurs in early childhood, and the endocrine disease develops during adolescence.

Figure 200

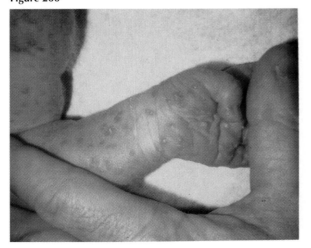

Figure 201

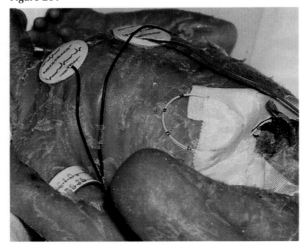

Congenital cutaneous candidiasis The presence of a generalized candidal dermatitis at birth is the result of intrauterine infection. Typically, erythematous papulovesicles and macules evolve into pustules and areas of superficial desquamation over a period of 6–8 days. The characteristic lesions frequently involve the palms and soles and may be accompanied by paronychias and true nail involvement. In contrast to neonatal can-

didiasis (acquired during passage through an infected birth canal), the diaper area and oral mucosa tend to be spared. If congenital candidiasis involves only the skin, the disease follows a benign course. Infants with low birth weight or respiratory distress may develop disseminated infection and require systemic therapy.

7

Bites and Infestations

Figure 202

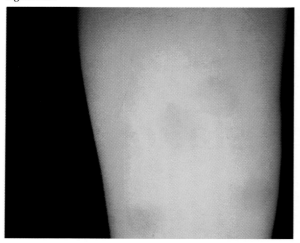

Figure 203

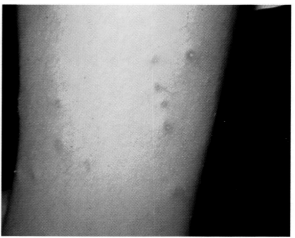

Insect "bites"   Many effects of metazoal parasitism are attributed to bites. Some metazoa (insects in a loose sense) do indeed bite, and others sting, but what we frequently designate as insect bite is attachment for feeding. The result of such attachment looks like a bite and is sooner or later attended by pain, itching, or stinging. True bites and stings, however, are instantly painful; many have immediate or late, more baleful effects; and most are generally inflicted in self-defense or seemingly wanton offense, not for feeding. Attachment for feeding is para-

sitism that may be silent for a while and then variably symptomatic. In a given region, common, indigenous metazoa that cause cutaneous effects by a bite, sting, or attachment for feeding may be recognized or guessed from signs and symptoms. These two illustrations are representative. Figure 202 may be guessed with reasonable correctness to be mosquito "bites," and Fig. 203, flea bites. We use quotation marks to suggest that the proboscis of a mosquito is not a true biting part. Fleas may nip.

Figure 204

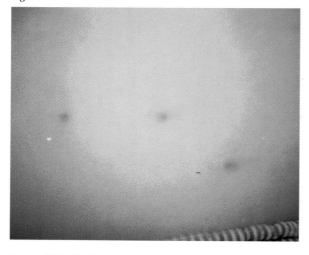

Figure 205

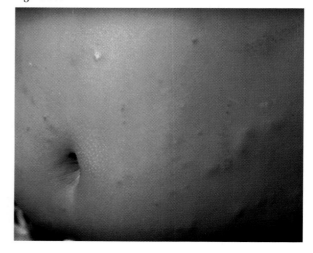

Insect "bites"   The mark of mosquito feeding is usually recognized easily because the season is right; the actual event is frequently seen as well as felt; often it is interrupted by a slap, which, when successful, results in a dead assailant; and the clinical and symptomatic consequences are familiar. Figure 202 shows the type of pruritic, urticarial, or edematous lesion caused by mosquitoes. Figure 203 and Figs. 204 and 205 are characteristic of "bites" of insects that feed, browse, and feed again.

Bedbugs and fleas are such insects. The marks tend to be aligned in rows of two or three. In the case of the mosquito, the lesions may be one, few, or many, depending on the insensitivity, foolhardiness, or defenselessness of the subject assailed. In the case of the bedbug, the number of lesions will depend on the number harbored and the immobility or restlessness and ineffable attractiveness of sleepers. Commonly, only one of two or more contiguous bedfellows is afflicted.

Figure 206

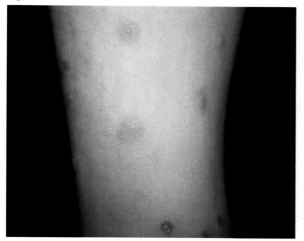

Insect "bites" (cont.)   When a subject has been bitten, stung, or fed upon, the consequent lesion may be typical at the time and in its course to resolution, or may be modified by scratching, secondary infection, or idiosyncratic host response. The lesions in Fig. 206 may well have been caused by mosquitoes, bedbugs, or fleas, but instead of the usual central punctum and surrounding erythema and edema, a summit of vesiculation has developed, probably signifying more-than-average host response as a result of previous sensitization.

Figure 207

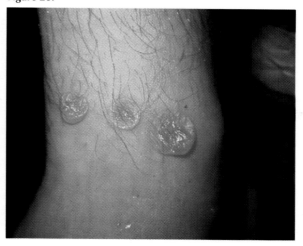

Dermatitis caused by the common carpet beetle   The common carpet beetle is not common in modern, well-sanitized homes, and even where it is abundant, effects from it are not common. Nevertheless, on occasion, the crawl of the insect on an unwary individual leaves its marks as wheals, papulovesicles, or bullae. This figure shows just such an event in the form of large, flaccid blisters. The three lesions in a line record the walk of a creature and the deposition of its irritant principle.

Figure 208

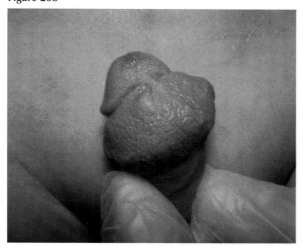

Insect "bites"   Insect assaults on ordinarily well-covered parts of the body are special. The body louse lives in the seams of garments and comes onto the body to feed. The marks of its sojourns are scratches produced by the itchy victim. Certain insects creep under clothes and bite when they reach a point of restriction like a garter or belt. Figure 208 shows bite marks and vast edema on the penis. The assaulting insect may have been an ordinary one that merely took advantage of a child left undressed and unguarded.

Figure 209

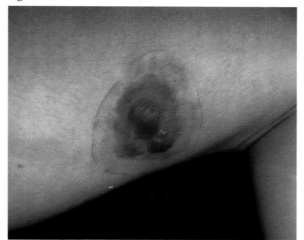

Spider bites   Spiders, timid creatures for all their fierce looks, would rather entertain insects in their parlors than attack humans. The tarantula is more dangerous in fable than in fact. Two spiders can deliver painful bites and serious venenation if frightened or cornered: the black widow spider (*Latrodectus mactans*) and the brown recluse spider (*Loxosceles reclusa*). The bite of the latter is illustrated here. It is a hemorrhagic bleb; in time it will become a necrotic ulcer. The patient will be severely sickened.

Figure 210

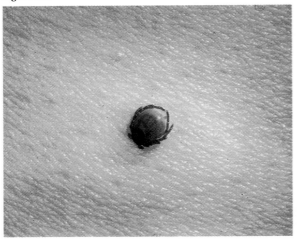

Ticks This figure shows an engorged deer tick attached to its human host. Ticks of the *Ixodes* species are vectors of Lyme disease as well as hemorrhagic fevers and viral encephalitis. Most tick bites are not painful and therefore may go unnoticed by patients for variable periods of time. A tick bite may appear as a red papule or may progress to erythema with local swelling, blistering, or ecchymosis. Chronic tick bite granulomas can develop that last for months to years.

Figure 211

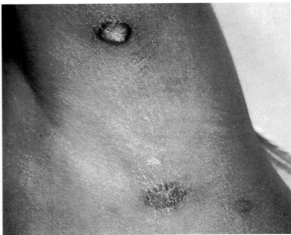

Tick "bite" Tick infestation occurs when the female soft or hard tick inserts her proboscis into the skin in order to withdraw blood. The site of attachment may develop into an erythematous nodule, and persistent pruritus may result if tick parts are left within the skin. Although most tick bites are insignificant, these insects may cause tick paralysis and are the vectors of Rocky Mountain spotted fever (Figs. 154 and 155) and erythema chronicum migrans (Lyme disease) (Figs. 74 and 75).

Figure 212

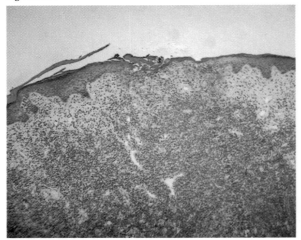

Histopathology of insect bites and stings Clinical and histopathologic responses to bites and stings of insects vary from urticarial edema to long-enduring inflammation. The latter is the more important because it consists of cellular infiltration in the dermis and may suggest malignancy. In this photomicrograph, one sees epidermal thinning and crusting, hemorrhage in the upper cutis, and a heavy infiltrate of pleomorphic cells that simulates a lymphoma.

Figure 213

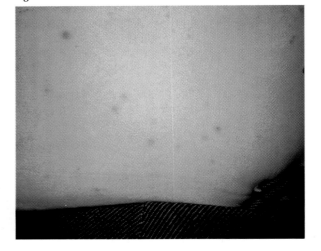

Scabies Infection of the skin by the human scabies mite *(Sarcoptes scabiei* var. *hominis)* is an extremely common skin disease of childhood. Numerous other species of mites that are obligatory parasites of dogs, cats, mice, and fowl or that subsist on food (cheese, grain, and other cereals) may also infest humans. This photograph shows a mild infestation with a mite ordinarily obligatory to dogs.

Figure 214

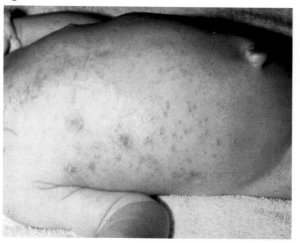

Figure 215

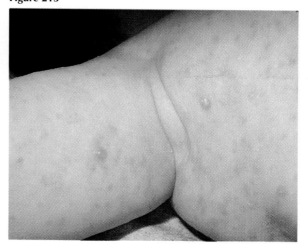

Scabies (cont.) This photograph shows infestation with the human itch mite. The infant with scabies illustrated here has numerous excoriated papules and a diffuse eczematous dermatitis. In infants, scabies frequently involves the entire cutaneous surface, including the face and scalp. Young infants without apparent pruritus may manifest extreme irritability.

Scabies Inflammatory nodular lesions involving the axillae and the diaper area are particularly typical of scabies in the very young child. These lesions may coexist with burrows, papules, vesicles, pustules, and areas of crusting. The nodules may persist for quite some time after the infestation is treated and do not reflect a persistent infestation.

Figure 216

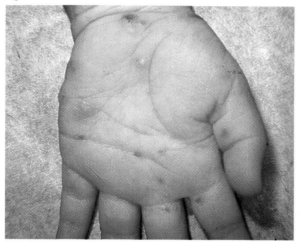

Figure 217

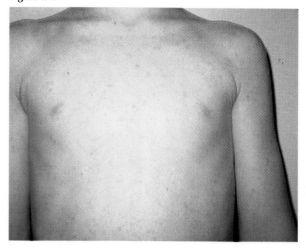

Scabies The location of primary lesions is often helpful in establishing the diagnosis of scabies. In older children and adolescents, the most common sites for the intensely pruritic lesions are the anterior axillary lines, the inner aspect of the upper arm, the areolae, the penis, the wrists and interdigital webs, and the ankles. In young children, the palms (Fig. 216) and soles are additional sites of predilection. Figure 217 is an illustration of the infestation in the anterior axillary lines. The undisturbed

lesion of scabies is a red papule that is a shallow burrow directly beneath the stratum corneum. It contains the gravid female and her young. When scabies is widespread and in typical areas of distribution, diagnosis can be made with surety on clinical grounds alone. In sporadic cases and when lesions are few, the top of a primary lesion may be gently shaved or scraped off into a drop of mineral oil and examined microscopically for the presence of mites.

Figure 218

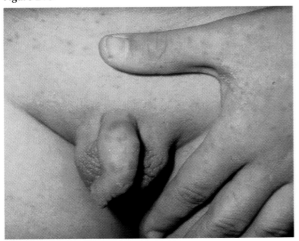

Figure 219

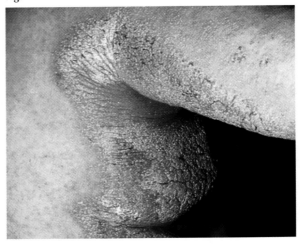

Scabies (cont.) Figure 218 shows typical lesions of scabies on the lower part of the abdomen, the penis, and the dorsum of the hand. The preferred treatment of scabies is a single overnight application of a 5% permethrin cream, repeated 1 week later. The application of any scabicide must be accompanied by the thorough laundering of all recently worn clothing and of bed linen, which may still contain mites or eggs. All close contacts should be treated.

Scabies This is a photograph of what is called Norwegian scabies. Individuals with this form of the disease develop thick areas of heavy crusting. Favored locations for the hyperkeratotic plaques include the elbows, knees, scalp, and buttocks. The areas of involvement contain numerous mites, and therefore the disease is highly contagious. Norwegian scabies occurs most commonly in patients with Down syndrome and among those who are debilitated or who suffer from an immune deficiency.

Figure 220

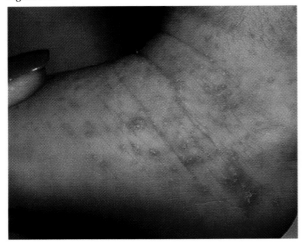

Figure 221

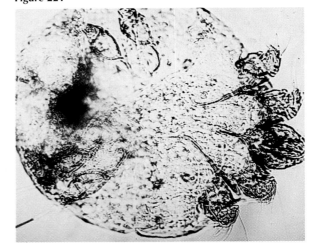

Scabies This figure illustrates burrows that are diagnostic of scabies. Burrows are represented by slightly raised white to light-brown linear lesions. The superficial part of the burrow has a scaly appearance, and at the distal end there may be a tiny black dot representing the mite, eggs, and/or fecal material (scybala) in a small vesicle.

Scabies This is a scabies mite. The mite has an ovoid body with four pairs of short legs. Eggs and feces (scybala) are deposited in the burrows by the female mite, and it is common to find all or some of these elements in a scraping of a burrow.

Figure 222

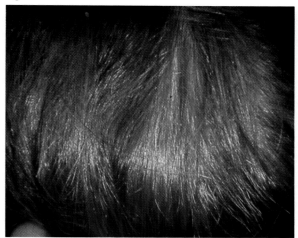

Figure 223

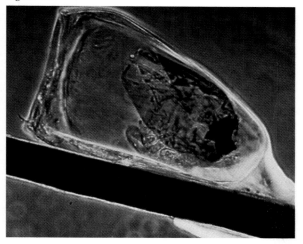

Pediculosis capitis The head louse is a wingless six-legged insect that is the smallest of the three human lice. It is adapted to live in the hair of the scalp only and lives by feeding on blood. The female louse lays approximately four eggs per day and has a life span of 2–4 weeks. It uses a gluey substance to attach the egg cases or nits to the hair. The diagnosis of pediculosis capitis is suggested by the presence of itching in the posterior scalp or signs of redness or folliculitis at the nape of the neck. Diagnosis is confirmed by the presence of nits, which, even when sparse, are easily recognized with hand-lens magnification. The reader is advised to use a hand lens on Fig. 222, which will reveal the nits well. The nit can also be recognized by one examining an infested hair under the microscope (Fig. 223). Treatment is simple and consists of either 1% lindane shampoo or a permethrin cream rinse. Remaining nits may be removed with a fine-toothed comb, aided by the application of an equal mixture of vinegar and water.

Figure 224

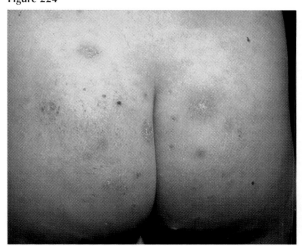

Figure 225

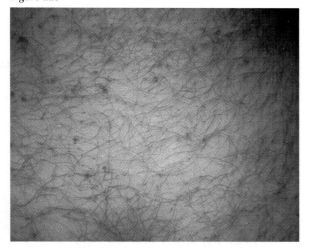

Pediculosis corporis The body louse belongs to the genus *Pediculus;* it is larger and broader than the head louse. Whereas the head louse infests the skin of the scalp, the body louse does not live on the body. It lives in the seams of undergarments and comes onto the body only to feed. Clinically, one sees marks of feeding and excoriations; the lice themselves can be found in the clothes. Treatment consists of disinfestation of clothing and bedding and the application of a pediculicide to the patient.

Pediculosis pubis The pubic louse *(Phthirus pubis)* is aptly called the crab louse. Examined under the microscope, this insect is broad like a crab and has legs that look like claws. On the skin, the louse looks like a brown fleck and may be mistaken for a freckle. Nits are also easily seen grossly, and better by hand-lens magnification. The illustration here is a good representation. Infestation may also occur in the eyelashes and axillary hair. Treatment consists of lindane shampoo or a variety of over-the-counter products that contain a pyrethrin.

Figure 226

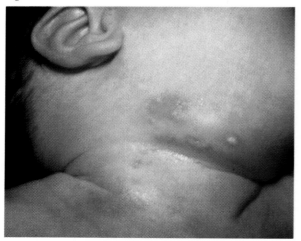

Figure 227

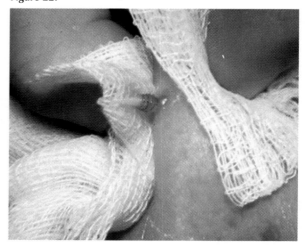

Myiasis The term for infestation with the larvae of flies is pronounced mī′yĕ-sĭs or mī-ī′ĕ-sĭs. In this condition, flies deposit fertilized ova upon neglected wounds or under onycholytic nails. The infestation is usually a sign of poor hygiene. *Dermatobia hominis, Wohlfahrtia vigil,* and several other species of botflies and warble flies may foster their young in this way. Figure 226

shows a cutaneous lesion but does not reveal the larvae, which can be better seen in movement in vivo by the naked eye. Figure 227 shows a larva clearly. In most cases, the larvae can be easily removed mechanically under local anesthesia. Antibiotics may be needed to treat secondary infection.

Figure 228

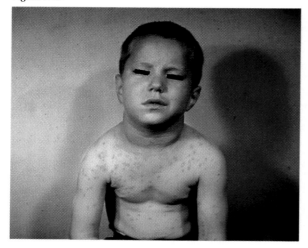

Figure 229

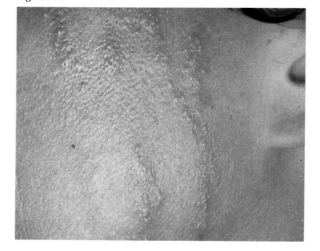

Caterpillar dermatitis The hairs of caterpillars and moths may produce pruritic or painful inflammatory skin lesions. The puss caterpillar and the brown-tail moth are the most common offenders. The toxin on the spines and hairs of these insects causes an irritant dermatitis. The resultant lesions, which are sometimes seen in linear array, may be papular or urticarial and are accompanied by itching or stinging. Systemic symptoms are rare but may occur. The hairs may be seen microscopically in skin scrapings. Treatment is purely symptomatic.

Dermatitis caused by blister beetles There are several species of beetles (order Coleoptera) that secrete onto their bodies cantharidin or some other vesicant substance. The crawl of the so-called blister beetles smears their irritant substances on the skin, causing the edema and blistering illustrated in the figure. Treatment with cool compresses and topical antibiotics to prevent superinfection is usually adequate.

Figure 230

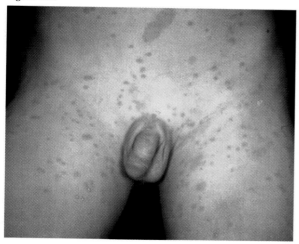

Figure 231

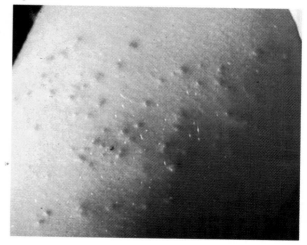

Seabather's eruption This eruption is an acute, pruritic dermatitis that occurs under covered areas after one bathes in seawater. Pruritus begins shortly after leaving the water, with the subsequent development of erythematous macules, papules, or urticarial lesions. Children may present with fever and chills. These intensely itchy lesions tend to resolve spontaneously over a period of 1 to 2 weeks. Recent reports have linked this eruption to the larvae of the phylum Cnidaria, which comprises jellyfish, corals, hydroids, and sea anemones.

Swimmer's itch This is an acute dermatitis produced by cercarial forms of schistosomes and primarily occurs in uncovered areas of the body. The eruption may be acquired in freshwater or saltwater. Like any intensely pruritic condition, excoriations and secondary infection are complications. Treatment consists of antipruritics, and antibiotics when superinfection occurs.

Figure 232

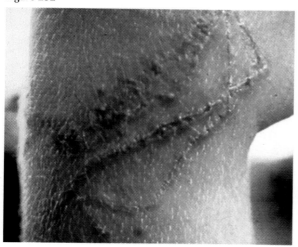

Figure 233

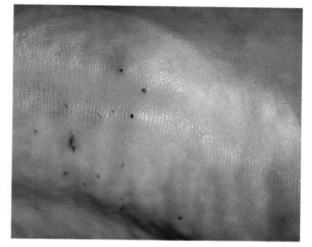

The sting of the Portuguese man-of-war One of the most painful effects on skin is the consequence of attack by oceanic hydrozoans known as Portuguese men-of-war, which are amazing for their size, brilliant color, and power to induce whealing. They have a small float that buoys them up and from which hang long tentacles. The wrap of these tentacles results in linear stripes, which look like whiplashes, caused not by the force of their swing but from deposition of urticariogenic and irritant substances.

The effect of contact with a sea urchin Sea urchins are a gastronomic delight when prepared properly, but a cutaneous torture when stepped on unprepared. The echinoids have spines that in some species are several inches long. Driven into skin when one steps or falls on or brushes against the creatures, the hard spines break and lodge in skin. Pain is inevitable, and secondary infection is nearly inevitable if they are left in. Nothing but tedious and meticulous extraction of every one of dozens, possibly scores, of spines is required for relief.

Figure 234

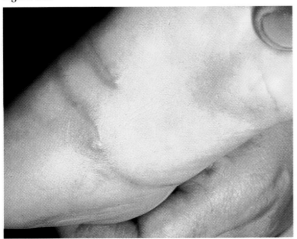

Figure 235

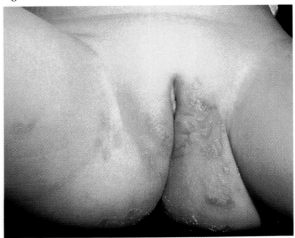

Larva migrans (creeping eruption)   Infestation of the skin with larvae of certain helminths, notably *Ancylostoma braziliense,* is common on the southern coast of the United States as well as in some other parts of the world. Helminths like *A. braziliense* infest the intestines of animals, particularly the dog, whose excreta contain larvae that have remarkable capacity to enter unbroken skin. Attaining the interior just below the stratum corneum, the immature forms move in a serpentine, erratic way, creating long channels. The larvae are sometimes barely discernible at the ends of the channels in the direction of travel. The feet, buttocks, arms, hands, and back are common sites of lodgment and lesions. The pictures show characteristic linear lesions on a foot (Fig. 234) and on buttocks and labia in an infant (Fig. 235) who was unwittingly placed on a contaminated beach or lawn. Treatment consists of the topical application of thiabendazole.

Figure 236

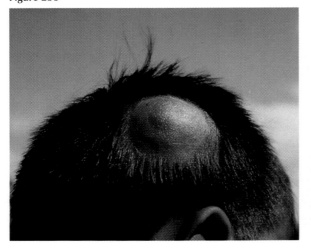

Figure 237

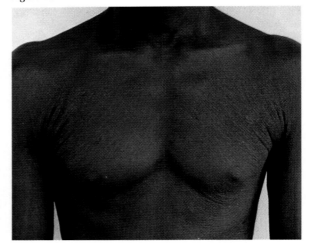

Onchocerciasis   *Onchocerca volvulus,* like *Tunga penetrans, Dracunculus medinensis, Wuchereria bancrofti,* and *Loa loa,* is limited to parts of the developing world. All these metazoa infest deeply and are difficult to eradicate. The filarial elephantiasis caused by *W. bancrofti,* the edema (Calabar swellings) about the eyes caused by the "African eye worm" *(Loa loa),* and the interdigital nodule, usually between toes, that harbors yards of the guinea worm *(D. medinensis)* are endemic to varying regions of Africa, South America, and Asia. Onchocerciasis is seen commonly in parts of Mexico. The metazoan that causes this disease is often found in the scalp and around the eyes, where infection may have serious consequences. Figure 236 is a lumpy lesion on the scalp, caused by the adult worm. Figure 237 shows less discernible lesions on the chest. These are caused by the organism in its microfilarial phase. The oral medication ivermectin is the drug of choice.

Allergic, Eczematous, Irritant, and Light-Related Dermatoses

Figure 238

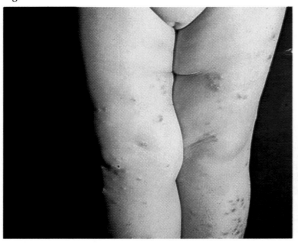

Figure 239

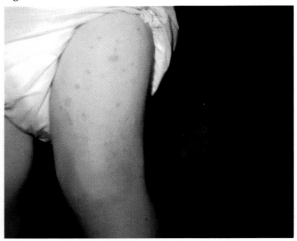

Papular urticaria   This is a pruritic dermatosis that is causally related to bites by mosquitoes, fleas, or other insects. Children with this common disorder tend to have recurrent episodes during the spring and summer months. The lesions consist of firm erythematous papules, sometimes with surrounding wheals. They favor exposed areas, especially the anterior lower extremities and lower arms. The individual papules are often excoriated and are sometimes impetiginized. The lesions tend to last for several days to weeks but will persist longer if chronically scratched or rubbed. Papular urticaria is more common among children with the atopic diathesis and represents a hypersensitivity reaction to the assaulting arthropod. Treatment consists of shake lotions, topical steroids, and antihistamines. The elimination of the offending insect from the household environment is helpful but will not prevent encounters during outdoor play.

Figure 240

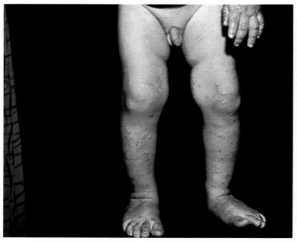

Figure 241

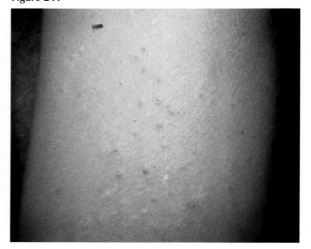

Prurigo mitis   This dermatosis occurs exclusively in children with the atopic diathesis, i.e., either a personal or a family history of atopic disease. The disease consists of chronic, pruritic papules that tend to favor the abdomen, extensor extremities, and buttocks. The lesions become excoriated, impetiginized, and lichenified over time. The relation between papular urticaria and prurigo mitis is somewhat unclear. Some observers believe that this condition begins with papular urticaria and is a chronic form of that disorder. In any case, children with prurigo mitis seem to have a more chronic and persistent dermatosis than those with simple papular urticaria.

Figure 242

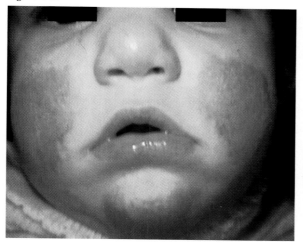

Figure 243

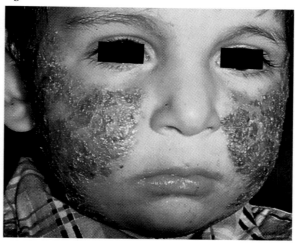

Atopic dermatitis This condition is the most common of all pediatric dermatoses. For the majority of patients, onset occurs during infancy. The classic clinical appearance in this age group is illustrated in Fig. 242. There are symmetrical patches of erythema, exudation, and scale involving the cheeks and chin. It is not unusual also to see widespread involvement of the trunk and extensor extremities during infancy; the diaper area is most often spared. Figure 243 shows similar distribution in an older child. In this case, impetiginization may be contributing to the crusted appearance of the lesions. Pruritus is a cardinal feature of atopic dermatitis and may be evidenced in the infant by irritability, scratching, and rubbing against nearby objects. Atopic dermatitis is an inherited disorder. Children with the disease most often have a family history of the atopic diathesis (atopic dermatitis, asthma, or allergic rhinitis) and may themselves manifest asthma or allergic respiratory disease.

Figure 244

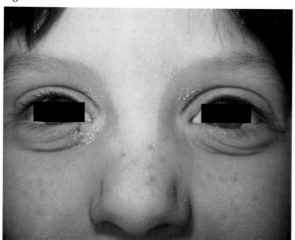

Figure 245

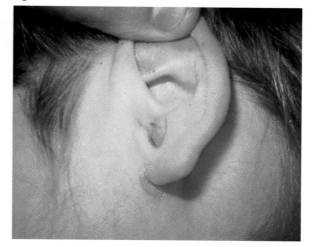

Atopic dermatitis When the diagnosis of atopic dermatitis is in doubt, the search for associated clinical findings is often helpful. Two such near-pathognomonic cutaneous signs of atopic dermatitis are pictured here. The Dennie-Morgan line (Fig. 244) is a double fold under the eye, which is seen in many children with atopic dermatitis. Figure 245 shows another telltale sign: a fissure at the junction of the pinna of the ear and the face.

Other associated findings related to atopic dermatitis include pityriasis alba (Figs. 254 and 255), keratosis pilaris (Figs. 277–278), lichen spinulosus (Figs. 341 and 342), and ichthyosis vulgaris (Figs. 433–435). Children with atopic dermatitis are also frequently noted to have hyperlinear palms and soles. Keratoconjunctivitis and cataracts may occur in the child with atopic dermatitis.

Figure 246

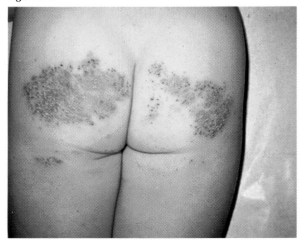

Figure 247

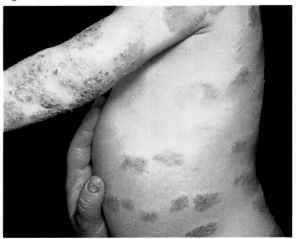

Atopic dermatitis (cont.)   During childhood, the most common locations of atopic dermatitis are the antecubital and popliteal fossae and the posterior neck. Pictured here are children in whom involvement is more widespread. The lesions show the characteristic erythema, oozing, and crusting of acute atopic dermatitis. This appearance correlates with the histopathology. Spongiosis and intracellular edema are cardinal features of acute lesions; chronic plaques show acanthosis and hyperkeratosis. The pathogenesis of atopic dermatitis remains a

mystery. Patients with the disease seem to have altered autonomic function and increased plasma histamine levels. Many have elevated levels of IgE, but some are completely normal in this respect. Finally, there is evidence of diminished cell-mediated immunity and polymorphonuclear chemotaxis in atopics. However, none of these observations has yet provided a basis for understanding the chronic and recurrent skin lesions of atopic dermatitis.

Figure 248

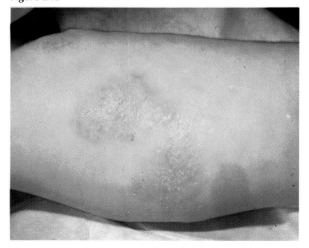

Figure 249

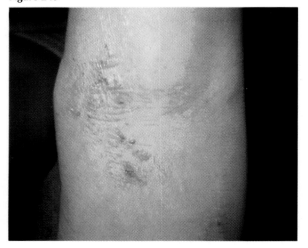

Atopic dermatitis   These are illustrations of atopic dermatitis on the elbow (Fig. 248) and in a popliteal space (Fig. 249) in a 5-year-old child. As mentioned above, the latter is a very common site for involvement in this age group. The majority of children with atopic dermatitis experience resolution of their disease and have normal skin as adults. However, the severe pruritus and the unpleasant appearance of the skin that accompany the exacerbations of this condition can be extremely troubling to parent and child alike. The role of diet in the treatment

of atopic dermatitis remains controversial. Despite evidence that some children with atopic dermatitis display a significant histamine response to some foods, it is fair to say that the majority of children with the disease do not respond to modifications of their diet. However, any foods that cause an obvious worsening of the condition should be avoided. Occasionally, food allergy in the atopic child may even be manifested by the rapid evolution of contact urticaria on the face and hands.

Figure 250

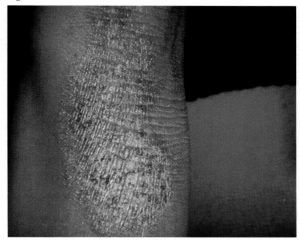

Figure 251

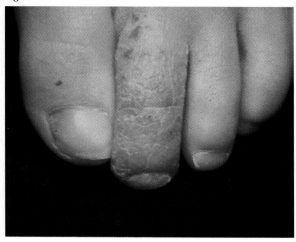

Atopic dermatitis   Figure 250 illustrates an area that is scaly and lichenified. Figure 251 shows atopic dermatitis involving one toe. The treatment of atopic dermatitis should include the establishment of a routine of skin care that maintains adequate hydration of the skin. Frequent bathing and the use of alkali soaps are to be avoided. Parents should be encouraged to apply a lubricating ointment to the child's skin several times a day. Topical corticosteroid ointments are currently the mainstay of medical management. Many children do well with proper use of the milder, non-fluorinated ointments, but some require stronger preparations for brief periods of time. The dangers of local atrophy and stria formation and of systemic absorption must be considered carefully with the use of the stronger formulations. The fluorinated corticosteroids should never be used on the face or in intertriginous areas. Important adjuncts to therapy include antihistamines and, occasionally, a brief course of oral antibiotics to reduce skin colonization with streptococcus and staphylococcus.

Figure 252

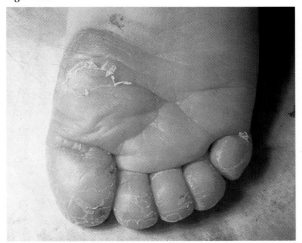

Figure 253

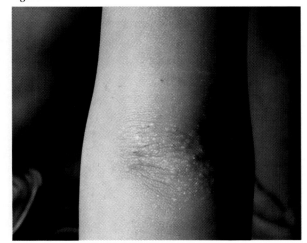

Juvenile plantar dermatitis   Figure 252 shows erythema and fissuring on the weight-bearing surface of the foot. This disorder, which tends to be worse in the winter months, is called *juvenile plantar dermatitis.* It is much more common in children with atopic dermatitis. Juvenile plantar dermatitis, which has also been called *wet-dry foot syndrome,* is caused by excessive sweating of the feet in occlusive footwear and rapid drying in a low-humidity environment. The use of emollient ointments is extremely helpful.

Summer prurigo   Illustrated here are fine, erythematous, and flesh-colored papules on the elbows. This pruritic eruption, termed summer prurigo or summertime pityriasis, occurs most commonly but not exclusively in children with the atopic diathesis. The rash is seen most frequently between the ages of 4 and 10 years and tends to recur seasonally in the late spring or early summer. Some children also have lesions on the knees and dorsa of the hands.

Figure 254

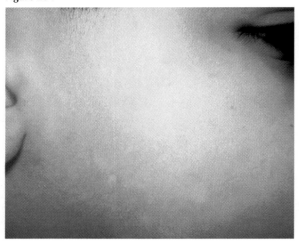

Figure 255

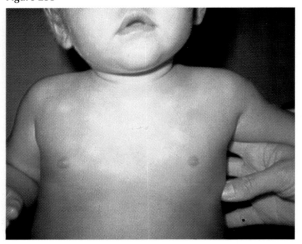

Pityriasis alba   This is a condition that is characterized by blotchy areas of hypopigmentation, with or without scale. The lesions are usually asymptomatic. In older children, the cheeks are a favored location; but in infants, the process may be more generalized. Both figures illustrate how the borders of the lesions tend to fade into the surrounding normal skin. This contrasts with vitiligo (Figs. 790–793), another common cause of pigment loss. In vitiligo, the areas of involvement tend to be a whiter white and are more sharply demarcated. Pityriasis alba is more common among children with atopic dermatitis and probably represents a form of postinflammatory hypopigmentation. There may or may not be a preceding inflammatory dermatosis in the same area. It is important to reassure parent and child that the loss of pigment is temporary and that complete restoration of normal skin color will occur. The use of a mild topical steroid may speed the process.

Figure 256

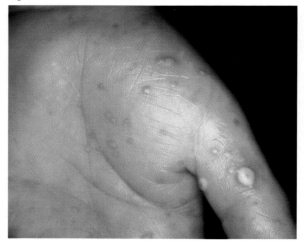

Figure 257

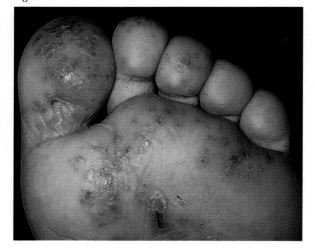

Pompholyx (dyshidrotic eczema)   This is a chronic, recurrent eruption of the hands and feet that is often accompanied by severe pruritus. It is considerably more common among individuals with an atopic history or with a family history of atopic disease. These photographs show a number of deep-seated vesicles and pustules on the palm and thumb. Small, firm vesicles along the sides of the fingers are a particularly common clinical sign. At times, bullae may occur. Patients who develop pompholyx often tend to have hyperhidrosis of the hands and feet. Some observers note that episodes of the disease are brought on by stress. Management of this condition is best achieved by the use of drying agents and topical corticosteroid creams or ointments with or without tar.

Figure 258

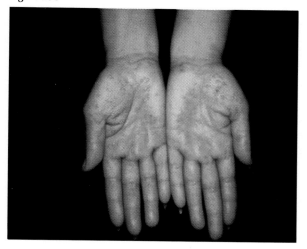

Figure 259

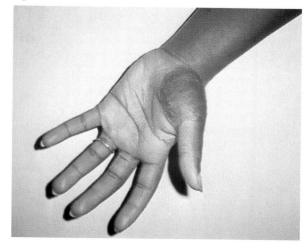

Palmoplantar pustulosis This chronic condition is characterized by erythematous plaques that are studded with multiple small pustules. The lesions are confined to the palms and soles, and onset may occur during childhood. The etiology of palmoplantar pustulosis is a mystery, and early theories that tried to correlate this disease with chronic occult infection (the so-called pustular bacterid) have largely been discarded. Although pustular eruptions of the palms and soles are seen in many patients with psoriasis, the patients with palmoplantar pustulosis do not

go on to develop psoriasis in other areas. Adolescents with palmoplantar pustulosis sometimes develop recurrent multifocal osteomyelitis. This is a chronic condition in which episodes of bone pain are found to be caused by localized areas of biopsy-proven osteomyelitis, usually in the long bones or sternum. Characteristically, repeated cultures of the bone marrow are negative. The osteomyelitis and pustular dermatosis tend to flare spontaneously, but the relationship between the two conditions is not known.

Figure 260

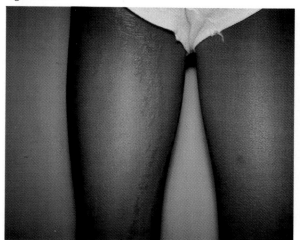

Figure 261

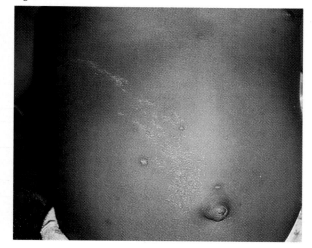

Lichen striatus This is a common and benign self-limited childhood dermatosis that is easily diagnosed from its classic appearance. Onset is usually between the ages of 3 and 10 years, and it is rare in young infants, adolescents, and adults. The lesions consist of pink, flesh-colored, or slightly hypopigmented flat-topped papules that evolve in a linear array following lines of Blaschko. As pictured in Fig. 260, the linear course of the

papules may eventually traverse the major part of an extremity. The area of involvement is often noted to become wider as it advances and may even include the nails. The lesions of lichen striatus are usually asymptomatic but may last 6 months to 1 year or even longer. The etiology of the condition is unknown. Treatment is not strictly necessary, but mild topical steroids tend to speed the process of resolution.

Figure 262

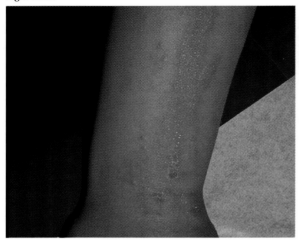

Figure 263

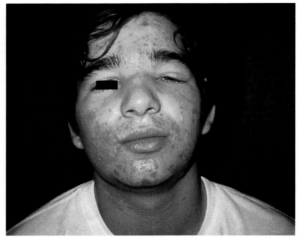

Allergic contact dermatitis This condition is a T-cell–mediated delayed hypersensitivity response to a variety of different antigens. Acute lesions are characterized by erythema, vesiculation, and oozing, whereas chronic areas of involvement may be dry and lichenified. The diagnosis of allergic contact dermatitis is a simple one when there is a clear history of exposure to an allergen or when the distribution of the lesions provides a strong clue. At other times, the identification of the causative agent can be very difficult. A number of different plants are capable of causing contact dermatitis. By far the most common are members of the genus *Toxicodendron:* poison ivy, oak, and sumac. These are illustrations of contact dermatitis from poison ivy, the most common single cause of contact dermatitis in childhood. The linear array of vesicles and bullae in Fig. 262 reflects the pattern in which the resin was transferred from leaf to skin. Figure 263 shows a more diffuse reaction. Children who experience recurrent episodes of this phytodermatitis should be encouraged to learn to recognize the causative plants.

Figure 264

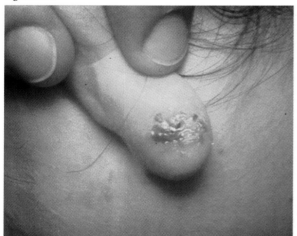

Figure 265

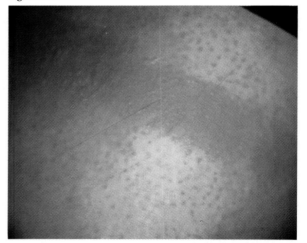

Allergic contact dermatitis These photographs illustrate two other common causes of allergic contact dermatitis. The young girl in Fig. 264 has developed an area of vesiculation and crusting because she is allergic to the nickel in her earrings. The same rash may develop under the metal buttons on blue jeans or beneath a wristwatch. Coating the surface of these metallic objects with clear nail polish will sometimes protect the skin from the allergen. In Fig. 265, a band of erythema and vesiculation has appeared on a thigh of a girl who has become sensitive to some component of rubber in an undergarment. Synthetic rubber contains many potential allergens, but the most common offenders are antioxidants and rubber accelerators. The treatment of allergic contact dermatitis is based on the successful identification and avoidance of the skin allergen. When the cause is not obvious, the use of a standard patch test kit may be of enormous benefit. The resolution of acute episodes of contact dermatitis is hastened by the application of topical corticosteroids; a brief course of oral prednisone is sometimes indicated in widespread disease.

Figure 266

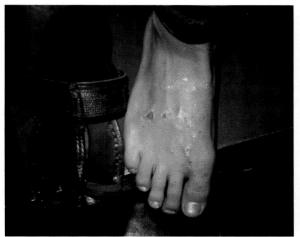

Figure 267

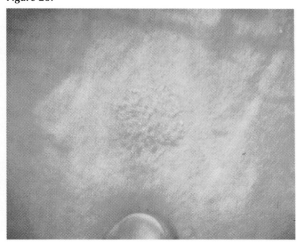

Allergic contact dermatitis (cont.) The allergic contact dermatitis in this figure was caused by a sandal. Note how the eruption conforms, like a patch test, to the design of the thongs. Shoe dermatitis should be considered in any eczematous eruption on the dorsum of the foot in a child. The agent responsible for the rash in this photograph was a tanning agent or dye. The other common causes of shoe dermatitis are rubber and rubber accelerators, adhesives, and leather. If the allergen is correctly identified by patch testing, it is possible to select footwear that is tolerable.

Allergic contact dermatitis The picture is of a patch test with resorcinol, positive in the form of a vesicular reaction at 48 hours in a person who has become sensitive to it. Resorcinol is a common substance used in dermatologic preparations and in proprietary formulations sold over the counter. The same sort of reaction would occur in a person sensitive to mercury, benzocaine, formaldehyde, paraphenylenediamine, and many other substances used in formal prescriptions and proprietaries.

Figure 268

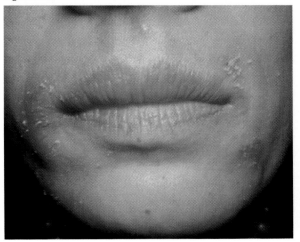

Figure 269

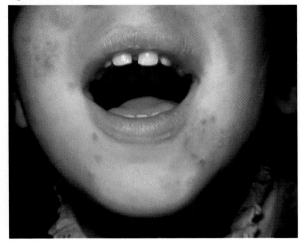

Allergic contact dermatitis Figure 268 illustrates the result of sensitization to an ingredient in lipstick. Lipstick cheilitis may be caused by indelible dyes, perfumes, or lanolin derivatives. The child in Fig. 269 has an allergic contact dermatitis resulting from the repeated application of a preparation containing neomycin. The development or worsening of an eczema-

tous eruption after the use of a topical medication, either prescribed or over-the-counter, should alert the physician to the possibility of a contact dermatitis (dermatitis medicamentosa). In addition to neomycin, common offenders are the stabilizer ethylenediamine and the paraben preservatives.

Figure 270

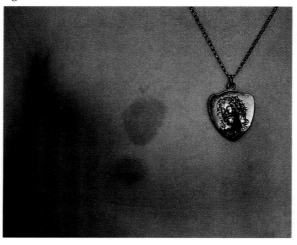

Allergic contact dermatitis (cont.)   Allergy to nickel is one of the most common causes of contact dermatitis in children. Infants may present with skin lesions corresponding to the location of snaps on their pajamas or other garments. Older children may show reactions to watches, chains, belt buckles, or earrings.

Figure 271

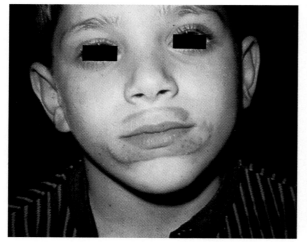

Figure 272

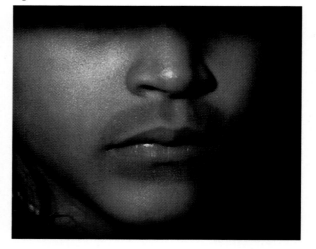

Cutaneous effects of primary irritation   Irritant contact dermatitis is an eczematous eruption that results from the application of an irritating substance to the skin. Examples would include strong acids or alkalis, harsh soaps, and bleaches. In these cases, T-cell–mediated allergy is not involved. The irritant in Fig. 271 is saliva. The child pictured here has developed a habit of licking his lips. Some children do this as compulsively as others suck their thumbs or bite their nails. Notice how the design of the inflammatory lesions conforms to the extent to which the lips can be drawn into the mouth or licked by the tongue. In Fig. 272, postinflammatory hyperpigmentation is shown in a child who has recovered from inflammation induced by chewing and blowing bubble gum.

Figure 273

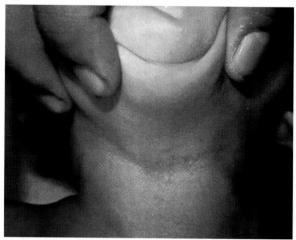

Figure 274

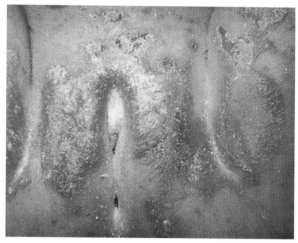

Intertrigo   Where skin is in natural apposition (for example, in the axillae, intergluteal folds, and neck folds) or where the skin is occluded, it is susceptible to the effects of wetness, higher temperature, friction, and accumulated debris. An area of slight erythema in the neck fold is illustrated here. The skin is superficially inflamed from excessive maceration of the stratum corneum, caused by retention of wetness from washing and insufficient drying or from retained sweat.

Irritant diaper dermatitis   The most common form of diaper dermatitis is related to the combination of moisture and friction. The result is illustrated in Fig. 274. Note that the areas of involvement are folds of skin that are in direct apposition to the diaper itself; the skin creases tend to be spared. The bright erythema and shiny appearance of the involved skin are typical. Rashes of this type must be differentiated from candidiasis, seborrheic dermatitis, and psoriasis.

Figure 275

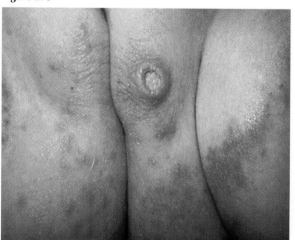

Figure 276

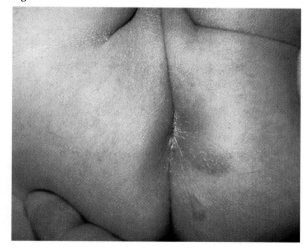

Erosive diaper dermatitis (dermatitis of Jacquet)   Inflammation that results from the precipitating factors of wetness, heat, friction, and debris in intertriginous places varies directly with the intensity and duration of those precipitating factors. The inflammation may be merely a slight erythema, a tumid, beefy redness with serous exudation, or an area of ulceration. The punched-out ulcer illustrated here is typical of the erosive diaper dermatitis of Jacquet. This severe irritant dermatitis responds to the use of barrier creams and mild topical steroids.

Granuloma gluteale infantum   This term refers to a granulomatous eruption of infancy that is usually confined to the diaper area but may also involve other intertriginous parts. The lesions are typically large nodules with a red or purplish hue; their alarming appearance may falsely suggest the presence of a neoplasm. The cause of this dermatosis seems to be a combination of local inflammation and, sometimes, cutaneous candidiasis. It may be aggravated by the use of fluorinated topical steroids.

Figure 277

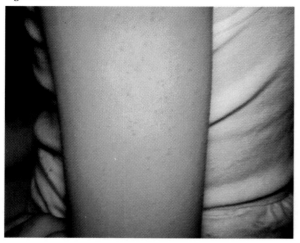

Figure 278

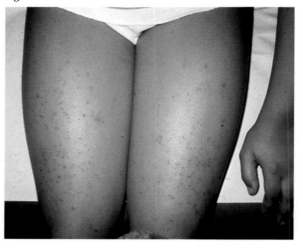

Keratosis pilaris   This is an asymptomatic condition that is often familial and is sometimes associated with atopic dermatitis or ichthyosis vulgaris. Pictured here are typical lesions in the two most common areas of involvement, the lateral aspect of the upper arms and the anterior thighs. The lesions are fine keratotic papules; each represents a plug in the upper part of a hair

follicle. The appearance of the involved areas is often likened to chicken skin or gooseflesh; the sensation on palpation is a grater-like roughness. Keratosis pilaris tends to worsen during the winter months and abates somewhat after puberty. Keratolytics and emollients are somewhat helpful.

Figure 279

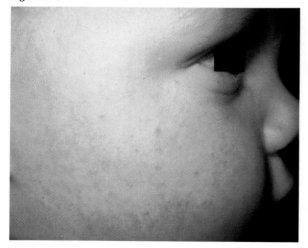

Figure 280

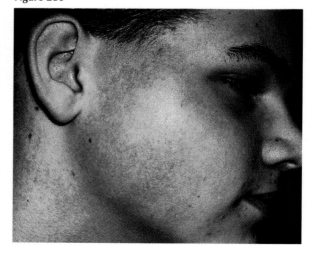

Keratosis pilaris   Children with keratosis pilaris sometimes develop the condition's typical follicular papules on the cheeks. When this occurs, there may also be erythema associated with the roughness. This condition is sometimes termed *keratosis pilaris rubra faciei*. Again, mild keratolytics are sometimes helpful.

Keratosis pilaris rubra faciei   This eruption is sometimes confused with infantile acne, in which comedones are found along with papules, pustules, and sometimes cysts. The prognosis of facial keratosis pilaris is good, although this condition may persist on the extremities.

Figure 281

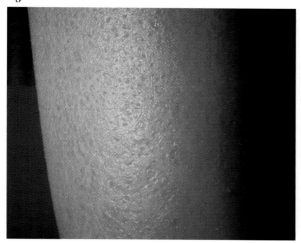

Xerosis   The accentuation of skin markings and fine scale illustrated here are typical of xerosis. The tendency toward dry skin tends to be inherited and is more common in families with a history of atopy. Low humidity, usually related to dry heat during the winter months, is an aggravating factor. Treatment of xerosis is aimed at rehydrating the stratum corneum. Emollients containing urea or lactic acid are particularly effective. Excessive bathing and the use of alkaline soaps must be avoided.

Figure 282

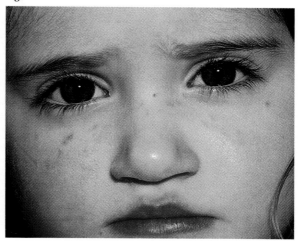

Naproxen-induced pseudoporphyria   Patients being treated with naproxen may experience an eruption characterized by the development of erythema, vesicles, and shallow atrophic scars after sun exposure. In many patients, frank vesicles are not appreciated. The acute eruption may persist for a few weeks after the medication has been stopped.

Figure 283

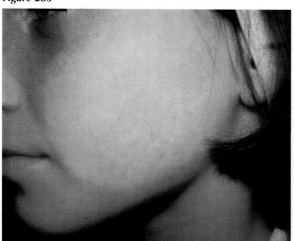

Polymorphous light eruption   Patients with this condition develop papules, papulovesicles, or erythematous plaques in response to sun exposure. The lesions erupt a few hours to several days after the subject has been exposed to sunlight and seem to be a response to the UVB (290–320 nm) part of the action spectrum. Lesions are most often located on the face, upper chest, and exposed parts of the extremities. Ocular inflammation and cheilitis may also occur. Among North American and Latin American Indians, polymorphous light eruption tends to

Figure 284

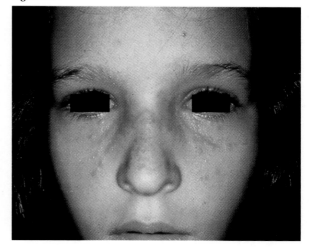

be a familial disease with childhood onset. Figure 283 shows an area of erythema and edema. The butterfly rash illustrated in Fig. 284 gives a sense that polymorphous light eruption can sometimes be difficult to differentiate from the cutaneous findings in systemic lupus erythematosus. Both immunofluorescence and serology are useful techniques in differentiating the two diseases. Sunscreens, antimalarial medications, topical corticosteroids, and psoralens with ultraviolet light (PUVA) are among the treatments used for polymorphous light eruption.

Figure 285

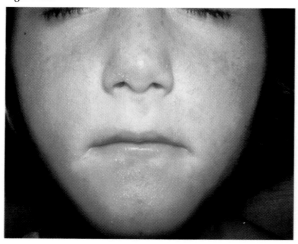

Figure 286

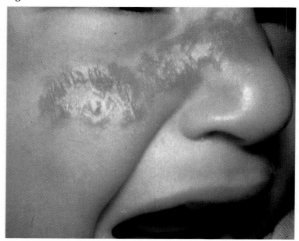

Photoallergic and phototoxic dermatitides   In addition to sunburn and polymorphous light eruption, there are several other abnormal cutaneous reactions in which sunlight is part of the causative mechanism. Among these are photoallergic (Fig. 285) and phototoxic (Fig. 286) dermatitides. In the former, sensitization and subsequent clinical reactions develop to a topically applied or internally administered substance that has been activated to allergenicity by sunlight. The topical halogenated sal-

icylanilides are among the most common causative agents in photoallergy. In phototoxic reactivity, no immunologic mechanism is involved, and the patient reacts as anyone would to a primary irritant. Phototoxic drugs and chemicals include some dyes, coal tar derivatives, and the psoralens. Drugs that may cause a phototoxic reaction include the sulfonamides, tetracyclines, and thiazides.

Figure 287

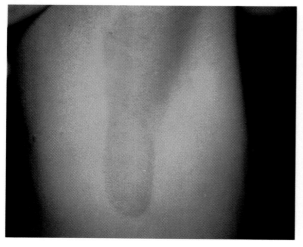

Figure 288

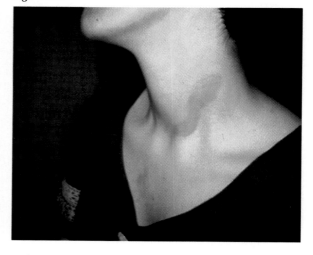

Phytophotodermatitis (berloque dermatitis)   This condition is a special kind of photoreaction in which the skin becomes slightly inflamed and quickly develops hyperpigmentation. The cutaneous changes are the result of contact with a photosensitizing chemical, followed immediately by sunlight. The most common causative agents are furocoumarins (psoralens). These figures illustrate the form of this condition that results from the application of a psoralen-containing perfume,

such as oil of bergamot. Note that the hyperpigmentation follows the exact distribution in which the perfume was applied. In addition to perfumes, a number of plants, grasses, fruits, and vegetables contain psoralen as a photosensitizer. The child who helps mother or father slice limes before a trip to the park may develop an identical eruption on the hands. Celery and parsley may present similar problems.

Figure 289

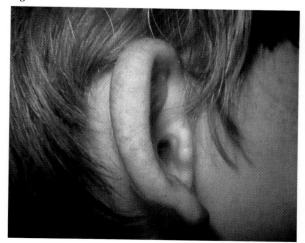

Figure 290

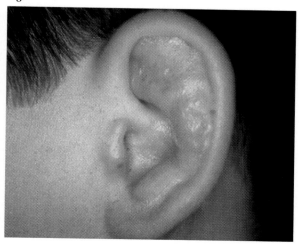

Actinic prurigo   This term refers to a disease with onset in early childhood. Patients develop an intensely pruritic eruption in response to sunlight. The papules, vesicles, and crusted plaques tend to favor areas of exposed skin but may become generalized. The disease process is most severe during the late spring and summer. Illustrated in both figures is the inflammatory pruritic dermatitis on a common location, the pinnae of the ears. The relationship between the disease called *actinic prurigo* (or Hutchinson's summer prurigo) and polymorphous light eruption (Figs. 283 and 284) has been an area of controversy. Some observers believe that the diseases are identical, but others feel that actinic prurigo is a distinct entity. Treatment for children with this clinical syndrome consists of maximal protection from sunlight. Topical steroids are of some benefit during exacerbations.

Papulosquamous, Lichenoid, and Perforating Disorders

Figure 291

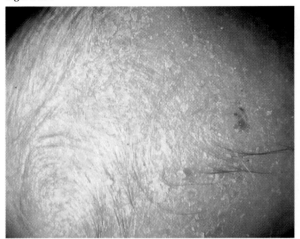

Figure 292

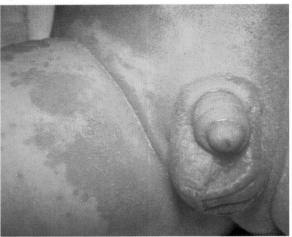

Seborrheic dermatitis　This term refers to a scaly, crusting, and erythematous eruption that favors areas where there are numerous sebaceous glands. It is most common in infancy (ages 2 to 12 weeks), when it tends to favor the scalp, diaper area, and intertriginous folds. Figure 291 is an illustration of the process in the scalp, where it is often referred to as cradle cap. Figure 292 shows seborrheic dermatitis in the diaper area. The photographs cannot convey the greasiness of the condition, and indeed at certain stages dry scaling rather than oiliness is predominant. A subset of infants with seborrheic dermatitis will go

on to develop atopic dermatitis, and it sometimes may be difficult to differentiate between these two conditions. Some basic principles are that the lesions of seborrheic dermatitis are usually well circumscribed, do not itch, and localize toward the scalp and intertriginous areas. The greasy red-orange scaliness of seborrheic dermatitis is somewhat helpful in differentiating this disorder from atopic dermatitis. Finally, seborrheic dermatitis has its onset early in infancy and usually resolves by 1 year of age; atopic dermatitis tends to begin later and to be more persistent.

Figure 293

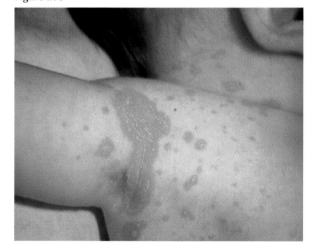

Figure 294

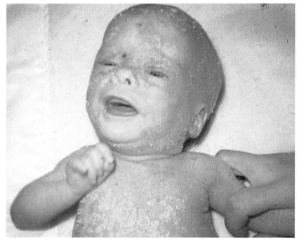

Seborrheic dermatitis　Figure 293 shows seborrheic dermatitis in and around the axilla. Note the circumscribed salmon-colored lesions and the greasy character of the scale. Figure 294 shows a more extensive process that is nearly generalized and drier in scaly appearance. The cause of this very common condition remains unknown. Although it favors areas with an increased number of sebaceous glands, there is no evidence that

seborrheic dermatitis is a disease of sebaceous glands or is related to excessive sebum production. Some studies have suggested that the lipid composition of sebum in seborrheic dermatitis may be abnormal. Bacteria and yeasts are often present in areas of involvement, but neither *Candida albicans* nor *Pityrosporum ovale* has been shown to be an etiologic agent.

Figure 295

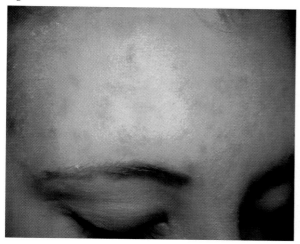

Figure 296

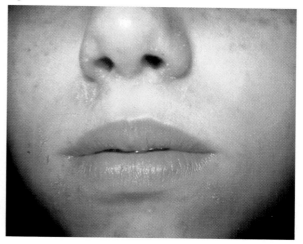

Seborrheic dermatitis　Seborrheic dermatitis, common during infancy, is relatively unusual during later childhood. It resurfaces as a problem during adolescence and then seems to become progressively more common through adult life. The generalized seborrheic dermatitis of infancy gives way to a process that primarily involves the scalp, forehead, tarsal margins of the eyelids (blepharitis), ears, and nasolabial folds. Itching or vague discomfort sometimes accompanies the low-grade inflammation. Flare-ups of the disease tend to occur during the

spring and fall seasons. Pictured in Fig. 295 are erythema and greasy scaling of the forehead and eyebrows. Figure 296 illustrates typical involvement of the nasolabial folds. Seborrheic dermatitis is easily controlled but not everlastingly curable. Treatment may consist of a sulfur and salicylic acid ointment or a mild topical steroid cream. The frequent use of tar shampoos is particularly helpful in the control of seborrheic dermatitis of the scalp.

Figure 297

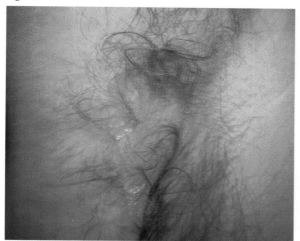

Figure 298

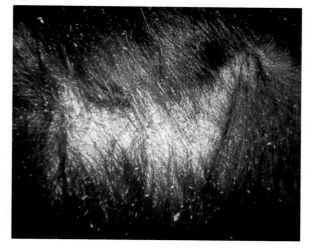

Seborrheic dermatitis　After puberty and in adulthood, seborrheic dermatitis occurs not only on the scalp and face but also on the chest, on the back, and in intertriginous spaces like the axillae, inframammary areas, groin, and intergluteal folds. Lesions on the chest and back are described as petaloid, i.e., flat and demarcated like petals; in intertriginous spaces, glistening redness is the appearance. This photograph shows the latter in an axilla.

Tinea amiantacea　This term requires etymological explanation. The *tinea* does not mean superficial fungal infection but rather a condition that resembles a superficial mycosis. *Amiantacea* means asbestos-like. The combination describes a superficial scaly process that recalls the crumbling exfoliation of asbestos. Such an appearance occurs in the scalp in some cases of seborrheic dermatitis, psoriasis, tinea capitis, and pityriasis sicca (dandruff). The term is discarded as soon as a better diagnosis is made.

Figure 299

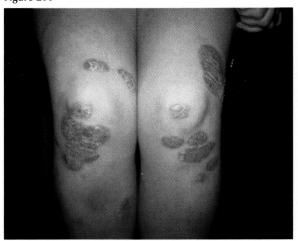

Figure 300

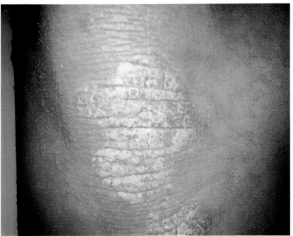

Psoriasis   More than one-quarter of all individuals with psoriasis develop their disease during childhood or adolescence. The degree of involvement is extremely variable; some children develop only a few localized plaques, while others suffer from generalized skin disease and severe arthritis. Pictured in Fig. 299 are the typical lesions of psoriasis; the plaques have a red-to-orange hue, are scaly, and are sharply demarcated from the surrounding skin. The symmetrical involvement of the knees is a common pattern; elbows and buttocks are other favored loca-

tions for plaques like these. The distinctive character of the scale is best appreciated in Fig. 300. The scale is usually described as silvery or micaceous (resembling the mineral mica). When the scale is removed, pinpoint areas of bleeding (Auspitz sign) are uncovered. Each lesion of psoriasis represents an area of rapid epidermal cell turnover. The thickening of the involved epidermis and the overlying parakeratosis translate into the raised and scaly appearance of the involved skin.

Figure 301

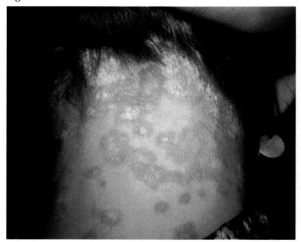

Figure 302

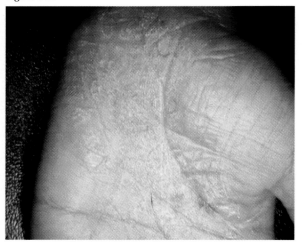

Psoriasis   In Fig. 301 we see typical areas of involvement on the glabrous skin of the neck and plaques of dense adherent scale in the scalp. Circumscribed areas of micaceous scale in the scalp are a common presenting sign of psoriasis. Figure 302 shows the scaling and thickening of the palms and soles that are very common in both children and adults with psoriasis. Therapy of psoriasis is based on the skillful use, either alone or in combination, of a number of therapeutic agents. The most effective are topical steroids, tars, keratolytics, ultraviolet light, and topical calcipotriol in older patients. Children with simple

plaque psoriasis can often be managed with short-contact anthralin preparations. When topical steroids are used, it is important to employ the least potent preparation that is effective and to avoid the use of fluorinated steroids on the face and in intertriginous areas. Preparations containing salicylic acid, a keratolytic, are especially useful for treatment of scalp psoriasis. Finally, careful exposure to sunlight during the summer months and artificial ultraviolet light at other times is enormously beneficial in selected patients with extensive involvement.

Figure 303

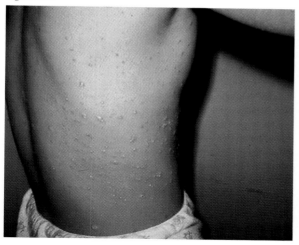

Figure 304

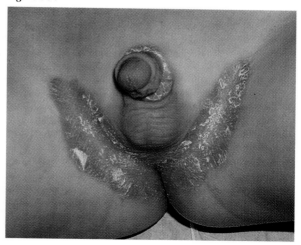

Psoriasis   Pictured here are two more representations of common forms of psoriasis. In Fig. 303 the lesions consist of numerous papules, each covered with the typical silvery scales of psoriasis. This form of the condition, termed *guttate psoriasis,* is more common in childhood and may have an explosive onset. There is often a history of an antecedent upper-respiratory infection, and streptococcal disease is of particular importance in triggering this eruption. The use of oral antibiotics that are

effective against streptococcus sometimes hastens the resolution of guttate psoriasis. Figure 304 illustrates psoriasis in the diaper area. When onset of the disease occurs during infancy, this is a very common area of involvement. It is postulated that the repeated irritation in this area constitutes a type of Koebner phenomenon. Scales are less in evidence because of the maceration that is inevitable in this location.

Figure 305

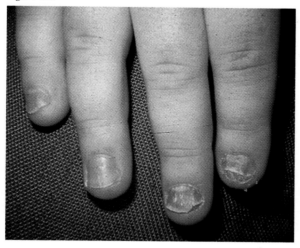

Figure 306

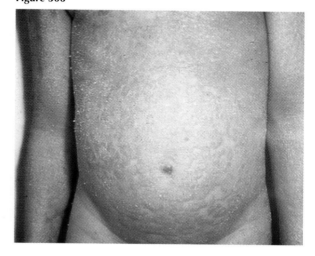

Psoriasis   Psoriasis of the nail plates is a frequent manifestation of the disease and exceedingly difficult to treat. The most characteristic and often the earliest change is the formation of numerous small pits in the surface of the nail plate. As the disease progresses, the nail becomes discolored, and there is subungual hyperkeratosis, onycholysis (separation of nail bed and nail plate), and onychomadesis (shedding). Figure 305 illustrates severe involvement with crumbling in two fingernails and minimal disease in the nails of the neighboring fingers. Figure

306 illustrates generalized psoriasis. Almost the entire body is covered with scaly lesions. Some such cases also go on to exfoliative erythroderma. The condition then is not only disfiguring and uncomfortable but also severely disruptive to cutaneous function. Problems arise with respect to heat regulation, sweating, and maintenance of electrolyte balance. Protein loss from excessive scaling is metabolically disruptive. Hospitalization and careful management of this condition are required.

Figure 307

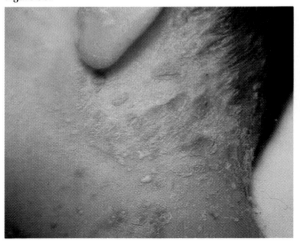

Figure 308

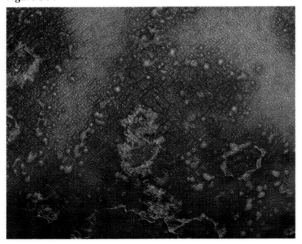

Psoriasis (cont.)   These figures illustrate pustular psoriasis. Both are examples of the disease in relatively mild form, but even in these the suppurative quality of the lesions can be appreciated. Severe pustular psoriasis, also known as the von Zumbusch form, is a rare and potentially life-threatening disease. Pustular psoriasis may be triggered by physical or emotional stress, a number of medications, or the abrupt discontinuation of steroid therapy. Patients with this form of the disease form develop shaking chills, fever, and leukocytosis. Numerous superficial pustules develop on psoriatic plaques and on uninvolved skin. Over a brief period of time, the pustules enlarge and become confluent; lakes of pus form. The process may eventuate in an exfoliative erythroderma. Hospitalization and careful supportive therapy are important aspects of treatment.

Figure 309

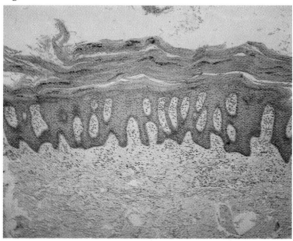

Figure 310

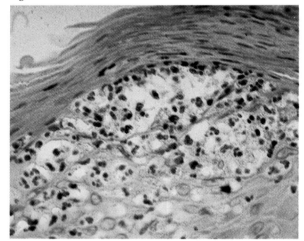

Histopathology of psoriasis   The microscopic picture of typical psoriasis is generally diagnostic. In Fig. 309, one sees a markedly thickened stratum corneum with retained nuclei (parakeratosis) and focal collections of degenerating neutrophils (microabscesses of Munro). The stratum granulosum has disappeared, and the rete ridges of the stratum malpighii are fairly uniform in length, club-shaped, and fused. The interdigitating dermal papillae reach very close to the surface, with thinning of the overlying epidermal suprapapillary plates. Often the papillae contain prominent, thin-walled blood vessels, which easily rupture when the surface scale is forcibly removed, resulting in minute bleeding points (Auspitz sign). In the migration of neutrophils toward the stratum corneum, as they seem to be released in intermittent bursts from the papillary vessels, accumulations of them may develop high in the malpighian layer, producing the so-called spongiform pustule of Kogoj, one of which is seen in Fig. 310.

Figure 311

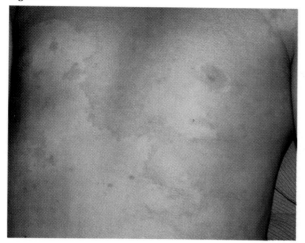

Figure 312

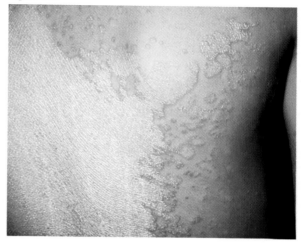

Pityriasis rubra pilaris   This is a chronic and often severe cutaneous disorder that may sometimes begin during childhood. Depending on the stage and location of the disease process, the appearance varies. The most unique distinguishing manifestation of this disease are the red-orange perifollicular keratotic papules that are usually located on the dorsal surfaces of the fingers and hands. The "nutmeg grater" appearance in these areas is virtually pathognomonic of pityriasis rubra pilaris. Fig-

ures 311 and 312 illustrate the disease process as it appears on the trunk. Here, follicular localization may be apparent early in the condition, but later, plaques of scaling, erythema, and edema are more usual. The condition may become generalized, but usually some islands of normal-appearing skin remain interspersed between involved areas. A similar erythema and scaling of the face and scalp may represent the initial presentation of pityriasis rubra pilaris.

Figure 313

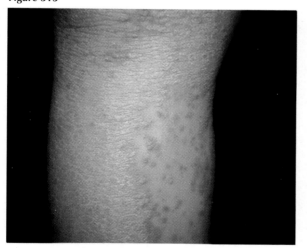

Figure 314

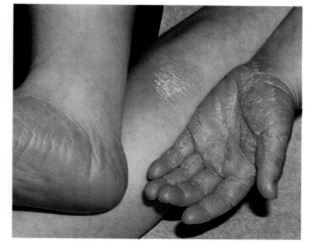

Pityriasis rubra pilaris   Figure 313 shows both discrete follicular papules and larger confluent, psoriasiform plaques on the leg. Palmoplantar involvement in pityriasis rubra pilaris is very common and can be disabling. Figure 314 illustrates the highly characteristic appearance of the condition on the palms. There is a diffuse hyperkeratosis that is symmetrical and covers the entire palmar surface. Similar changes may be present on the soles of the feet, and dystrophy of both fingernails and toenails may

be prominent. Pityriasis rubra pilaris in children has been divided into subtypes based on natural history and clinical appearance. The *classic* juvenile form affects children in the first 2 years of life and often tends to become generalized and severe. The *circumscribed* juvenile type presents with patches of follicular papules and displays a lesser tendency toward progression to generalized disease. Finally, the *atypical* juvenile form is the rarest, has the poorest prognosis, and tends to be familial.

Figure 315

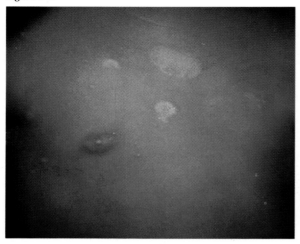

Figure 316

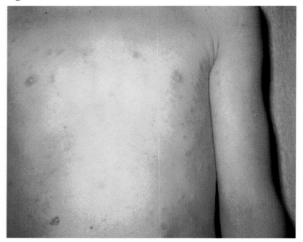

Pityriasis rosea　This benign and self-limited eruption occurs most often in the spring and autumn. Most patients are adolescents and young adults, but the disorder is not unusual in children and may even occur during infancy. In its classic form, pityriasis rosea follows a specific and predictable clinical course. The first, solitary lesion is a circle or oval of erythema and scaling. As it develops to its full size of 2–3 cm, this so-called herald patch may easily be mistaken for a lesion of tinea corporis. The chest and upper thigh are common locations for the herald patch, but any area may be involved. A typical her-

ald patch is shown in Fig. 315. Within a period of 5–15 days, additional lesions begin to develop. Patients develop numerous round-to-oval pink-orange macules that are 3–10 mm in diameter. Each has an edge of fine scaling, the characteristic "collarette." Larger, round-to-oval patches may also be present. The lesions of pityriasis rosea tend to cluster on the trunk and proximal extremities and often are most numerous in the axillae. The generalized process is illustrated in Fig. 316. The duration of the total process is 6–9 weeks.

Figure 317

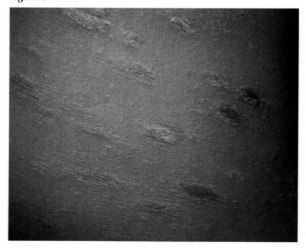

Figure 318

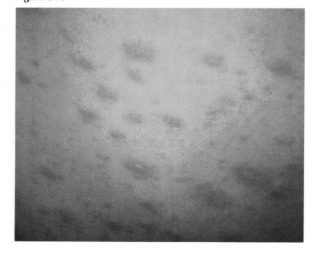

Pityriasis rosea　These figures illustrate well-developed lesions of pityriasis rosea in the mid-course of the condition. In Fig. 317, the fine rim of scale on the periphery of each lesion may be noted. In addition, one can appreciate the parallel array of the individual macules. On the back and chest, this tendency of the lesions to follow skin lines (the so-called Christmas tree distribution) is usually most obvious. A number of atypical forms of pityriasis may occur, and these variations in both mor-

phology and distribution seem to be more common during childhood. In particular, papules, pustules, and even vesicles may occur, and their presence may suggest a number of other cutaneous disorders. However, a careful search will usually lead to one or several of the typical papulosquamous lesions. In addition, lesions may extend to involve the face, and there may be relative sparing of the trunk. In some cases, the process is confined to intertriginous areas.

Figure 319

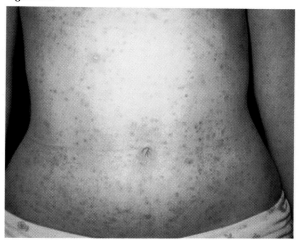

Figure 320

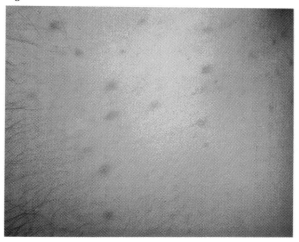

Pityriasis lichenoides chronica (guttate parapsoriasis)
The term *parapsoriasis* is used to describe a number of unrelated dermatologic conditions that are also unrelated to psoriasis. Pityriasis lichenoides chronica is a chronic disorder that is relatively unusual in children. It consists of superficial lesions that evolve from papules into oval pink-brown papulosquamous lesions. There may be an adherent scale overlying the individual lesions, and there is sometimes mild pruritus. Involvement

tends to favor the trunk and proximal extremities, although it may become more widespread. Many cases of pityriasis lichenoides chronica are initially diagnosed as pityriasis rosea. However, the persistent course of this disease, with remissions and exacerbations, eventually distinguishes it. A number of treatment modalities have been tried, but none has been consistently successful. Pityriasis lichenoides chronica has no systemic manifestations.

Figure 321

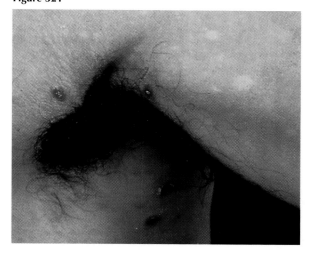

Figure 322

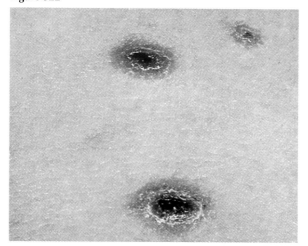

Pityriasis lichenoides et varioliformis acuta (PLEVA, Mucha-Habermann disease) This is a troubling papulosquamous disorder of acute onset that occurs in both children and young adults. The individual lesions go though a distinctive process of evolution over a period of weeks. Each begins as an erythematous papule. The lesion enlarges to a brownish 2–3 mm oval and then develops a central area of vesiculation or a hemorrhagic or necrotic crust. Lesions of this type are depicted in both photographs. Involvement tends to favor the anterior trunk

and proximal extremities. The axilla, as in Fig. 321, is a particularly common location. Facial and palm and sole involvement is relatively rare, and pruritus is usually absent. The condition has no systemic manifestations and tends to resolve gradually over a period of 4–6 months. However, some childhood cases last considerably longer, and scarring and pigmentary changes frequently occur. It appears that the resolution of this process can be hastened by a course of oral erythromycin. The mechanism of action of the drug in this situation is not known.

Figure 323

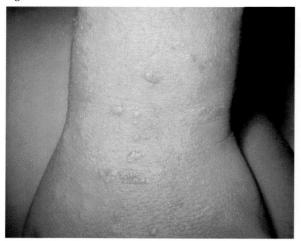

Figure 324

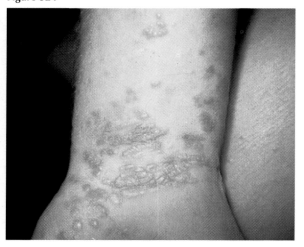

Lichen planus This condition is a pruritic eruption of unknown etiology. It is not uncommon in childhood. These illustrations are of the most representative lesions of lichen planus on a most common site, the wrists. The primary lesion consists of a flat-topped, polygonal, violaceous papule 2–6 mm in diameter. The characteristic shiny appearance of the individual papules is seen best in Fig. 324. The same figure illustrates the tendency for the solitary lesions to form confluent plaques. Exaggerated surface markings in the overlying skin (Wickham's

striae) may also be evident but are difficult to appreciate from these photographs. The forearms, the middle of the back, and the anterior surfaces of the lower extremities are other common locations. On the legs, lesions may become markedly hypertrophic and plaque-like. Diagnosis can sometimes be confirmed by the presence of oral lesions. Typically there are small white papules in a reticular pattern on the buccal mucosa. The tongue, lips, and palate may also be involved.

Figure 325

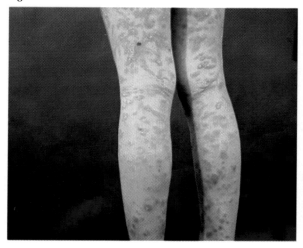

Figure 326

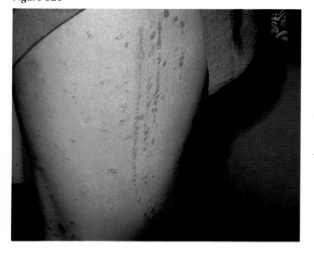

Lichen planus The clinical severity of lichen planus varies from a few mildly pruritic lesions in some cases to extensive and severe involvement of the skin and mucous membranes with intractable itching in others. The latter situation is illustrated in Fig. 325. Children with limited disease often respond well to the local application of topical corticosteroids. However, when the process is generalized, a short course of systemic steroids

may be necessary and will sometimes yield a dramatic improvement. Lichen planus tends to be a problem of long duration, with periods of remission and exacerbation. Figure 326 illustrates the tendency for new lesions to form in a scratch or abrasion. The so-called Koebner phenomenon is highly characteristic of lichen planus, and some evidence of "Koebnerization" is seen in almost every patient with this disorder.

Figure 327

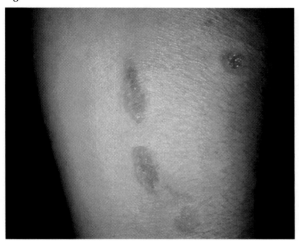

Figure 328

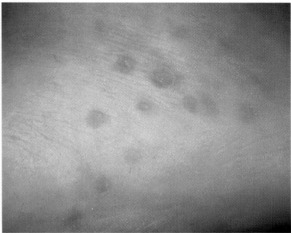

Lichen planus Most often, the lesions of lichen planus are small purplish papules, solitary or confluent, with exaggerated surface markings. There are, however, several variants. Some lesions develop adherent scales, sometimes vesiculation occurs, and, rarely, necrosis and scarring may occur upon resolution. The lesions in Fig. 327 are larger and more inflammatory than usual; there is a suggestion of vesiculation and necrosis. The vesicular and bullous forms of lichen planus must sometimes be differentiated from other bullous disorders. Figure 328, closely examined, shows a suggestion of scaling. Although the etiology of lichen planus remains a mystery, the clinician must bear in mind that certain lichenoid drug eruptions may be clinically indistinguishable from true lichen planus. The most common agents are gold salts and antimalarial agents. Topical exposure to paraphenylenediamine may have the same result.

Figure 329

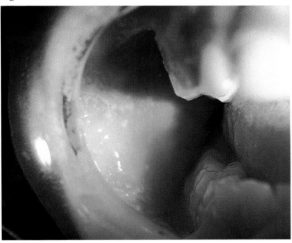

Figure 330

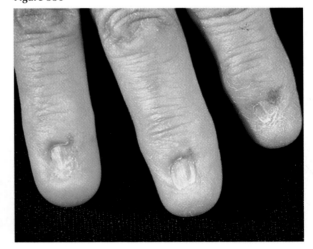

Lichen planus More than one-half of patients with cutaneous lesions will have oral mucosal involvement, although mucosal involvement may occur without any skin lesions. The oral lesions are most commonly found on the buccal mucosa and the lips. The lesions are characteristically white reticulated patches, although bullae, erosions, and ulcers may be seen. Erosive lesions may be quite painful.

Lichen planus A small percentage of patients with lichen planus develop nail involvement. The severity varies. Some children develop only mild thinning or ridging of the nail plate. Others have a severe nail dystrophy, with pterygium formation and complete and permanent nail loss. A case where the nails are destroyed is pictured here. Rarely, there may even be severe lichen planus of the fingernails and toenails without skin involvement. In any case, attempts to treat the severe forms of nail disease in lichen planus are rarely successful.

Figure 331

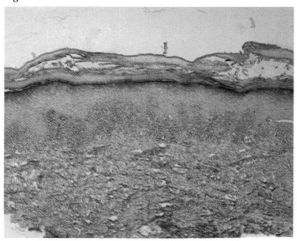

Histopathology of lichen planus Typical cases of lichen planus are clinically and histologically distinctive. Microscopically, the stratum corneum is hyperkeratotic (not parakeratotic), overlying a stratum granulosum that is thickened. The entire epidermis (suprapapillary plates and rete ridges) is hyperplastic in a plate-like manner. The dermoepidermal interface is blurred by a subepidermal band of mononuclear inflammatory cells.

Figure 332

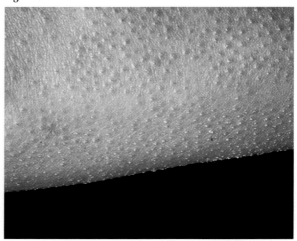

Lichen planopilaris (follicular lichen planus) This is a variant of lichen planus in which the primary involvement occurs around hair follicles. It is more common in females. Patients with this form of disease are also likely to have the more typical flat-topped papules and mucosal lesions as well. Pictured here are numerous rough follicular papules on an extremity. Lichen planopilaris can be a severe and disfiguring disorder when it involves the scalp. In such cases, either a temporary or permanent scarring alopecia may develop.

Figure 333

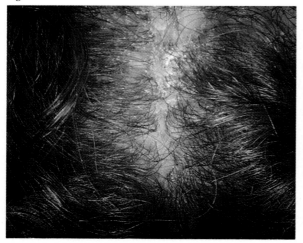

Lichen planopilaris (follicular lichen planus) This figure shows a scalp with a scarring alopecia, follicular spines, and erythema. This condition is progressive and may be very difficult to treat, although the use of potent topical corticosteroids may be useful.

Figure 334

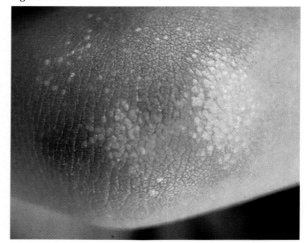

Lichen nitidus This is an unusual and distinctive dermatosis that has its peak incidence during childhood. The individual papules, as pictured here, are smaller than 1 mm in diameter. They are flat and shiny, with a round or polygonal shape. The lesions usually cluster, and an occasional linear grouping suggests that they occur in areas of trauma (the Koebner phenomenon). Lichen nitidus is occasionally seen in association with lichen planus. However, the marked differences in both histopathology and natural history indicate that they are different diseases.

Figure 335

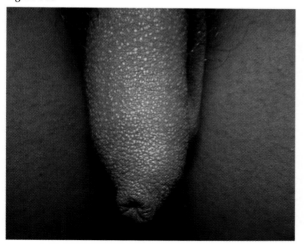

Lichen nitidus   In this illustration, the shiny character of the lesions of lichen nitidus is more appreciable. The penis is a site of predilection for this condition, as are the abdomen and upper extremities. The lesions of lichen nitidus are usually asymptomatic, but pruritus may occur. They may clear spontaneously in a short period of time, or they may last for months or years. There is no known effective treatment for the condition itself; itching can be treated symptomatically with antihistamines and mild topical steroids.

Figure 336

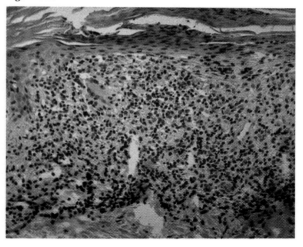

Histopathology of lichen nitidus   Lichen nitidus is characterized microscopically by a thickened stratum corneum that is parakeratotic; the stratum granulosum is gone; the stratum malpighii is thinned. A band-like infiltrate of cells hugs the overlying epidermis, but it is discontinuous and is somewhat granulomatous, as can be judged from the giant cell on the left.

Figure 337

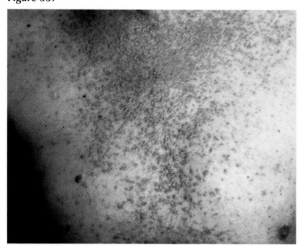

Figure 338

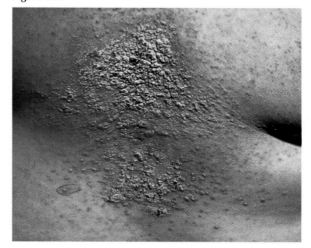

Darier's disease (keratosis follicularis)   This autosomal dominant disorder usually begins during mid-childhood. The primary lesion is a small, crusted papule; in some areas these coalesce to form hyperkeratotic, greasy plaques. The lesions tend to favor the so-called seborrheic areas, and the upper back and chest, as shown in Fig. 337, are the most common locations. In more severe cases there is extensive scalp and facial involvement, and there are moist, erythematous vegetating plaques in the flexures (Fig. 338). Small, warty papules on the dorsa of the hands are a common finding. The lesions tend to worsen in the summer; both humidity and ultraviolet light have a negative effect on the disease process. Nail involvement is characteristic of Darier's disease and may include red or white longitudinal streaks, thinning or thickening of the nail plate, and subungual hyperkeratosis. The severity of Darier's disease varies greatly among members of the same affected family. The use of synthetic retinoids in the most severe cases must be balanced against the problems of long-term toxicity.

Figure 339

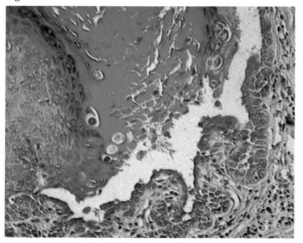

Figure 340

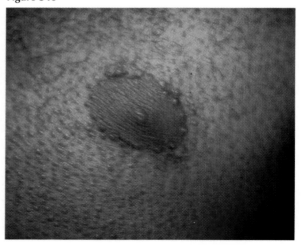

Histopathology of Darier's disease (keratosis follicularis)
Keratosis follicularis is a misnomer, because the lesions are not
exclusively follicular. The stratum corneum is thickened, elevated above the adjacent surface, and invaginated to form a plug.
In the latter, one finds keratinized cells (grains) and large round
cells with clear halos *(corps ronds)*. The subjacent stratum
malpighii is acanthotic, usually papillomatous, and marked by
slits (lacunae).

Infundibulofolliculitis   The intraepidermal portion of the pilosebaceous apparatus is called the infundibulum. In microscopy, its vaguely funnel shape can be appreciated. Inflammation of the hair follicle at different levels and by different
causes, microbial or inanimate, produces different pictures. At
the level of the hair bulb, abscesses or furuncles are the usual
lesions; above that level, pustules develop; and still higher, about
the infundibulum, inflammatory papules (as pictured) are the
lesions.

Figure 341

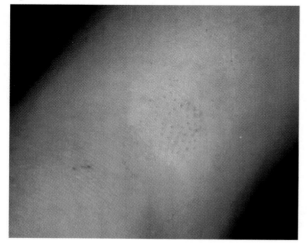

Figure 342

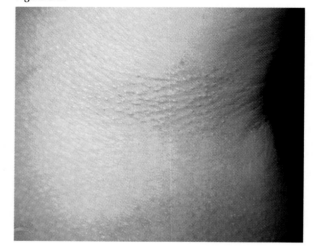

Lichen spinulosus   This condition consists of a small aggre-
gation of keratotic papules at the openings of the hair follicles.
The follicular hyperkeratosis is so marked that the involved area
has an appreciable spiny texture. The typical circular or oval
plaque is present in Fig. 341. The same process in a more lin-

ear arrangement is shown in Fig. 342. Lichen spinulosus is probably most common among children with atopic dermatitis. Effective treatment may be achieved by use of topical preparations containing keratolytics, such as small percentages of
salicylic acid (2–3%) and urea (10–20%).

Figure 343

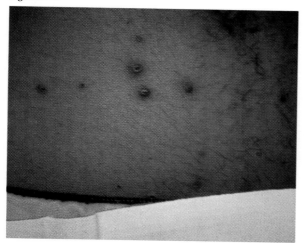

Figure 344

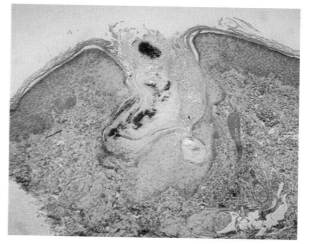

Perforating folliculitis This eruption consists of numerous small erythematous follicular papules with central keratotic plugging. The lesions, which vary in size from 2 to 8 mm, are usually located on the buttocks and thighs. The cause of this eruption is unknown; irritation of the hair follicle is probably the primary process. At various times, perforating folliculitis has been ascribed to the wearing of tight garments or to some chemical in clothing.

Histopathology of perforating folliculitis In contrast to types of folliculitis that are acute inflammatory processes, perforating folliculitis is a disorder of keratinization. A plug of horn, together with some basophilic debris, is seen within the distended upper portion of a pilosebaceous unit. The follicular epithelium is thinned almost to nothing at the lower left edge of the plug, and the surrounding connective tissue is only moderately inflamed.

Figure 345

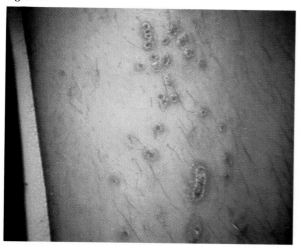

Figure 346

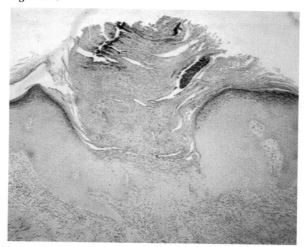

Reactive perforating collagenosis This rare disease usually has its onset during infancy and early childhood. Autosomal recessive, dominant, sporadic, and acquired forms have been reported. The lesions, as shown here, consist of small erythematous papules that gradually increase in size and develop a central hyperkeratotic plug. In some cases, the linear array of lesions suggests that they are induced by trauma—the so-called Koebner phenomenon. Pruritus is an occasional feature. Lesions usually last 6–8 weeks and then resolve, only to be followed by the eruption of fresh papules.

Histopathology of reactive perforating collagenosis This rare condition is secondary to trauma of a kind that damages collagen in localized areas in the upper cutis. The injured collagen is slowly extruded to the surface by a process of transepithelial elimination, often with scarring. During the active stage, a plug of horn and debris, sometimes a crust, forms on the surface and sits in a cup-shaped depression of the subjacent epidermis. Mild dermal inflammation is present.

Figure 347

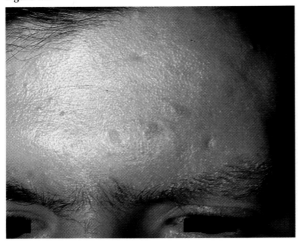

Figure 348

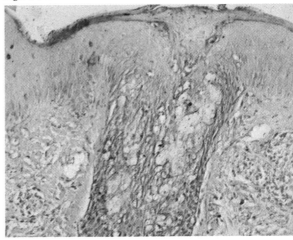

Follicular mucinosis (alopecia mucinosa) This is an uncommon disorder of unknown etiology that affects both children and adults. The lesions, which are usually located on the head and neck, vary in clinical appearance. Most often, as illustrated here, there are grouped flesh-colored papules. There may also be erythematous plaques with follicular accentuation and scale. When the disorder affects the scalp, it causes areas of permanent alopecia. In children, this disease tends to resolve spontaneously. Rarely, however, an association with lymphoma may occur.

Histopathology of follicular mucinosis Follicular mucinosis (alopecia mucinosa), as it occurs in children, is usually a self-limited disease. The pilosebaceous unit is not destroyed but assumes an edematous or even cystic appearance by accumulation of acid mucopolysaccharide (mainly hyaluronic acid), which here stains blue against a pink background. Digestion with testicular hyaluronidase eliminates the positive staining.

Figure 349

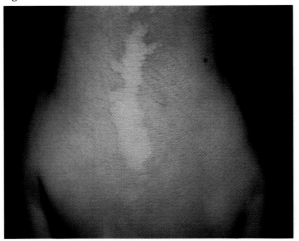

Figure 350

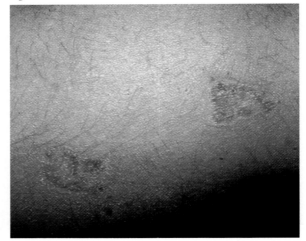

Porokeratosis (porokeratosis of Mibelli) This is a rare autosomal dominant dermatosis with unique clinical and histologic findings. Lesions usually develop during childhood and favor the hands, forearms, and face. Each lesion begins as a papule and evolves into an irregular atrophic plaque. A well-developed plaque is pictured in Fig. 349. The elevated and hyperpigmented border, with a fine groove running throughout, is somewhat difficult to appreciate in this photograph. This border, which corresponds to the histologic cornoid lamella, is the

most diagnostic clinical feature. Note the two lesions in Fig. 350. Here one can begin to appreciate the raised hyperkeratotic border that surrounds each circinate plaque. In some cases, lesions are arranged in a linear array. There are two other forms of porokeratosis: the disseminated superficial actinic type (numerous small lesions on sun-exposed skin) and porokeratosis palmaris et plantaris disseminata (an autosomal dominant syndrome that begins on the palms and soles).

Figure 351

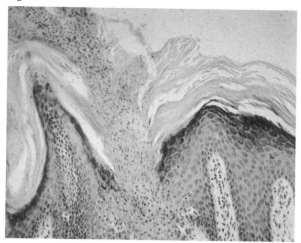

Histopathology of porokeratosis This classic condition develops in childhood or early adult life, usually as a ringed lesion whose elevated margin constitutes the active area, where the biopsy specimen is best taken. That margin consists of a vertical or oblique column of thickened parakeratotic horn (the cornoid lamella) seated in a small depression of hyperplastic stratum malpighii. At the base of the cornoid lamella, the stratum granulosum is attenuated or absent.

Figure 352

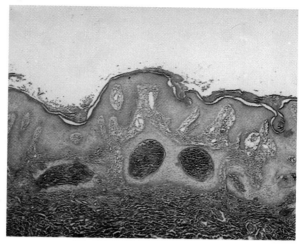

Histopathology of elastosis perforans serpiginosa This condition may resemble porokeratosis clinically when both have ringed lesions with elevated borders. Microscopically, in elastosis perforans serpiginosa, hyperplasia of elastic fibers develops in the papillae. Some of the elastica is eliminated by transepithelial expulsion. In this photomicrograph, one sees within an acanthotic stratum malpighii three masses of degenerating elastic tissue and debris en route to the surface.

Figure 353

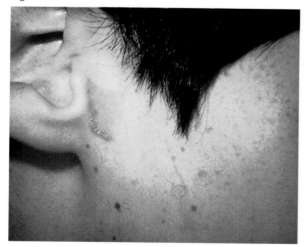

Elastosis perforans serpiginosa This rare disorder is characterized by small, cone-shaped, hyperkeratotic papules that are arranged in annular or circinate patterns. The lesions are usually localized; involvement in two common locations, the side of the face and the nape of the neck, is illustrated here. The process may also be disseminated. The underlying histologic process is the transepidermal elimination of elastic tissue. An association with heritable disorders such as Ehlers-Danlos syn-

Figure 354

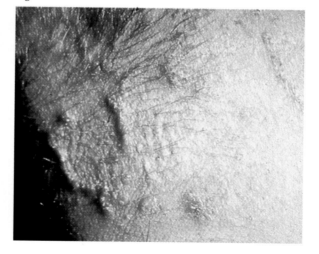

drome, Marfan syndrome, pseudoxanthoma elasticum, osteogenesis imperfecta, Rothmund-Thomson syndrome, and Down syndrome has been reported. Elastosis perforans serpiginosa may also occur as a side effect of treatment with penicillamine. In most patients, there is no effective therapy. Attempts at surgical removal are complicated by the high incidence of recurrence and scar formation.

10

Nutritional and Metabolic Disorders

Figure 355

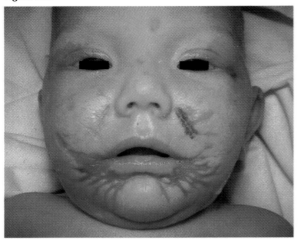

Figure 356

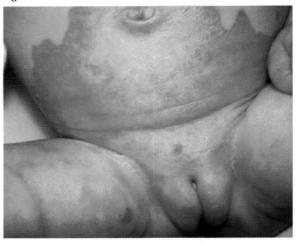

Acrodermatitis enteropathica   This syndrome results from inadequate absorption or dietary intake of zinc. Figure 355 shows erythema, crusting, and fissuring of the perioral skin and cheeks. The eruption that is pictured here may be preceded by blisters. Other features of acrodermatitis enteropathica include stomatitis, paronychia, and alopecia.

Acrodermatitis enteropathica   The diaper area that is seen in this figure is diffusely erythematous and has a sharply marginated border on the abdomen. Acrodermatitis enteropathica may be inherited in an autosomal recessive fashion. This form of the disease seems to be related to an inability to absorb zinc.

Figure 357

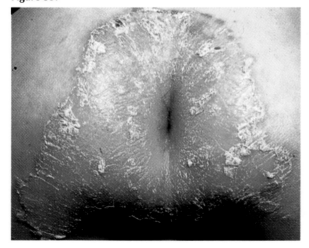

Figure 358

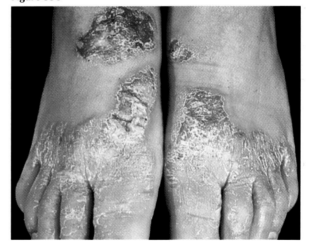

Acrodermatitis enteropathica   Figure 357 shows a highly characteristic picture of the cutaneous changes of acrodermatitis enteropathica about the anus, the buttocks, and on the perineum. Note how psoriasiform this lesion and those on the feet in Fig. 358 are. The full-blown picture of acrodermatitis enteropathica goes far beyond the typical changes of skin and hair. Affected children have severe diarrhea, growth retardation, and irritability. Without treatment, the disease follows a progressive course and may even be fatal. The crucial relationship between

acrodermatitis enteropathica and zinc deficiency was discovered in 1973. The child with suspected acrodermatitis enteropathica should be evaluated for a low zinc level, or a low alkaline phosphatase level when zinc levels are normal or low-normal. (Blood must be drawn in plastic, non–rubber stoppered tubes to avoid the possibility of zinc contamination.) Treatment with dietary zinc supplementation leads to a dramatic resolution of all symptoms and must be maintained indefinitely.

Figure 359

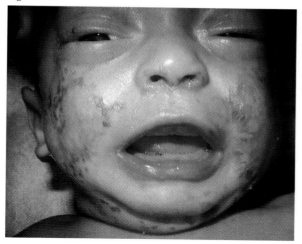

Acrodermatitis enteropathica Acquired acrodermatitis enteropathica is seen in infants who have received parenteral alimentation lacking sufficient zinc and, rarely, in breast-fed premature infants, who have larger zinc requirements. Occasionally, acrodermatitis enteropathica in a full-term breast-fed infant may be the result of low levels of zinc in the breast milk.

Figure 360

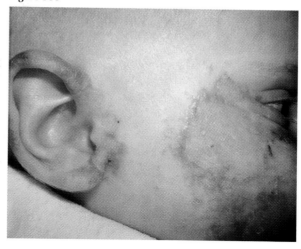

Acrodermatitis enteropathica The patient with acquired acrodermatitis enteropathica requires temporary zinc replacement. The differential diagnosis of this eruption includes psoriasis, biotin and multiple carboxylase deficiencies, essential fatty acid deficiencies, and cystic fibrosis.

Figure 361

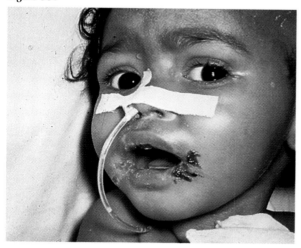

Cutaneous expressions of kwashiorkor Kwashiorkor is a type of protein energy malnutrition. It is seen most commonly in developing countries, and onset tends to occur after weaning. At that time, the balance of protein and carbohydrate in breast milk is replaced by a diet that contains almost exclusively carbohydrates. The initial signs are diarrhea, irritability, and edema of the hands and feet. Small dark patches appear at pressure points of the elbows, ankles, wrists, and knees, and then spread. The patches have a sharp border and tend to peel; the superficial desquamation in these areas is often likened to the

Figure 362

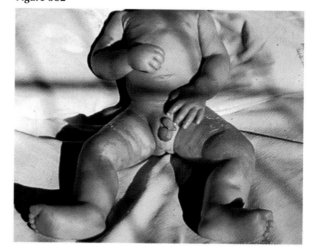

appearance of flaking paint or enamel. As the condition progresses, there develops a generalized red-brown discoloration. Other findings include fissuring at the edges of the mouth (Fig. 361) and the development of coarse, hypopigmented hair. Photosensitivity and easy bruising may also be present. The child with severe kwashiorkor appears extremely apathetic and has generalized edema. Pictured in Fig. 362 is a child with areas of desquamation and anasarca. Kwashiorkor carries a high mortality rate. With timely dietary intervention, it can often be reversed.

Figure 363

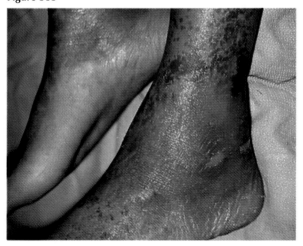

Figure 364

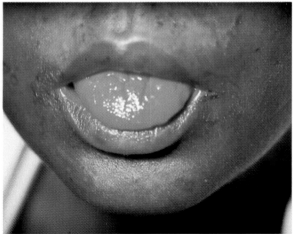

Cutaneous expressions of pellagra Pellagra is a disease caused by inadequate dietary intake of niacin. It is now seen in parts of the world where dietary intake of tryptophan, an amino acid precursor of niacin, is inadequate. In particular, diets that consist largely or exclusively of maize or millet predispose to this disease. The signs and symptoms of pellagra are often remembered by the mnemonic four Ds: dermatitis, diarrhea, dementia, and death. The classic cutaneous changes are inflama- tion, hyperpigmentation, and scaling in symmetric distribution and in areas exposed to heat or sunlight. Typical areas of involvement are the hands and forearms, legs and feet, and face and neck. Figure 363 shows moderate changes on the feet and legs. Figure 364 shows the scaling dermatitis on the face and an angular cheilitis. Edema and inflammation of the tongue are also common features of pellagra. The addition of supplemental niacin to the diet brings a quick resolution to the disease.

Figure 365

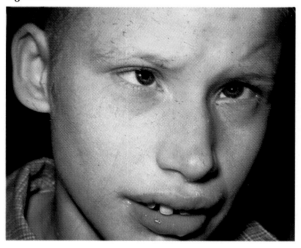

Figure 366

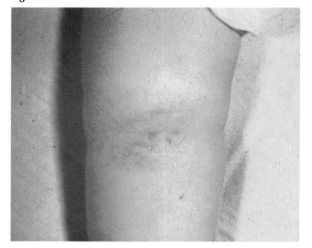

Cutaneous expressions of phenylketonuria This is a rare metabolic disorder that is inherited in autosomal recessive fashion. Children with the disease have a defect in the enzyme phenylalanine hydroxylase and are unable to convert phenyl- alanine to tyrosine. There are several associated cutaneous changes. Affected individuals have fairer skin and lighter- colored hair than their normal siblings; Caucasians with the disease typically have blond hair and blue eyes. Because the melanocytes of patients with phenylketonuria are less able to manufacture melanin, patients tend to sunburn easily. In addi- tion, an eczematous dermatitis is a common component of phenylketonuria. The lesions may resemble atopic dermatitis in morphology and distribution, as in these figures. In other pa- tients, the dermatitis is more widespread. Treatment of this dis- ease consists of dietary restriction of phenylalanine. The early institution of this diet limits the possibility of severe intellec- tual impairment, which is the most significant aspect of the disease.

Figure 367

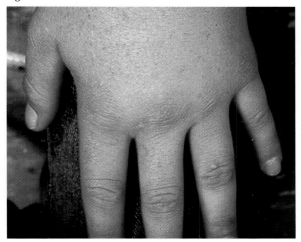

Figure 368

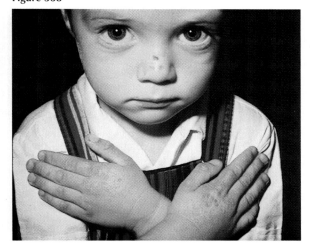

Cutaneous expressions of erythropoietic protoporphyria
This is among the more common porphyrias; onset is usually during early childhood. The typical presentation of this disease features the development of pruritus and burning of the skin in areas of recent sun exposure. These sensations may be accompanied by erythema, edema, and vesiculation. Over time, superficial scarring and a waxy thickening of the involved areas develop. These changes, as seen on the hands and feet, are illustrated here. The bridge of the nose is another common area

of involvement. Children with erythropoietic protoporphyria have inherited a deficiency of the enzyme ferrochelatase, which normally converts protoporphyrin to heme. The disease can be readily diagnosed from the combination of the clinical findings outlined above and an elevated free erythrocyte protoporphyrin level. The most serious complication is the development of hepatic involvement. Treatment of the skin disease consists of avoidance of the sun and oral therapy with beta-carotene.

Figure 369

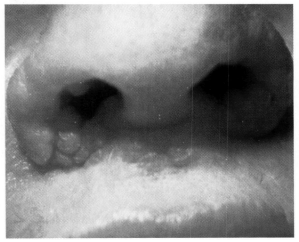

Figure 370

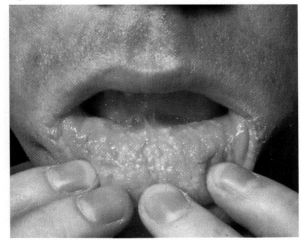

Lipoid proteinosis (hyalinosis cutis et mucosae) This is a rare autosomal recessive disease that is caused by the deposition of hyaline material in the skin and mucous membranes. Laryngeal involvement may be present from birth and eventually produces a characteristic hoarseness in every affected individual. Cutaneous disease begins during the first 2 years of life and consists of papules, nodules, and areas of thickening and hy-

perkeratosis. The cutaneous lesions on the alae nasi and in the choanae are shown in Fig. 369. In Fig. 370, the mucosal surface of the lower lip is extensively involved with the characteristic papules. Not shown here are the numerous small papules that dot the free margins of the eyelids. The disorder is attributed to a defect in glycoprotein metabolism, but the exact mechanism is unknown.

Figure 371

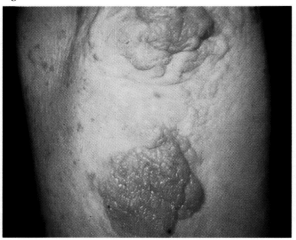

Lipoid proteinosis   Pictured here are a plaque and lesions of smaller sizes on and around the elbow. Most children with lipoid proteinosis continue to develop additional lesions during adult life. The most serious sequelae are caused by lesions in the mouth and oropharynx. The tongue may become thick and bound down, and dysphagia and respiratory obstruction may result from lesions in the pharynx and larynx. Finally, intracranial calcifications are a common feature of lipoid proteinosis. For most patients, these are asymptomatic, but seizure disorders may occur.

Figure 372

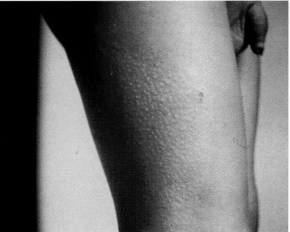

Hurler's syndrome   This inherited condition results in the accumulation of chondroitin sulfate B in the skin and other organ systems. Dwarfism and an unusual facial appearance are also aspects of the disease. This photograph is an excellent representation of shagreen skin, an appearance that is also seen in tuberous sclerosis. *Shagreen* refers to a type of leather that is embossed with knobs by processing and then variably stained.

Figure 373

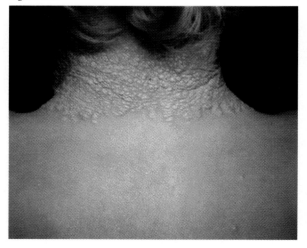

Xanthomatosis   Xanthomas are papules or nodules of the skin or mucous membranes that contain lipids. The appearance of xanthomas during childhood should prompt a thorough search for underlying systemic disease. The yellowish papules seen in Fig. 373 are a form of planar xanthoma. These may occur on any part of the body and may be an indicator of a hereditary lipoproteinemia, diabetes mellitus, or liver disease. Multiple myeloma and histiocytosis X are less common etiologies. The patient pictured here has biliary cirrhosis.

Figure 374

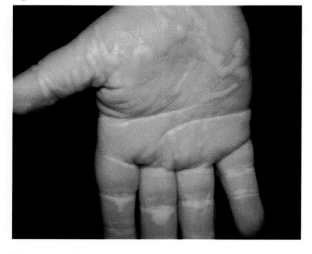

Xanthomatosis   The lesions illustrated here are typical of xanthoma striatum palmare, a form of planar xanthoma. This patient also has biliary cirrhosis. Note how the yellowish papules and plaques follow the creases of the fingers and the palmar folds. The familial hyperlipidemias, particularly types II, III, and V, may present with an identical clinical picture. Patients with these disorders are at high risk for ischemic heart disease.

Figure 375

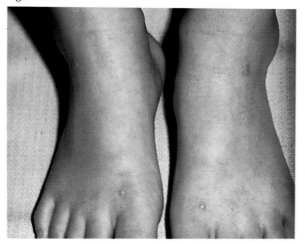

Xanthomatosis These small papules on the dorsa of the feet are also xanthomas. The patient is a 4-year-old child with type II hyperlipoproteinemia. This is an autosomal dominant condition in which there may be massive elevations in serum cholesterol. Individuals with this disease often develop ischemic heart disease during young adulthood. The recognition of the cutaneous lesions is important in identifying children who may require dietary or medical management of their hypercholesterolemia.

Figure 376

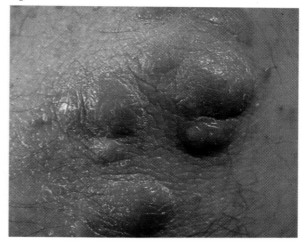

Xanthomatosis These yellow-red nodules, which often occur on the elbows and knees, are termed *tuberous xanthomas*. They may also be found in other areas where ordinary trauma is common, e.g., buttocks, knuckles, and heels. Similar lesions that overlie extensor tendons are sometimes called *tendon xanthomas*. Lesions of this sort are almost always caused by a hyperlipoproteinemia and should prompt investigation of serum cholesterol and triglycerides. Types II, IV, and V are those most commonly associated with tuberous and tendon xanthomas.

Figure 377

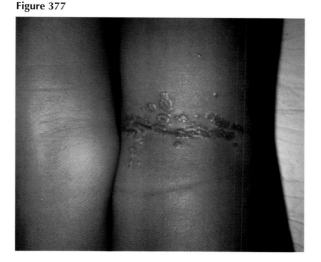

Xanthomatosis Not all xanthomatoses are rooted in abnormalities of cholesterol metabolism or other systemic disease. In this illustration, xanthomatous papules that developed in a lymphedematous leg are shown. Since serum lipids are normal, local causes stemming from the lymphatic obstruction must account for the lesions. The condition does not have the serious import of those xanthomatoses associated with abnormalities of serum lipids.

Figure 378

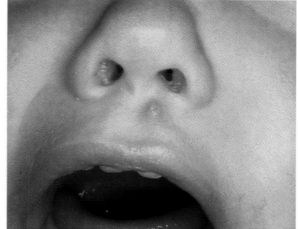

Calcinosis cutis When calcification occurs in the skin, it may represent an isolated local event, or it may be a sign of an underlying systemic disease. The lesion pictured here is a solitary nodular calcification. These sometimes result from local trauma, such as an insect bite, or from the rupture of an epidermal cyst (dystrophic calcinosis cutis). When such nodules occur on the face of an infant, they are usually idiopathic and of no medical significance.

Figure 379

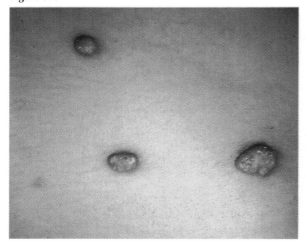

Figure 380

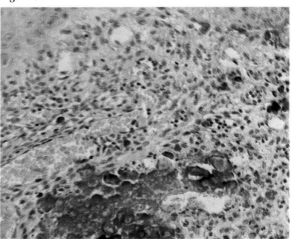

Calcinosis cutis   The nodular calcifications pictured here also turned out to be idiopathic. However, grouped calcifications like these may also be seen in children with CRST syndrome (calcinosis cutis, Raynaud's phenomenon, sclerodactyly, telangiectasia) or dermatomyositis. Pseudoxanthoma elasticum and Ehlers-Danlos syndrome are other causes. The so-called metastatic calcinosis cutis, with widespread precipitation of calcium salts, is a sign of abnormal calcium metabolism and may result from parathyroid tumors, chronic renal failure, or vitamin D intoxication.

Histopathology of calcinosis cutis   Insoluble salts of calcium may be deposited ectopically in soft tissues (in skin uncommonly) as a result of obviously deranged calcium-phosphorus metabolism (in parathyroidism, renal disease, etc.), following trauma (ossifying myositis), in association with abnormal or altered tissue (scleroderma), or for no apparent reason. Which is the case illustrated. Calcium salts are seen as amorphous basophilic material surrounded by a pronounced cellular response.

11

Genodermatoses

Figure 381

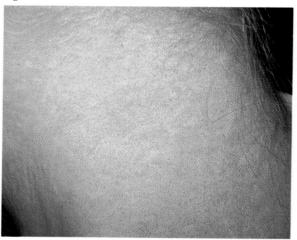

Figure 382

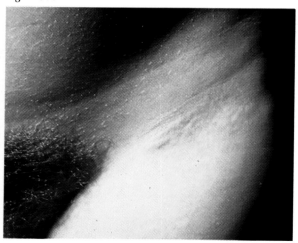

Pseudoxanthoma elasticum   This is a generalized condition in which elastic fibers are degenerative. Clinical signs of the phenomenon can be recognized in the skin and eyes. In the skin, patches of yellowish discoloration and general laxness or redundancy develop on the neck ("chicken skin"), in the axillae, and in other places, such as the fossae of limbs and the inguinal folds, where considerable movement of skin is normal. In the eye, the so-called angioid streaks can be seen. They represent the result

of faulty elastic fibers in Bruch's membrane and generally precede the cutaneous changes. These eye changes frequently result in the loss of central vision and sometimes result in blindness. Gastrointestinal hemorrhage is the most serious acute consequence, but slower structural damage in various organs may result in hypertension, coronary artery occlusion, diabetes mellitus, thyroid dyscrasia, or ectopic calcinosis. The disease may be inherited in autosomal recessive or autosomal dominant fashion.

Figure 383

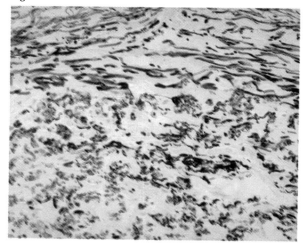

Figure 384

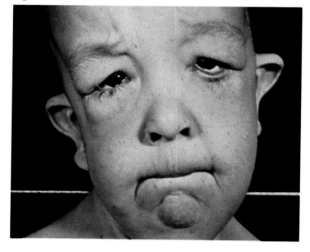

Histopathology of pseudoxanthoma elasticum   The diagnosis of pseudoxanthoma elasticum is confirmable by biopsy. The elastic fibers of the midcutis are abnormal both morphologically and tinctorially. This is easily appreciated with this stain for elastic tissue. The slightly wavy fibers high in the photomicrograph are normal; the deeper fibers are disrupted and granular. When stained with hematoxylin and eosin, they are basophilic, indicating calcification.

Cutis laxa   In this condition, elastic fibers are decreased in number by an unknown mechanism. As seen in this patient, the skin hangs in folds and produces an appearance of premature aging. Because elastic fibers are affected in all organ systems, intestinal and urinary bladder diverticulae, rectal prolapse, inguinal hernias, and pulmonary emphysema frequently occur. The last of these is associated with significant mortality. The most common and severe form is inherited in autosomal recessive fashion.

Figure 385

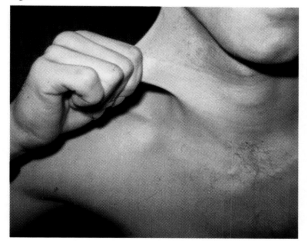

Figure 386

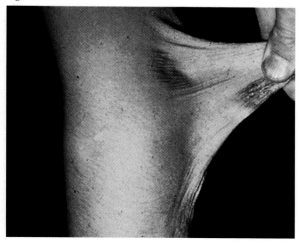

Ehlers-Danlos syndrome This syndrome is actually a collection of 11 discrete conditions with the common features of hyperextensible skin and joints, easy bruising, defective wound healing, and blood vessel fragility. Distinct abnormalities in collagen synthesis have been identified in some of the varieties of Ehlers-Danlos syndrome. The result of the anomaly is extreme stretchability but unimpaired elasticity (i.e., the ability to return to normal after stretching). The photographs illustrate

the phenomenon; Fig. 385 shows skin of the neck and Fig. 386 of the elbow extended several times more than normal skin can be pulled out. Depending on the type, inheritance may be autosomal dominant, autosomal recessive, or X-linked recessive. Gastrointestinal perforation and rupture of a large artery are the most severe complications of this syndrome. Premature birth (probably due to fragility of the fetal membranes) is a common event in patients with Ehlers-Danlos syndrome.

Figure 387

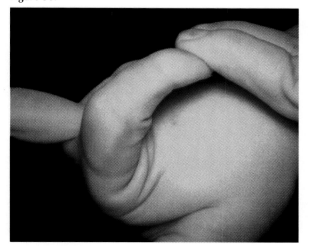

Figure 388

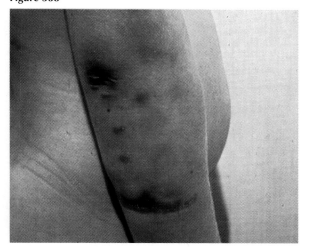

Ehlers-Danlos syndrome In these illustrations, more of the hyperextensible phenomena and the consequences of functional abnormality of elastic fibers and collagen are shown. Figure 387 shows hyperextensibility of joints, from which it may be inferred that skin, ligament, tendon, and to some extent bone are also abnormally stretchable. Another way in which softness of muscle and related structures can be appreciated is in the feel of a handshake with a patient who has Ehlers-Danlos syndrome.

No matter how hard one presses, there is a feeling that one is not quite through with the handshake, so compressible is the hand. Figure 388 illustrates the result of incisions and shearing trauma in the skin of a patient with Ehlers-Danlos syndrome. The result is hemorrhage, failure of healing by primary intention, and finally broad, friable scars. Small "pseudotumors" on the elbows and knees are actually calcified herniations of fat through the dermis.

Figure 389

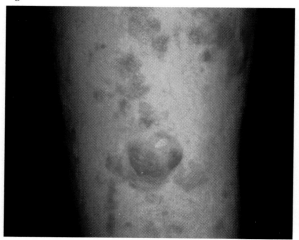

Focal dermal hypoplasia (Goltz syndrome) This is a combination of disordered structure of ectodermal and mesenchymal tissue of both skin and bone. The syndrome is transmitted in an X-linked dominant fashion. The most common cutaneous lesions are linear or reticulate areas of hypoplasia with telangiectasia, atrophy, and abnormal pigmentation. Figure 389 shows some such patches as well as the nodular fat tumors that are typically present.

Figure 390

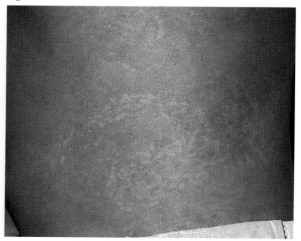

Focal dermal hypoplasia (Goltz syndrome) This figure shows the whorled nature of the lesions on the trunk following the lines of Blaschko. Ulcers may be present initially in areas of congenital absence of skin and heal with atrophy. The range of clinical presentation varies from a minor process on the limbs to extensive distortion of the skin and bony skeleton.

Figure 391

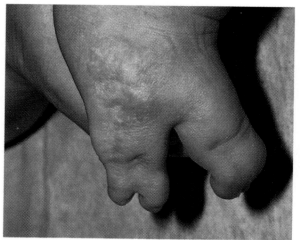

Focal dermal hypoplasia (Goltz syndrome) When bone is involved, syndactyly, polydactyly, oligodactyly with lobster claw deformity (as seen in this figure), skeletal asymmetry, and scoliosis may occur. Ocular abnormalities include colobomas, microphthalmia, and strabismus.

Figure 392

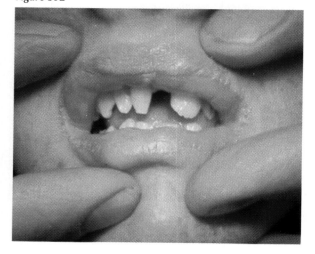

Focal dermal hypoplasia (Goltz syndrome) This figure illustrates the frequent involvement of the perioral skin and teeth. Patients may present with hypodontia, oligodontia, or small teeth with dysplastic enamel. Papillomas may be present on the lips or in the axillae, periumbilical area, or perineum.

Figure 393

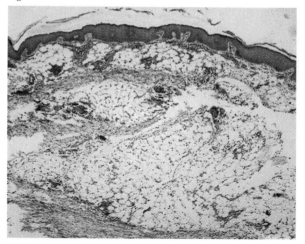

Histopathology of focal dermal hypoplasia Of the many abnormalities in this complex syndrome, the histologically specific one is the almost total absence of dermis. In this photomicrograph one sees the adipose tissue, which normally is limited to the subcutis, lying under the epidermis, separated from it by an almost imperceptible bit of connective tissue. A similar picture may be seen in nevus lipomatosus, which, however, can be distinguished clinically.

Figure 394

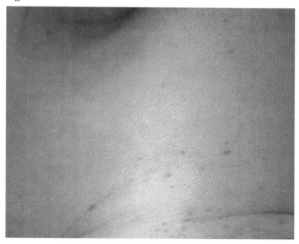

Cutaneous expressions of the Wiskott-Aldrich syndrome This is another severe immunologic defect with X-linked recessive inheritance. The classic symptoms of this disease, which occurs only in males, are thrombocytopenia, recurrent infection, and a generalized eczematous or exfoliative dermatitis. Children with this disorder have impaired humoral and cell-mediated immunity, with deficient IgM and elevated IgA, and are at risk for sepsis and hemorrhage. The figure shows the kind of petechiae that are evidence of the persistent thrombocytopenia.

Figure 395

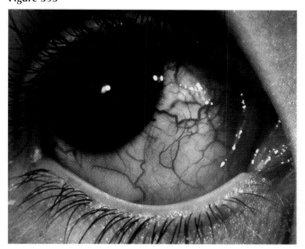

Cutaneous expressions of ataxia-telangiectasia This autosomal recessive disorder affects the skin and the immunologic and central nervous systems. The onset of the disease, during early childhood, is characterized by the combination of progressive cerebellar ataxia and telangiectasias. The earliest site of telangiectasia is usually the bulbar conjunctiva, as pictured in Fig. 395. These vascular lesions also involve the neck, upper chest, face, and, as illustrated in Fig. 396, the pinna of the ear. Later cuta-

Figure 396

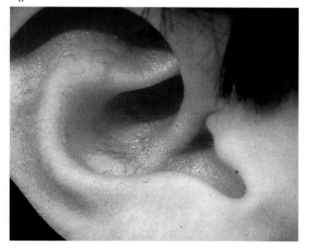

changes include blotchy hyper- and hypopigmentation, café-au-lait spots, hirsutism, a generalized eczematous dermatitis, and granulomatous skin lesions. There may be premature graying of the hair. The immunologic abnormalities include decreased levels of IgA and IgE and defective cell-mediated immunity. Children with ataxia-telangiectasia suffer from recurrent sinopulmonary infection and may die from bronchiectasis and respiratory failure. Lymphoreticular malignancies are an additional complication.

Figure 397

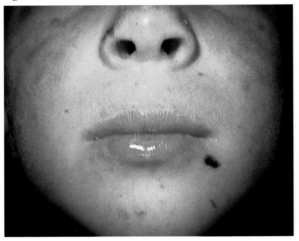

Figure 398

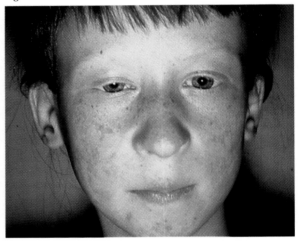

Cutaneous expressions of Bloom's syndrome   The princi-pal cutaneous manifestations of this autosomal recessive syn-drome are erythema and telangiectasias of the cheeks and pho-tosensitivity. Café-au-lait spots and acanthosis nigricans may also be present. Children with Bloom's syndrome are small at birth and have severe growth retardation throughout life. They also have recurrent respiratory infections and a strong tendency to develop malignancy. This rare disease is attributed to chro-mosomal abnormalities and defects in DNA repair. Chromo-some analysis is invariably abnormal.

Cutaneous expressions of poikiloderma congenitale (Roth-mund-Thomson syndrome)   This rare inherited condition be-gins during infancy with typically progressive skin changes. Erythema and edema of the facial skin are rapidly followed by the development of atrophy and telangiectasia. The same process occurs on the buttocks and extremities. Cataracts de-velop in many patients, and these often become apparent dur-ing infancy or early childhood. Skeletal deformities and short stature are other occasional features of this disease.

Figure 399

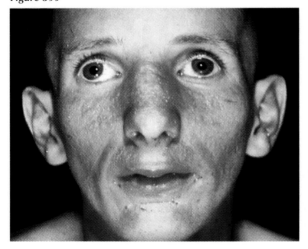

Figure 400

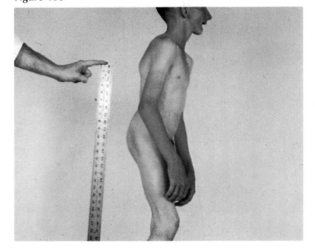

Cutaneous expressions of Cockayne's syndrome   This is another rare autosomal recessive condition, characterized by skin changes and dwarfism. During the second year of life, pa-tients develop a scaly photoeruption on the face and upper neck. This resolves with hyperpigmentation. The scaling photoder-matitis and typical bird-like facies of this syndrome are illus-trated in Fig. 399. In addition to dwarfism (Fig. 400), affected

individuals may demonstrate sensorineural deafness, micro-cephaly, and severe mental retardation. Optic atrophy and reti-nal degeneration may also be present. Characteristic intracra-nial calcifications are a feature of Cockayne's syndrome that may aid in confirmation of the diagnosis. The disorder has been attributed to a defect in DNA repair.

Figure 401

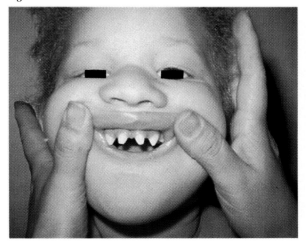

Figure 402

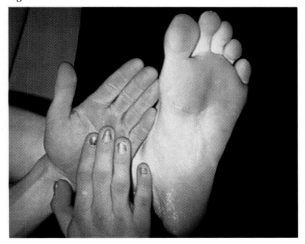

Congenital ectodermal dysplasia Embryonic underdevelopment of the ectoderm is seen in two syndromes: anhidrotic and hidrotic ectodermal dysplasia. Figure 401 shows the faulty dentition and pathognomonic facies in the more severe anhidrotic type. This syndrome, which occurs almost exclusively in boys, may include alopecia, nail dystrophy, stunted growth, and severe mental retardation. Severe hyperthermia during warm weather is the result of the absence of normal perspiration, and therapy should be aimed at regulation of environmental temperature, decreased exercise, and cool clothing. The hidrotic type affects males and females equally and is generally less severe. There is no abnormal sweating. Dystrophic nails, which may be distorted in size, shape, color, or consistency, are the hallmark of the syndrome. Patients tend to have sparse body and scalp hair. The nail dystrophy may be accompanied by severe hyperkeratosis of the palms and soles, as seen in Fig. 402. Topical keratolytics are of some help to affected individuals.

Figure 403

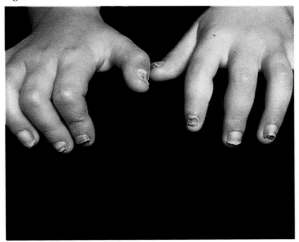

Figure 404

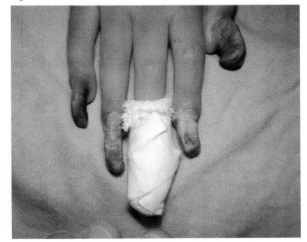

Pachyonychia congenita This condition is a heritable syndrome in which there is severe dyskeratinization of a special sort that especially affects nails, palms and soles, and the mucous membranes of the lips and mouth. The nail changes are distinctive in their discoloration, hardness, excessive growth, and attachment to hyperkeratotic nail beds: Fig. 403 shows such nails, in which scleronychia and binding to the nail beds can be appreciated; Fig. 404 shows nails excessively overgrown to the point of onychogryphosis. Not shown is a hyperkeratotic process on palms and soles that can be as bad as in nails. Also not shown is leukokeratosis of lips and tongue, a condition that severely disturbs function and is cosmetically distressing, to say the least. Aside from these major sites of hypertrophic dyskeratinization, there are other places and kinds of abnormality, which are shown on the next page.

Figure 405

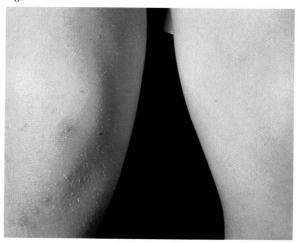

Figure 406

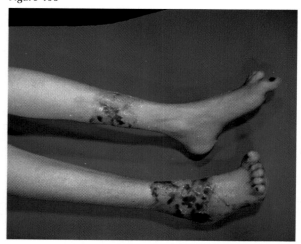

Pachyonychia congenita (cont.)   On the expanse of the body, especially on the buttocks and extremities, the dyskeratinization of pachyonychia congenita may take the form of what might be considered to be keratosis pilaris, except that forcible removal of the follicular keratotic plugs leaves cavities that have a tendency to bleed. This phenomenon is pictured in Fig. 405. More serious than follicular keratosis is a tendency to bulla formation on the

lower part of the legs in a form that suggests epidermolysis bullosa. Figure 406 shows how severe this part of the syndrome can be. Rooted as the entire condition is in a hereditary dyscrasia, there is no reasonable management of it. In the most severe instances of distortion of the nails, extirpation of the nail beds, even amputation of distal phalanges, may be required in order to achieve some degree of adequate function of the fingers.

Figure 407

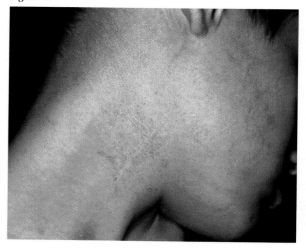

Figure 408

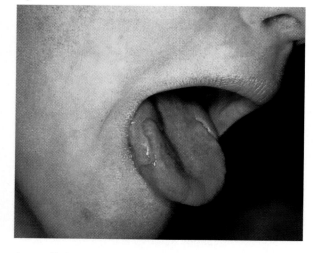

Dyskeratosis congenita   This is another congenital and hereditary condition that is also rare, different from other dyskeratinizations, and distinctive. Its marks are skin changes in the form of atrophy and dyschromia, atrophic dysplasia of nails, and a kind of leukoplakia. In Fig. 407 those skin changes are shown as mottled or retiform poikiloderma. The face, neck, and upper part of the body are characteristically involved. The process goes on to fine atrophy and hypo- and hyperpigmenta-

tion until the poikilodermatous character of the changes becomes established. The kind of process that occurs on mucous membranes is shown in Fig. 408. There are two lesions on the tongue that are gray and hypertrophic. The buccal mucosa and the mucosa of the urethra and anus may also be affected. Aside from the cutaneous and mucosal effects, abnormalities such as those seen in Fanconi's syndrome may be associated with this condition.

Figure 409

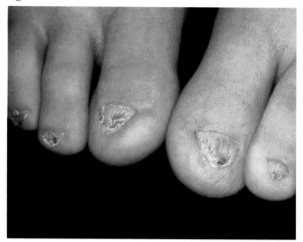

Figure 410

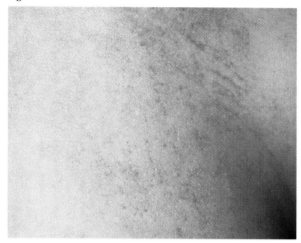

Dyskeratosis congenita   Here are more possible cutaneous changes in dyskeratosis congenita: Fig. 409 shows hypoplastic nail changes that are characteristic. Note how different they are from those of pachyonychia congenita (Fig. 403). Instead of overgrowth, there is underdevelopment. Details of the cutaneous changes on glabrous skin in and about the groin are shown in Fig. 410. Note how similar they are to those on the neck and face. In addition to what has been illustrated, hyperhidrosis of

palms and soles, conjunctivitis, esophageal strictures, intestinal diverticula, mental retardation, and anemia may be part of the syndrome. Malignant degeneration in the leukoplakia of the mucous membranes is a possibility. It is obvious that therapy for the condition is meager. Palliation of symptoms to whatever extent possible and observation for supervention of malignancy and its treatment are all that can be done.

Figure 411

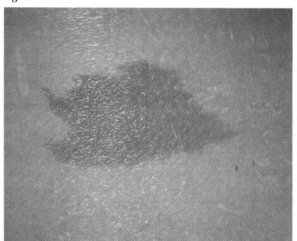

Figure 412

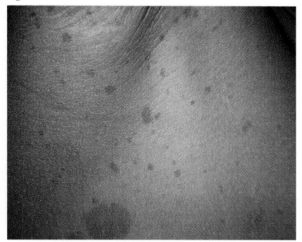

Neurofibromatosis (von Recklinghausen's disease)   This autosomal dominant disorder includes a number of distinctive cutaneous findings and a wide variety of neurologic manifestations. Figure 411 shows a café-au-lait spot. Solitary lesions of this type are common in normal individuals; most patients with neurofibromatosis have more than a single macule. The presence of more than six lesions that are larger than 1.5 cm in diameter is often considered to be a pathognomonic sign of the disease. In Fig. 412 there are several macules of hyperpigmen-

tation in the axilla. Axillary freckling, also called *Crowe's sign,* is a unique finding in neurofibromatosis. Pigmented hamartomas of the iris, termed *Lisch nodules,* are also present in almost all patients with this condition. Optic gliomas may also be seen. The inheritance of neurofibromatosis is complicated by a highly variable range of expression among those affected. A single family may include some individuals with only cutaneous involvement and others with numerous neurofibromas or severe neurologic disease. Spontaneous mutations are also common.

Figure 413

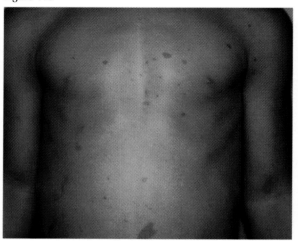

Figure 414

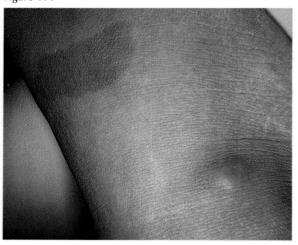

Neurofibromatosis (von Recklinghausen's disease) (cont.)
These are more illustrations of the pigmentary anomalies and tumors in the skin of patients with neurofibromatosis. Figure 413 shows several café-au-lait spots and small tumors. Figure 414 shows a large café-au-lait spot on the left and a barely discernible tumor on the right. Neurofibromas have variable consistency. The soft lesions can be pushed into the surrounding skin, a process called "buttonholing." Neurofibromas usually begin to develop during puberty and may cause severe cosmetic disfigurement. Pruritus of the skin that overlies the neurofibroma is a common complaint, and the itching is aggravated by exertion or a warm environment. Malignant degeneration of a benign neurofibroma is a constant concern. In addition, patients with the disease are prone to developing neurofibrosarcomas or malignant schwannomas de novo. Selective surgical removal of neurofibromas, in order to improve either appearance or function, is feasible.

Figure 415

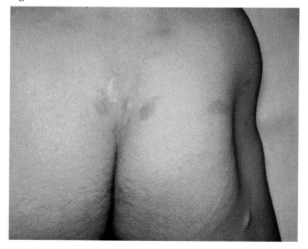

Figure 416

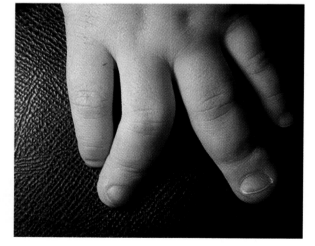

Neurofibromatosis (von Recklinghausen's disease) Figure 415 shows three café-au-lait spots and a small, soft neurofibroma. The enlargement in Fig. 416 was found to be due to a neurofibroma in the palm and along the length of the digits. Intellectual handicap, speech impediment, and seizures are frequent manifestations of classic, or von Recklinghausen, neurofibromatosis. Although this form of neurofibromatosis tends to be progressive, it is entirely unpredictable. There is no single aspect of the clinical course that allows the physician to foresee the evolution of other features.

Figure 417

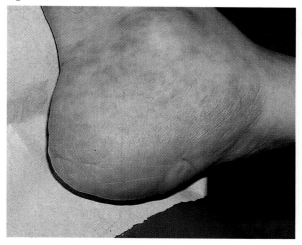

Neurofibromatosis (von Recklinghausen's disease) These subcutaneous tumors are congenital and are pathognomonic for neurofibromatosis type I. Plexiform neurofibromas may sometimes be subtle, initially presenting only as a patch of hyperpigmentation and/or hypertrichosis. With time they can grow quite large.

Figure 418

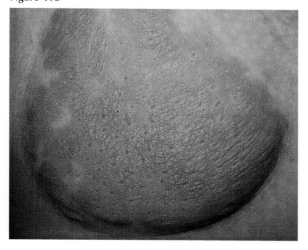

Neurofibromatosis (von Recklinghausen's disease) Larger lesions are described as having a "bag of worms" consistency and may be cosmetically disabling. Plexiform neurofibromas may also present as firm nodules attached to nerves. Tumors around nerves may cause pain, muscle weakness, or atrophy.

Figure 419

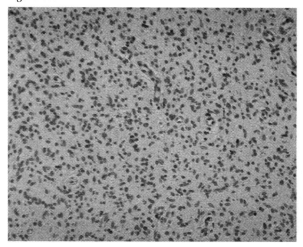

Histopathology of neurofibromas Neurofibromas, whether solitary or numerous (as in patients with von Recklinghausen's disease), may show more or less histologic resemblance to peripheral nerves, especially in deeper lesions obviously related to nerves. Often the pattern is neuroid, at times grossly plexiform. In most cutaneous lesions like the one shown here, one merely sees cells with oval nuclei and without plasma membranes, arranged randomly in a pink fibrillar background.

Figure 420

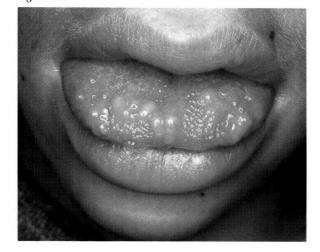

Mucosal neuroma syndrome The presence of numerous small neuromas of the lips, tongue, and oral mucosa is a marker for a unique autosomal dominant condition. This syndrome, now termed *multiple endocrine neoplasia type 2B,* carries a very high risk for malignancy. Eighty percent of affected individuals will develop medullary thyroid carcinoma. Pheochromocytoma may also occur. This patient developed both tumors, and had the marfanoid habitus that is frequently seen in patients with the disorder.

Figure 421

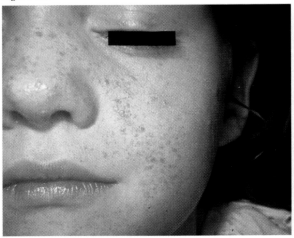

Figure 422

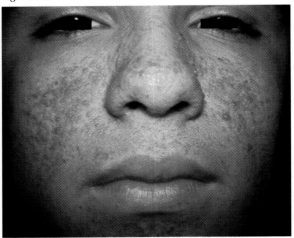

Tuberous sclerosis   This is an autosomal dominant disease with widely variable penetrance; its main effects are on the skin, central nervous system, eye, kidney, and heart. These photographs illustrate one of the most common cutaneous manifestations: adenoma sebaceum. The pink-to-red dome-shaped papules usually appear between the ages of 2 and 6 years. The lesions of adenoma sebaceum may be symmetrically distributed over the entire face but are usually most concentrated on the

cheeks. Histologically, the individual papules are angiofibromas. The extent of cutaneous involvement is not generally predictive of the severity of the disease. Patients who are severely affected suffer from seizure disorders and mental retardation. Other findings of tuberous sclerosis include retinal and renal hamartomas, cerebral nodules and calcifications, and cardiac rhabdomyosarcomas.

Figure 423

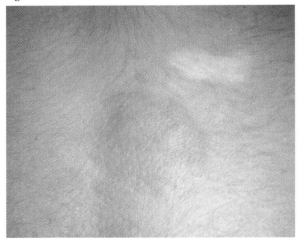

Figure 424

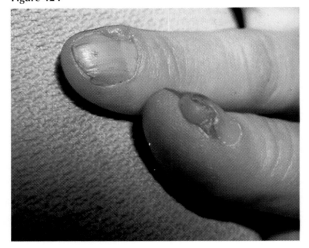

Tuberous sclerosis   Two cutaneous manifestations of the syndrome are shown in Fig. 423. Above and to the right is a hypopigmented macule, which sometimes takes the shape of an ash leaf. Hypopigmented macules may occur in healthy infants, but the appearance of several such lesions should prompt a search for other manifestations of tuberous sclerosis in the patient and family members. The so-called ash-leaf spots are the earliest cutaneous manifestation of the syndrome; they either are present at

birth or evolve during infancy. Wood's light examination may sometimes reveal hypopigmented macules whose presence is otherwise not obvious. In the midline in the same photograph is a shagreen patch, an area of cutaneous thickening with a pebbled surface. Histologically, this lesion, which is frequently seen in children with tuberous sclerosis, is a form of connective tissue nevus. In Fig. 424 there are subungual and periungual fibromas. These firm lesions arise from the nail beds, usually after puberty.

Figure 425

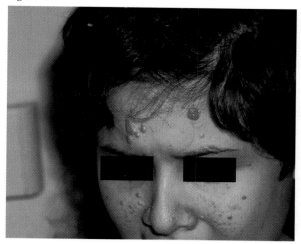

Tuberous sclerosis Another cutaneous finding in tuberous sclerosis is firm fibrous plaques that are located on the forehead, scalp, and cheeks. These lesions, which may be present at birth, are different from angiofibromas in that there is no vascular dilatation associated with the dermal fibrosis.

Figure 426

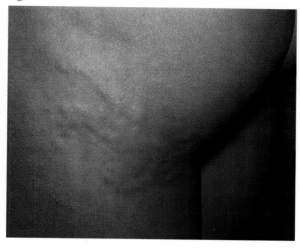

Buschke-Ollendorf syndrome This autosomal dominant syndrome is characterized by the presence of connective tissue nevi of the skin and a radiologic abnormality known as osteopoikilosis. The connective tissue nevi are yellowish plaques that tend to appear before puberty and are present on the trunk, buttocks, and arms. Osteopoikilosis is an asymptomatic bony abnormality that presents as round opacities within the carpal and tarsal bones, the phalanges, the epiphyses and metaphyses of the long bones, and the pelvis.

Figure 427

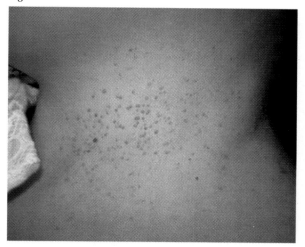

Basal cell nevus syndrome Patients with this autosomal dominant syndrome develop multiple basal cell carcinomas and cysts within the mandible. Additional findings include hypertelorism, a variety of other skeletal abnormalities, and calcification of the falx cerebri. Shown in this figure is an example of multiple basal cell carcinomas that are unusually small.

Figure 428

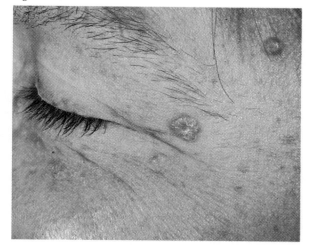

Basal cell nevus syndrome Most patients with this syndrome have more conventional basal cell carcinomas in the form of pearly telangiectatic nodules, sometimes with ulceration, as is shown in this figure. Basal cell carcinomas usually develop in these patients after puberty, although they may occur in childhood.

Figure 429

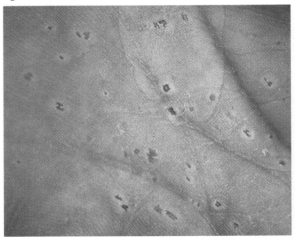

Figure 430

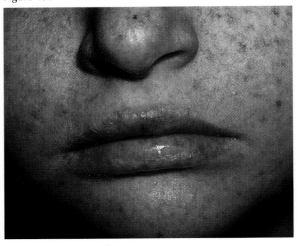

Basal cell nevus syndrome (cont.)   This figure shows the palmar pitting that appears during puberty in individuals with this syndrome. Rapidly enlarging basal cell carcinomas must be treated early on with the conventional surgical modalities in order to minimize disfigurement and avoid loss of function. Patients with this syndrome are also at risk for medulloblastoma. This grave complication tends to occur in early childhood.

Xeroderma pigmentosum   This rare autosomal recessive disease is caused by an inability to repair DNA that has been damaged by ultraviolet light. There are at least eight different molecular defects. Freckling develops on sun-exposed skin at a very early age, along with xerosis, scaling, and telangiectasia. Speckled hypo- and hyperpigmentation are also typical, as seen in Figs. 430, 431, and 432.

Figure 431

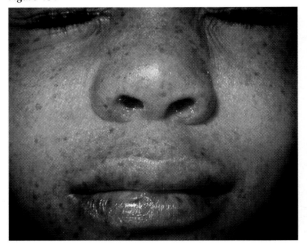

Figure 432

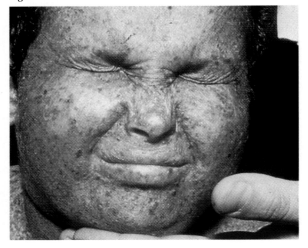

Xeroderma pigmentosum   Patients with this disease also tend to get hyperkeratoses and changes consistent with actinic keratoses. In early childhood, patients with xeroderma pigmentosum begin to develop cutaneous malignancies: basal cell and squamous cell carcinomas and, less commonly, melanomas. The mortality from this disease is caused by destructive local growth of tumors and by metastases. In addition, patients may suffer from severe neurologic dysfunction, including mental retardation. Although no treatment is available, individuals with this disease benefit from a lifestyle that allows minimal exposure to sunlight.

12

Ichthyoses and Disorders of Keratinization

Figure 433

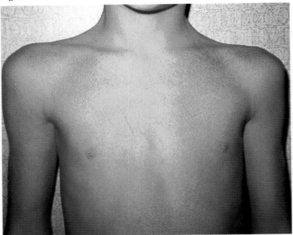

Figure 434

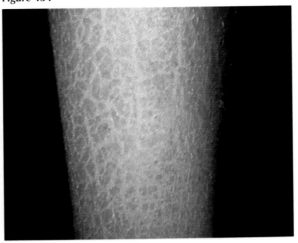

Ichthyosis vulgaris This is the mildest and most common form of ichthyosis, with an incidence in school-aged children as high as 1:250. It is inherited as an autosomal dominant trait and is present in a significant percentage of individuals with atopic dermatitis. It is not present at birth. The clinical appearance of this ichthyosis varies, depending on location. Figure 433 illustrates the fine, bran-like scaling on the upper chest. On the anterior lower leg, there are often larger, plate-like scales that resemble the skin of a fish (Fig. 434). Facial involvement is usually minimal, and flexural areas are typically spared. Children with ichthyosis vulgaris are likely to have increased skin markings on the palms and soles and a high incidence of keratosis pilaris (see Figs. 277–279). Ichthyosis vulgaris tends to worsen in winter, when there is less sweating and lower humidity.

Figure 435

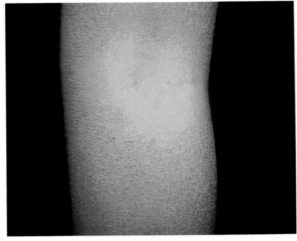

Figure 436

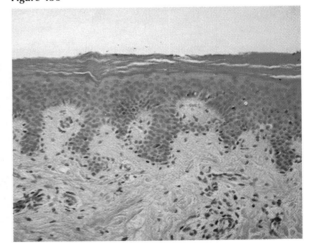

Ichthyosis vulgaris This figure illustrates the fine scaling of ichthyosis vulgaris and the conspicuous sparing of the flexures. Treatment of ichthyosis vulgaris entails the use of emollients and creams and ointments containing urea and lactic acid. Excessive bathing and the use of alkaline soaps should be avoided. The exacerbation that frequently occurs in winter months can be lessened if a humidifier is used in the child's room.

Histopathology of ichthyosis vulgaris The histopathologic picture of ichthyosis vulgaris of autosomal dominant inheritance is diagnostic. In this illustration, one sees the stratum corneum to be dense and moderately hyperkeratotic, and the stratum malpighii to be essentially normal except for the absence of a stratum granulosum. This combination of hyperkeratosis (without parakeratosis) and absence of the granular layer is unique to this type of ichthyosis.

Figure 437

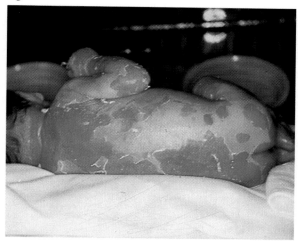

Figure 438

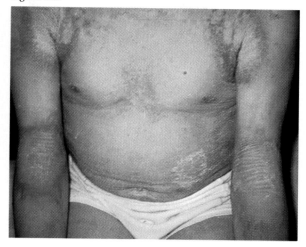

Bullous congenital ichthyosiform erythroderma (epidermolytic hyperkeratosis) This condition is a rare, chronic, and often severe genodermatosis that is inherited in an autosomal dominant fashion. The appearance of bullous ichthyosis in the newborn is illustrated in Fig. 437. Typically, there are large areas of denuded skin, and sometimes there are intact blisters. The differentiation from epidermolysis bullosa can usually be made by positive family history, the presence of subtle areas of hyperkeratosis, and, most important, the characteristic skin biopsy (see Fig. 444). The genetic defect lies in mutations in genes encoding keratins 1 and 10. Treatment in the newborn period should focus on gentle handling to avoid new blister formation, the maintenance of fluid and electrolyte balance, and the prevention of bacterial superinfection.

Figure 439

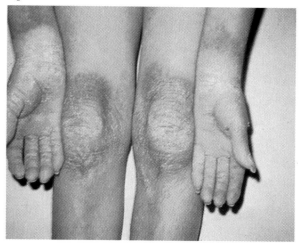

Figure 440

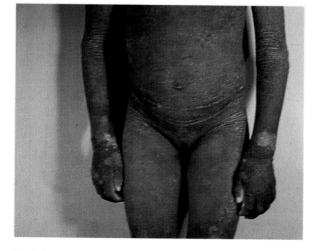

Bullous congenital ichthyosiform erythroderma (epidermolytic hyperkeratosis) Over time, the generalized blistering resolves, and widespread areas of thick hyperkeratosis and scale develop. In Fig. 438 there is a mixed picture; focal erosions are present on the arms and abdomen, and there are areas of thick, discolored, furrowed hyperkeratosis. Note the predilection, which is not seen in ichthyosis vulgaris, for the antecubital fossae and intertriginous spaces. Figure 439 shows the process in typical areas: the palms, wrists, and knees. For some patients, severe involvement of the palms and soles creates a particular disability. Figure 440 shows bullous ichthyosis in its most severe and generalized form. Patients with this kind of extensive disease face a very difficult set of problems.

Figure 441

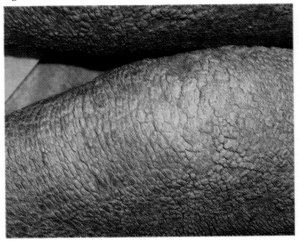

Figure 442

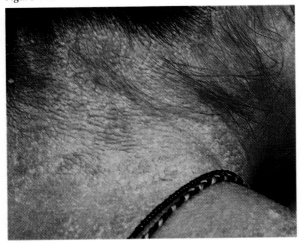

Bullous congenital ichthyosiform erythroderma (epidermolytic hyperkeratosis) (cont.) Bacterial colonization of this thickened and furrowed skin may result in an extremely unpleasant body odor. The foul smell, along with the disfigurement caused by the disease itself, may interfere enormously with social adaptation. Finally, some children remain prone to mechan-

ically induced blisters in areas of friction or trauma. Antibacterial soaps are of some help in reducing odor. Treatment with keratolytics will often induce painful superficial erosions, and the use of oral retinoids, with all of their side effects, has met with little success. Fortunately, in many patients the disease tends to localize to smaller, usually flexural, areas with advancing age.

Figure 443

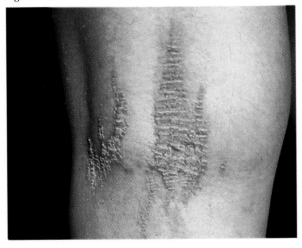

Figure 444

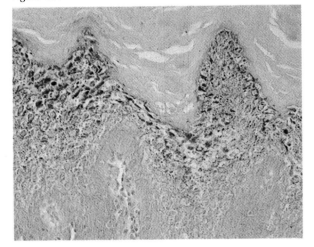

Bullous congenital ichthyosiform erythroderma (epidermolytic hyperkeratosis) This photograph shows a localized lesion in the popliteal space. Note the degree of hyperkeratosis and the sculptured character of the skin markings. When there is only local involvement, the clinical picture can be indistinguishable from epidermal nevus. Patients with minimal involvement, like this, may have relatives with severe generalized disease. Prenatal diagnosis is now possible.

Histopathology of bullous congenital ichthyosiform erythroderma (epidermolytic hyperkeratosis) The histopathologic pattern seen in bullous ichthyosis distinguishes it from the other ichthyoses. It is termed *epidermolytic hyperkeratosis,* or *granular degeneration.* A compact and hyperkeratotic stratum corneum overlies an abnormal upper spinous and granular cell layer. At this level there is a form of intracellular vacuolization and numerous clumped keratohyaline granules. Electron microscopy reveals excessive tonofilaments and keratohyaline granules.

Figure 445

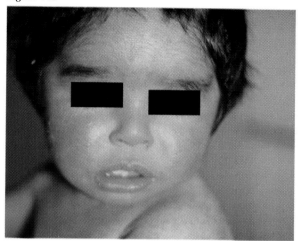

Figure 446

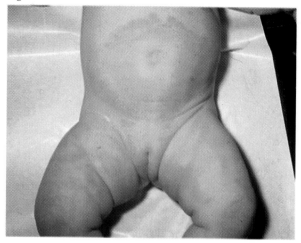

Non-bullous congenital ichthyosiform erythroderma This rare autosomal recessive condition may present with a collodion membrane at birth. The severity of the disease during infancy and later childhood is extremely variable. The most typical appearance features widespread scaling and moderate to severe erythroderma. The children with most severe involvement may experience difficulty with temperature regulation. Improvement sometimes occurs at puberty.

Erythrokeratoderma variabilis This is a rare autosomal dominant condition characterized by migratory areas of erythema and distinct plaques of hyperkeratosis. From an early beginning in infancy, there occur figurate and rapidly (within days) shifting areas of bright erythema on the face, anterior trunk, buttocks, and extensor aspects of the limbs. These may be brought on by changes in environmental temperature. In addition, there are fixed and localized hyperkeratotic plaques.

Figure 447

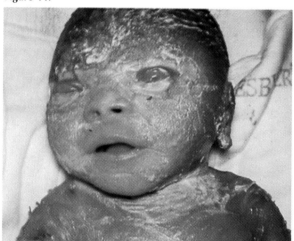

Figure 448

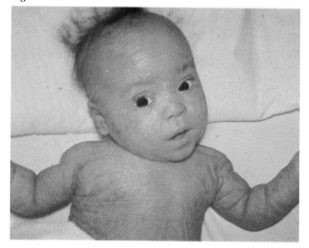

Lamellar ichthyosis *Collodion baby* is a descriptive term for the child who is born encased in a taut, parchment-like membrane, accompanied by ectropion and eclabium. The outcome of this process is unpredictable. A small group of infants shed their membrane and develop completely normal skin; their condition is termed *lamellar exfoliation of the newborn*. Some go on to develop nonbullous congenital ichthyosiform erythroderma, or Netherton's syndrome, or Conradi's disease (see Figs. 455–460). Still others, like the infant in Fig. 447, have the

chronic and severe autosomal recessive disease lamellar ichthyosis. Collodion babies, irrespective of the cause, are very often born prematurely. In addition, they are at risk for cutaneous infection, sepsis, pneumonia, and hypernatremic dehydration and require careful supportive therapy. The infant in Fig. 448 was formerly a collodion baby and has gradually sloughed his membrane. When the baby is several months of age, one can detect the beginnings of generalized hyperkeratosis and scaling. His underlying disease is lamellar ichthyosis.

Figure 449

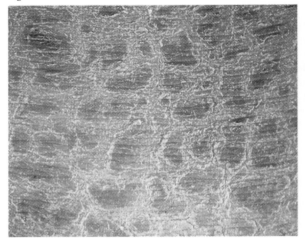

Lamellar ichthyosis (cont.) This figure shows in detail the kind of ichthyosis that gradually becomes established after the disappearance of the collodion membrane. Note the mosaic pattern of the scales and tendency of the edges of the scale to curl away from the surface. The scales are sometimes compared with armored plates. Bulla formation does not occur in this condition.

Figure 450

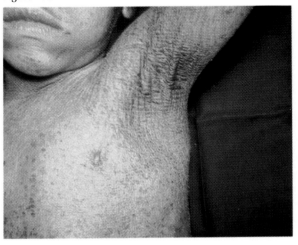

Lamellar ichthyosis Note that the entire skin surface, including the face, is affected by the hyperkeratotic, scaly, dyschromic dyskeratinization. Involvement tends to be most severe in flexural areas, as in the axilla pictured here. Topical therapy with the α-hydroxy acids, such as lactic acid, is somewhat helpful in reducing the amount of scale and improving appearance.

Figure 451

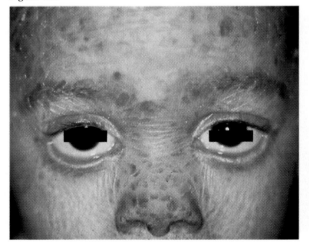

Figure 452

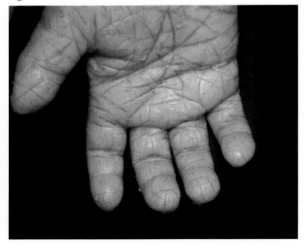

Lamellar ichthyosis The child in Fig. 451 has the severe degree of involvement that is an almost invariable feature of lamellar ichthyosis. Note the ectropion and tightness of the facial skin as a result of hyperkeratosis. The same compromised mobility of skin obtains on other parts of the body. Figure 452 illustrates involvement of the palms with thick hyperkeratosis and deep grooves. Not pictured here are the changes that may involve hair and nails. Scaliness of the scalp may be accompanied by partial hair loss. In addition, the nails may be ridged or thickened, and there may be thick subungual hyperkeratosis. Defects in keratinocyte transglutaminase have been reported in patients with lamellar ichthyosis.

Figure 453

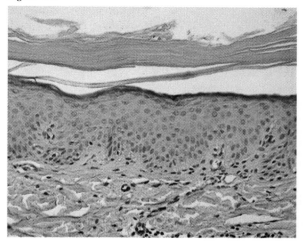

Figure 454

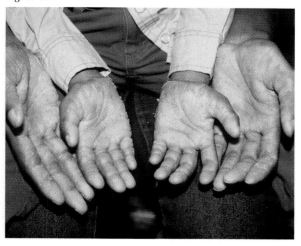

Histopathology of lamellar ichthyosis In lamellar ichthyosis there is merely a variable degree of hyperkeratosis. The thickened stratum corneum is generally dense (and here shows an artificial separation from the subjacent stratum malpighii), and the stratum granulosum may be somewhat thickened, which is in marked contrast to its absence in ichthyosis vulgaris. The condition cannot be distinguished by microscopy from the X-linked variety of ichthyosis.

Palmoplantar keratoderma There is a long list of genodermatoses that include thickening of the palms and soles as either the principal or an associated abnormality. The most common among all of these is Unna-Thost palmoplantar keratoderma. The autosomal dominant inheritance of this condition is illustrated by the mother-son involvement shown here. Treatment consists of the use of keratolytic agents to remove callus.

Figure 455

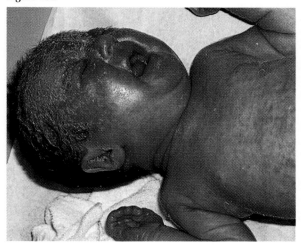

Figure 456

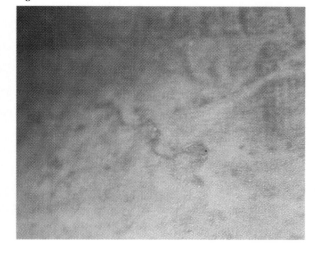

Netherton's syndrome This rare autosomal recessive syndrome manifests itself in a unique ichthyosis and hair shaft abnormality. At birth, these patients may have a generalized ichthyosiform erythroderma sometimes resembling generalized seborrheic dermatitis, as seen in Fig. 455. Severe hypernatremic dehydration is common. The most distinctive cutaneous feature is termed *ichthyosis linearis circumflexa,* a collection of circi-

nate, erythematous, and hyperkeratotic lesions with a very characteristic double-edged scale along the margin (Fig. 456). Patients with Netherton's syndrome tend to have an atopic diathesis, with some combination of asthma, allergic rhinitis, and eczematous dermatitis. Finally, there is a tendency toward impaired cellular immunity and developmental delay.

Figure 457

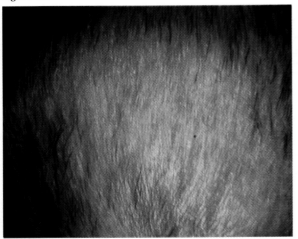

Figure 458

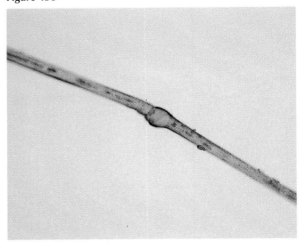

Netherton's syndrome (cont.)   The associated hair abnormality is seen in Fig. 457. Microscopic examination of these "bamboo hairs" (Fig. 458) most often reveals a hair shaft abnormality termed *trichorrhexis invaginata,* a ball-and-socket insertion of the distal hair shaft into the proximal hair. There may

also be pili torti (Fig. 837) or trichorrhexis nodosa (Fig. 835). The hair disorder is not evident at birth and may sometimes be first found upon examination of eyebrow hairs. The hair disorder tends to correct itself with the passage of time.

Figure 459

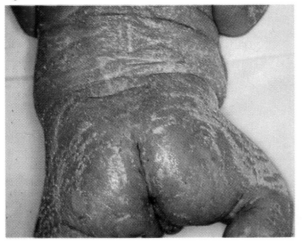

Figure 460

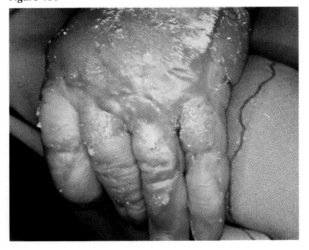

Cutaneous manifestations of Conradi's disease   Conradi's disease, or chondrodysplasia punctata, is actually a group of related syndromes that have differing prognoses and modes of inheritance. Skin changes are seen in some of the patients with each of the disease subtypes. The newborn may present as a collodion baby (see Fig. 447). In early infancy, there develops a generalized, whorled ichthyosiform erythroderma, as illustrated in these two photographs. Over time, the areas of ichthyosis are replaced by blotchy hyperpigmentation and then,

sometimes, by follicular atrophoderma. Patchy alopecia also may occur. Systemic features of chondrodysplasia punctata include stippling of the epiphyses, shortening of the femur and humerus, congenital cataracts, and saddle nose. The autosomal recessive form, also termed *rhizomelic dwarfism,* is most severe and usually causes psychomotor retardation and seizures. Those patients with the autosomal dominant disease (Conradi-Hunermann syndrome) have a generally better prognosis.

Figure 461

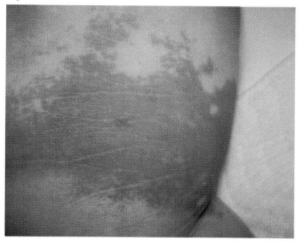

Figure 462

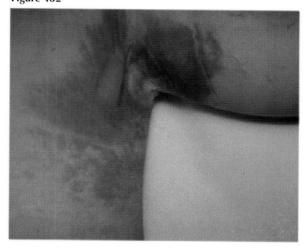

Cutaneous manifestations of Sjögren-Larsson syndrome
This is a rare autosomal recessive genodermatosis that is characterized by spasticity, mental retardation, and congenital ichthyosis. A combination of scaling and erythroderma is seen in the newborn. Over time, the ichthyosis tends to localize to the lower abdomen (Fig. 461) and flexural areas (Fig. 462).

There may be mild involvement of the palms and soles. The combination of spasticity and psychomotor developmental delay is often quite severe and may be accompanied by a seizure disorder. A specific retinal lesion, the so-called glistening dots, is present in almost all patients with Sjögren-Larsson syndrome after 1 year of age.

Figure 463

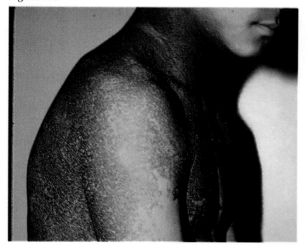

Figure 464

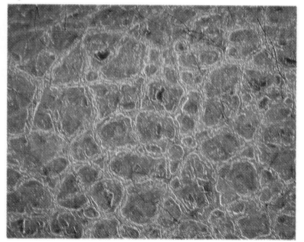

Recessive X-linked ichthyosis This disorder is characterized by ichthyosis that begins at or shortly after birth and persists through adult life. The "dirty" brown and tightly adherent scales are illustrated in both photographs. The scaling tends to favor the trunk and the extensor surfaces of the extremities. There is relative sparing of the face and flexural areas. The palms and soles are also spared, and the hair and teeth are normal. Most patients note marked improvement during the summer months, probably related to improved skin hydration. Asymptomatic

corneal opacities on the posterior membrane serve as an adult marker for this disease. In addition, there is a significant incidence of cryptorchidism in individuals with this syndrome. The locus for this rare genodermatosis is now known to be on the distal short arm of the X chromosome, and the disease is inherited in X-linked recessive fashion. The underlying metabolic disorder is a deficiency in the enzyme steroid sulfatase. Diagnosis can be confirmed by serum lipoprotein electrophoresis.

Figure 465

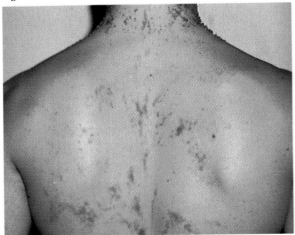

Figure 466

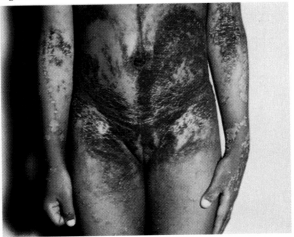

Linear epidermal nevus (systematized type) Widespread epidermal nevi occur, with the lesions following the lines of Blaschko. This condition was formerly termed *ichthyosis hystrix*. Patients with extensive lesions are especially prone to abnormalities in a variety of other organ systems—the epidermal nevus syndrome. Associated cutaneous lesions include hemangiomas, café-au-lait spots, and areas of hypopigmentation. Mental retardation and a seizure disorder may also be present. Skeletal ab-

normalities seen in the epidermal nevus syndrome include limb hypertrophy, bone cysts, and incomplete formation of certain bones. A higher-than-normal incidence of malignancy, particularly Wilms' tumor, has also been associated with this disorder. All children with epidermal nevi should have a careful physical examination, and laboratory evaluation should be pursued as indicated. Occasionally, patients with epidermal nevi are genetic mosaics for bullous congenital ichthyosiform erythroderma.

Figure 467

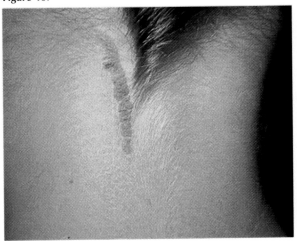

Figure 468

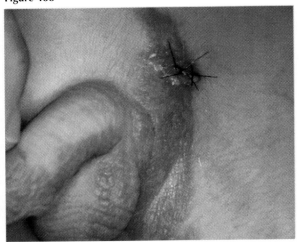

Linear epidermal nevus The lesion consists of verrucous, hyperkeratotic papules that are closely grouped in a linear array following the lines of Blaschko. Epidermal nevi are often present at birth but may arise during the first year of life, and occasionally later. They may occur on the head and neck, trunk, or extremities. Lesions of the appearance illustrated in this figure are sometimes termed *nevus unius lateris*. Epidermal nevus has no malignant potential, except for the rare development of basal cell carcinoma in a preexisting lesion. Surgical treatment is required only when indicated for cosmetic considerations.

Inflammatory linear verrucous epidermal nevus (ILVEN) This linear array of pruritic papules arises most often during childhood. The lesions are erythematous and scaling and are usually localized to the lower extremities or perineum. Sometimes this entity may be difficult to distinguish from psoriasis. The persistence of inflammation in one anatomic area and the absence of psoriatic lesions elsewhere favor the diagnosis of ILVEN. Histologically, it may resemble psoriasis or nonspecific chronic dermatitis.

Figure 469

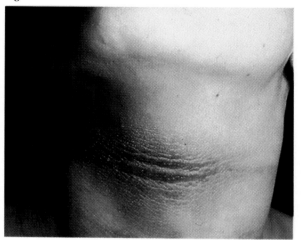

Figure 470

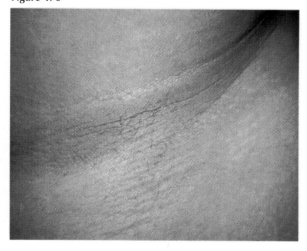

Acanthosis nigricans   This is a descriptive term for a velvety or varicose brown-to-black area of hyperkeratosis. The axilla is the most common location, but lesions are also seen on the posterior neck and in the groin. Less commonly, there is involvement in the antecubital and popliteal fossae, on the knuckles, and in other, nonflexural areas. Onset may occur during child-hood or adult life. The histologic pattern is that of hyperkeratosis and papillomatosis; the brownish discoloration seems to be caused by these surface changes rather than by any local increase in the amount of melanin. Illustrated here are lesions of acanthosis nigricans on the anterior neck and in the axilla.

Figure 471

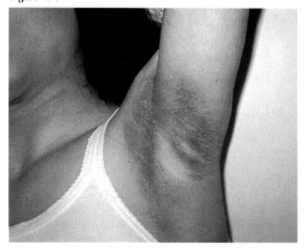

Figure 472

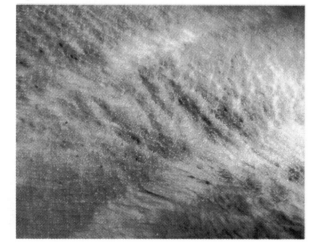

Acanthosis nigricans   On the basis of the varying etiologies, acanthosis nigricans is divided into several types. The title *benign acanthosis nigricans* is used to describe an autosomal dominant genodermatosis. The condition may develop at birth or during childhood and often intensifies after puberty. A second type, which heralds the presence of an associated malignancy (usually adenocarcinoma), is extremely rare during childhood. The term *pseudoacanthosis nigricans* refers to the form that is directly related to obesity. It is not unusual to see this condition on the nape of the neck or in the axilla and groin in an obese adolescent. This form of acanthosis nigricans frequently abates or resolves completely with dieting and weight loss. Finally, acanthosis nigricans may occur as a manifestation of several unrelated syndromes. These include Rud's syndrome, Bloom's syndrome, and Crouzon's syndrome. The relationship between acanthosis nigricans and insulin-resistant diabetes mellitus is discussed in the legend to Fig. 670.

Figure 473

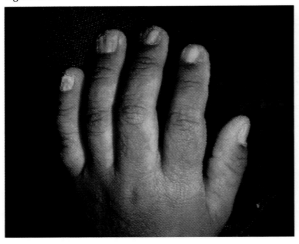

Figure 474

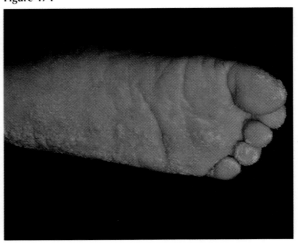

KID syndrome The keratitis-ichthyosis-deafness (KID) syndrome is a multisystem disorder that, in its most severe forms, may be disabling. Cutaneous changes consist of thick keratoderma of the palms and soles, keratotic plaques on the face and extremities, and a diffuse ichthyosis with follicular accentuation. Abnormal keratinization may be present at birth. Alope-cia, nail dystrophy, and hypoplastic teeth are all part of this disorder. The hearing impairment in this disease is progressive and due to neurosensory deafness. Keratitis begins during childhood and is accompanied by neovascularization. Visual loss may be severe. Recurrent and atypical cutaneous infections may also be seen in KID syndrome.

Figure 475

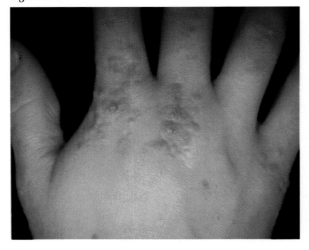

Figure 476

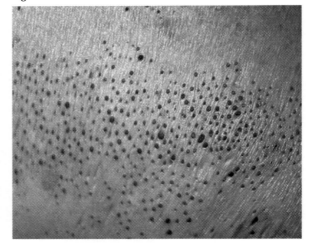

Acrokeratosis verruciformis This autosomal dominant disorder is characterized by numerous flat-topped or verrucous hyperkeratotic papules that are usually localized to the dorsa of the hands and feet. They tend to recur after surgical removal. Histologically, there are distinctive elevations of the epidermis that resemble church spires. It should be noted that patients with Darier's disease (see Figs. 337 and 338) may have identical acral lesions.

Nevus comedonicus The lesions in this condition consist of numerous clustered papules, each with a dark, central hyperkeratotic plug. The individual papules are clinically and histologically identical to the comedones seen in acne vulgaris. However, these nevoid plaques, which are often linear in configuration, do not necessarily occur in the ordinary sites of predilection of comedonal acne. Lesions may be single or multiple, and palm and sole involvement occurs. This may be a form of epidermal nevus.

13

Urticarial, Purpuric, and Vascular Reactions

Figure 477

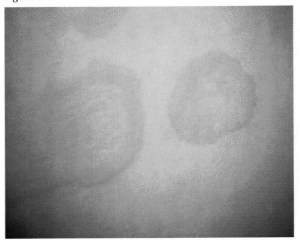

Figure 478

Urticaria   A wheal is an edematous papule that may enlarge to form a pink, sharply circumscribed, elevated plaque. The typical lesions of urticaria, pictured here, have a suggestion of central clearing. By definition, the individual lesions of urticaria evolve quickly and resolve within 24–48 hours. They are usually accompanied by severe pruritus. The most common etiologies of urticaria are medications, foods, and viral and bacterial infections. Autoimmune disease and malignancy are extremely rare causes. In the child with chronic urticaria, it is often difficult or impossible to identify a single cause.

Cholinergic urticaria   This type of urticaria is causally related to elevation in body temperature and sweating. The lesions usually develop rapidly after the beginning of exercise and resolve rapidly and spontaneously with cooling. The urticaria that develops in this condition has a typical appearance, illustrated here. The lesions consist of red or flesh-colored papules 2–3 mm in diameter that are surrounded by an ill-defined erythematous macule. The use of antihistamines will decrease the frequency and severity of attacks. Doxepin may also be effective.

Figure 479

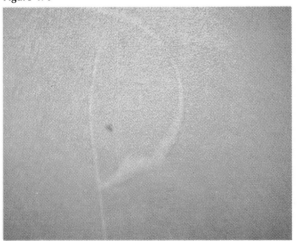

Figure 480

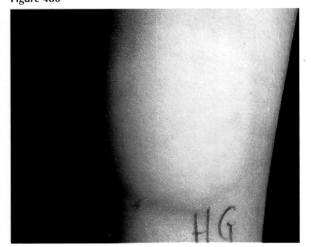

Physical urticarias   There are urticarias in which stroking, pressure, cold, heat, or sun exposure is causative. Figure 479 is whealing in linear form produced by stroking the skin with a degree of force that would ordinarily cause nothing more than transient erythema. The phenomenon, called *dermographism,* is present in a small percentage of normal individuals. Figure 480 is a huge wheal produced by resting an ice cube on the forearm. Cold-induced urticaria may be acquired or inherited. In the

most common, acquired form, patients develop lesions shortly after ingesting cold foods or liquids or shortly after exposure to a drop in environmental temperature. Patients with this form of sensitivity are at risk for laryngeal edema or circulatory collapse as a result of significant cold exposure. Antihistamines or doxepin is of some help in preventing attacks. In a very rare syndrome, contact of the skin with water, without respect to its temperature, produces wheals (aquagenic urticaria).

Figure 481

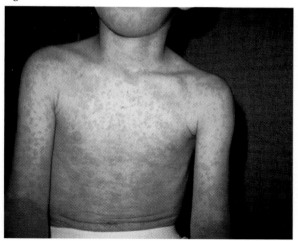

Figure 482

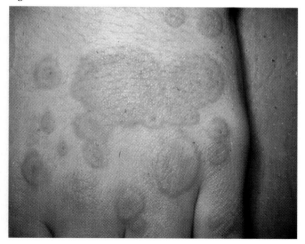

Erythema multiforme This disorder is termed *multiforme* because the morphology of its lesions is so variable. The primary lesion is most often an erythematous macule that evolves into a papule. Early in the course, these lesions may easily be mistaken for urticaria. As the lesions enlarge, they form round or irregularly shaped plaques. The central area may blister or become dusky in color; this change represents the necrosis of keratinocytes in areas of active involvement. Concentric circles of erythema and dark gray discoloration may evolve, forming the

typical "target" lesion of erythema multiforme. The "target" lesions may coalesce and develop annular or serpiginous borders. Figure 481 is an overview of a severe case. Figure 482 is a close-up of the target-like quality of the variably sized and shaped plaques. Note the redness and edema at the border and the duskier appearance at the center. Erythema multiforme tends to be acral in distribution, and the dorsum of the hand is a particularly common location.

Figure 483

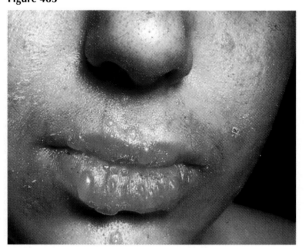

Figure 484

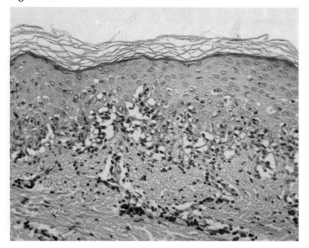

Erythema multiforme The type of bulla that may occur in erythema multiforme is shown here. Mucosal lesions are not uncommon. Erythema multiforme is a self-healing disease, with an average duration of about 2 weeks. Herpes simplex infection is by far the most common etiologic agent. Finally, a wide variety of drugs, most commonly the sulfonamides, may cause this syndrome.

Histopathology of erythema multiforme The term *erythema multiforme* is used differently by different authors, but all agree that an eruption that lasts only a few weeks and has iris (target) lesions is probably the disease in classic form. In the microscope, such lesions, prior to blister formation, generally show damage to the dermoepidermal junction with the formation of individual eosin-staining keratinocytes. The mild dermal inflammation is of mononuclear cells.

Figure 485

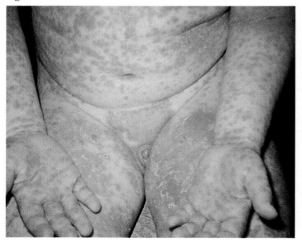

Figure 486

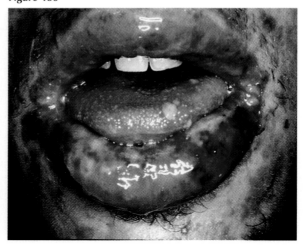

Stevens-Johnson syndrome   Drugs are the major etiologic factor in the development of erythema multiforme major. The most common agents are sulfonamides, anticonvulsants, and nonsteroidal anti-inflammatory drugs. *Mycoplasma pneumoniae* has been implicated as the most commonly associated infectious agent. The cutaneous lesions include fixed erythematous macules, target lesions, and bullae. There may be progression to widespread erythema and denudation, leaving

underlying erosions (Fig. 485). At least two mucous membranes are involved in this syndrome. The oral cavity is almost always involved, with bullae, ulcerations, and crusting most commonly presenting on the lips, buccal mucosa, and palate (Fig. 486). The bulbar conjunctiva and anogenital mucosa may also be involved. Tracheal and bronchial involvement may result in breathing difficulty. Ocular involvement may result in scarring of the conjunctivae or corneas.

Figure 487

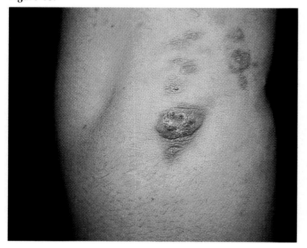

Figure 488

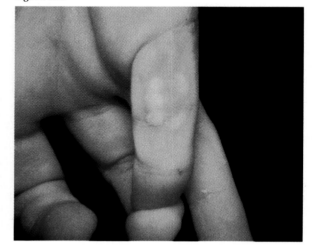

Erythema elevatum diutinum   This is a rare skin disease that is characterized by purple or yellowish papules, nodules, and plaques that tend to cluster on the hands, feet, and extensor surfaces of the extremities. The skin overlying joints is a favored location. The distribution is usually symmetrical, and the disease tends to be chronic. Lesions of erythema elevatum diutinum

may be asymptomatic but in some cases are painful. Figure 487 shows typical nodules and plaques on the elbow, and yellowish papules on the finger are seen in Fig. 488. The etiology of this chronic leukocytoclastic vasculitis remains unknown, but an immune-complex etiology has been suggested. Dapsone is one mode of treatment.

Figure 489

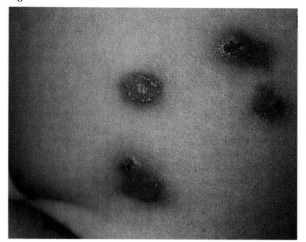

Figure 490

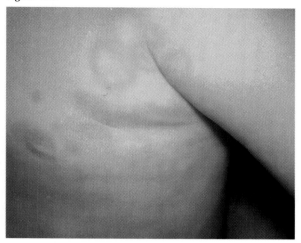

Sweet's syndrome (acute febrile neutrophilic dermatosis) This syndrome is characterized by painful, raised, erythematous plaques and nodules. The cutaneous eruption is accompanied by spiking fevers and a neutrophilic leukocytosis. This condition is seen most commonly in middle-aged women, but it does occur in children. Skin biopsy reveals a widespread infiltrate of polymorphonuclear leukocytes throughout the dermis. Sweet's syndrome is often associated with either malignancy or antecedent infection. Systemic corticosteroids are the treatment of choice.

Erythema annulare centrifugum This is an erythematous and edematous lesion that gradually enlarges to form annular, polycyclic, and gyrate shapes. The lesions tend to resolve spontaneously but may reappear. Erythema annulare centrifugum has been attributed to a wide variety of causes. In some cases, it is temporally related to the development of malignancy and resolves with treatment or removal of the tumor. In other patients, the disease has been related to superficial fungal infections and a wide variety of viral and bacterial diseases.

Figure 491

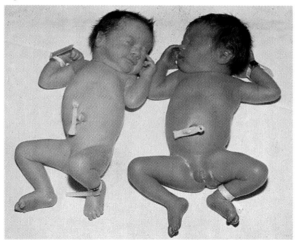

Figure 492

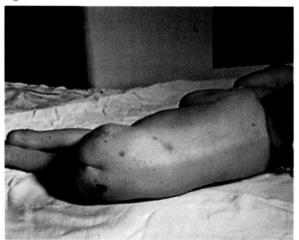

Twin-to-twin "transfusion" Twins who develop with some form of common circulation in utero may show a temporary difference of cutaneous color related to oddities of hemodynamics. In the photograph one sees twin neonates, of whom the one on the right is uniformly and abnormally erythematous, whereas the other is abnormally pallid. The one looks plethoric; the other, anemic. In the course of time, restoration of normal blood counts and color will develop in both.

Harlequin dyschromia The word *harlequin* connotes, among other things, the quality of being parti-colored. Here we see an infant in whom the left half of the trunk is pale and the right half red. The anomaly is transient and depends on circulatory derangement by gravity. If this child were to be turned onto its left side, which is now pale, that side would become red and the right side, now red, would become pale. This phenomenon is much more common among preterm infants.

Figure 493

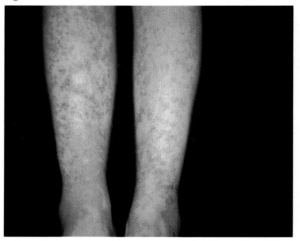

Figure 494

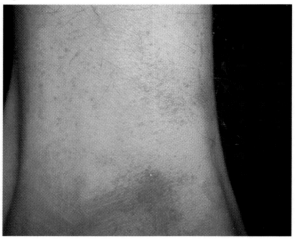

Purpura Hemorrhage into the skin takes many forms in structure, shape, and color. What we generally designate as purpura are macular lesions that may be punctate (petechial) or diffuse and red purple in color (ecchymotic). The causes are numerous. Most common among the benign pigmented purpuras is Schamberg's disease, a disorder of unknown etiology. Affected children have numerous discrete patches of petechiae on the lower extremities. The individual lesions evolve into typical brown-orange macules containing "cayenne pepper" spots. Fresh petechiae occur at other sites. More significant causes of purpura include septicemia (see Figs. 575–578), a wide variety of hematologic disorders, and vasculitis. Palpable purpura is, in fact, the hallmark of leukocytoclastic vasculitis, which may be a manifestation of bacterial or viral infection, drug allergy, connective tissue disease, or cryoglobulinemia. Henoch-Schönlein purpura, a common cause of childhood leukocytoclastic vasculitis, is discussed in Figs. 499–501.

Figure 495

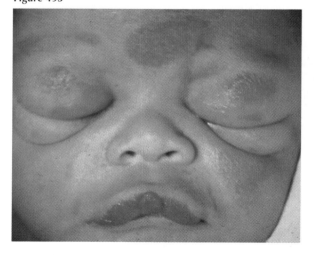

Figure 496

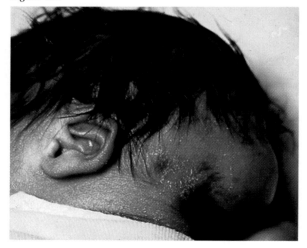

Traumatic purpura These photographs show hemorrhage into the skin occasioned by difficult passage of newborns through the birth canal. Such events are common, and as long as the hemorrhage is into skin alone, no great or lasting harm results. In Fig. 495 one sees edema and ecchymosis that resulted from molding of the head in a prolonged but spontaneous delivery. Figure 496 shows a hematoma of considerable size from a similar event. Modern obstetrics, which encompasses prenatal study of the maternal pelvis, ultrasonography, sedation, muscle relaxants, anesthesia during delivery, and cesarean section when indicated, has tended to make serious traumatic purpura of this sort less common. Nevertheless, in severe cases of traumatic hemorrhage of this kind, imaging studies for the possibility of skull fracture are good practice.

Figure 497

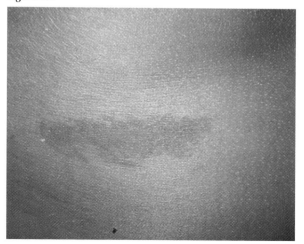

Figure 498

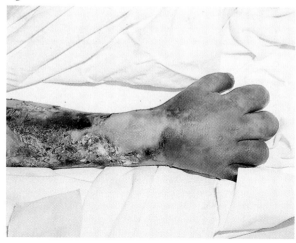

Traumatic purpura   Throughout life, hard knocks in the physical sense are the lot of us all. Rupture of capillaries is thus exceedingly common, and more extensive rupture of arterioles, vesicles, arteries, or veins is common enough. Petechiae, ecchymoses, vibices, and hematomas are banal, nearly everyday events. The black eye and contusions are in everyone's experience. Illustrated here is a traumatic ecchymosis that may well represent a hickey ("passion purpura").

Purpura fulminans   This condition is a rare and exceedingly serious consequence of certain acute infectious diseases. Scarlet fever of bygone days, meningococcal meningitis, severe varicella, and congenital protein C deficiency have been known to be complicated by fulminating purpura that went on to gangrene, extreme toxicity, shock, and death. The cause of the condition seems to be necrotizing vasculitis attended by defects of clotting (disseminated intravascular coagulation).

Figure 499

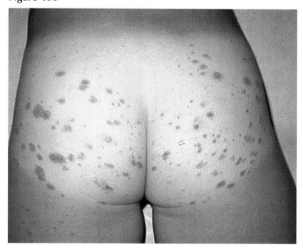

Figure 500

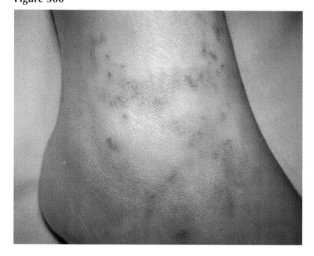

Henoch-Schönlein purpura   Palpable purpura is but one aspect of a syndrome that is marked also by attacks of arthralgia, abdominal pain, and hematuria. The entire complex of visible cutaneous purpura, arthralgia, and visceral signs and symptoms results from a widespread IgA-related vasculitis. In addition to purpura, as shown in Fig. 499 on the buttocks and in Fig. 500 around an ankle, the skin may show edematous plaques, vesicles, and even necroses. Without the cutaneous signs, arthralgia

might mislead one to consider rheumatic fever; abdominal pain might suggest an acute surgical abdomen and lead to unnecessary laparotomy; and hematuria might mislead to diagnoses like glomerulonephritis or nephrolithiasis. Good clinical judgment, however, will confirm the diagnosis of Henoch-Schönlein purpura. The cause of this condition is not known. The prognosis is usually good, except for the rare child who goes on to develop chronic nephritis.

Figure 501

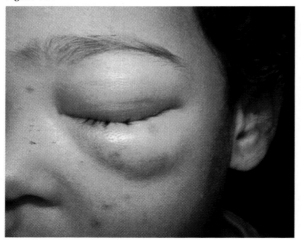

Figure 502

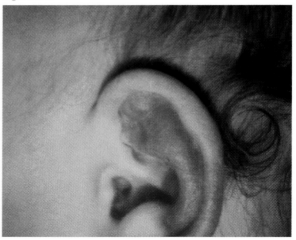

Henoch-Schönlein purpura (cont.) This picture is a good representation of both the purpuric elements and the edema that may appear in the Henoch-Schönlein syndrome. In itself, without signs and symptoms of hemorrhagic consequences or edema in joints, gut, or kidneys, many another diagnosis would have to be differentially considered in an appearance like this.

Idiopathic thrombocytopenic purpura This autoimmune condition is triggered by causes unknown and is manifest by intracutaneous bleeding. The purpura takes the form of petechiae and ecchymoses not only in the skin, where it is obvious, but also in the oropharyngeal mucous membranes, the nose, and the gastrointestinal tract. The illustration here is of ecchymosis in the pinna of an ear.

Figure 503

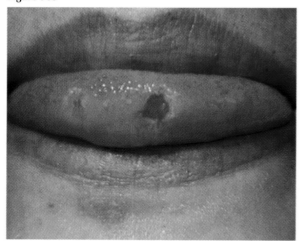

Figure 504

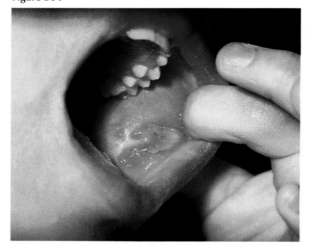

Aphthous stomatitis This very common condition is characterized by recurrent episodes of painful ulceration on the lip, tongue, or buccal surfaces. The individual lesions quickly evolve from erythematous macules to papules, and then to yellowish ulcerations with a surrounding pink or red halo. The etiology is not known, and the ulcers heal in 7 to 10 days without scarring. Whereas a solitary lesion is the cause of only temporary, minor discomfort, there are some individuals who develop deeper and larger ulcers, or numerous erosions. For them, aphthous stomatitis can be a severe problem.

Behçet's syndrome This rare disease is characterized by a classic triad of recurrent ulcerations of the oral mucosa, genital ulcers, and eye involvement. The oral ulcers, one of which is pictured here, tend to be larger, more numerous, and more frequently recurrent than those of simple aphthous stomatitis. Genital lesions occur on the penis and scrotum in males, and on the vulva in females. These frequently recurrent ulcers tend to heal with scarring. The various forms of eye involvement include uveitis and keratoconjunctivitis and may eventuate in blindness.

Figure 505

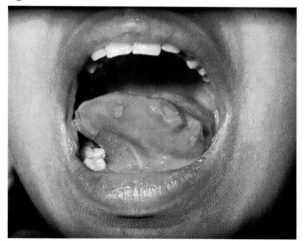

Figure 506

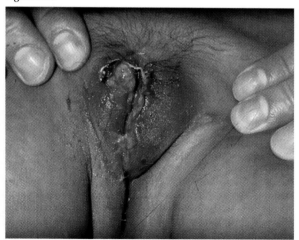

Behçet's syndrome The sharply marginated oral ulcers of this syndrome are pictured in Fig. 505. Figure 506 shows the typical genital lesions. Other cutaneous lesions may be widespread and include papules, vesicles, abscesses, and lesions of erythema nodosum. In addition to the eyes and skin, a number of other organ systems may become involved. Severe chronic arthritis and thrombophlebitis are common occurrences. Gastrointestinal disease ranges from mild abdominal discomfort to chronic diarrhea and an ulcerative colitis–like illness. Neurologic manifestations, including recurrent meningoencephalitis and brain stem lesions, are often the most serious and can be life threatening. Diagnosis of Behçet's syndrome is based on the presence of the typical clinical findings. The disease is difficult to treat, but immunosuppressive drugs and corticosteroids are the most frequently used therapies.

14

Bullous, Pustular, and Ulcerating Diseases

Figure 507

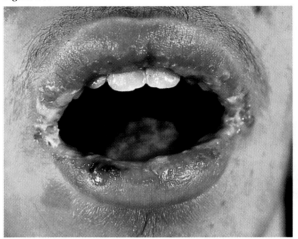

Figure 508

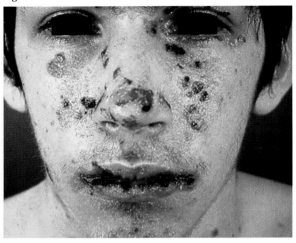

Pemphigus vulgaris Pemphigus vulgaris is a rare autoimmune, bullous disease that occasionally occurs during childhood. The disease affects both the skin and mucous membranes and can be life threatening. The typical lesions of pemphigus vulgaris are pictured here. Erosions of the lips, gums, tongue, and palate, as pictured in Fig. 507, are a common presenting symptom and may be misdiagnosed early in the course of the disease.

The difficulty in chewing and swallowing that may occur can become a significant complication. Cutaneous lesions consist of flaccid weeping blisters that quickly erode to leave large denuded areas of skin. Nikolsky's sign, the extension of blistering by lateral finger pressure, is seen in the presence of widespread disease. Figure 508 shows the kind of crusting that develops as the roofs of blisters of pemphigus vulgaris disintegrate.

Figure 509

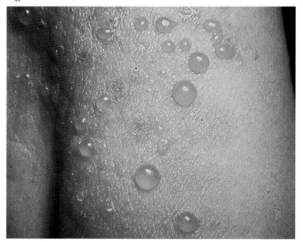

Figure 510

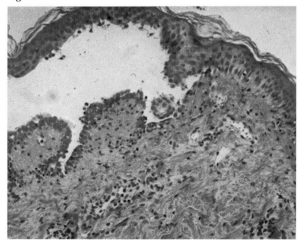

Pemphigus vulgaris The blisters of pemphigus vulgaris may arise on an erythematous base, or on normal-appearing skin, as pictured here. A variety of modalities have been employed in the treatment of this disease. The patient who is seriously ill requires hospitalization. For most patients, the most rapid and effective treatment remains high-dose systemic steroids. Patients undergoing this form of therapy are at high risk for infection and must be followed with extreme care. Immunosuppressive agents such as azathioprine, gold, and plasmapheresis are other useful therapies.

Histopathology of pemphigus vulgaris Biopsy analysis of a lesion of pemphigus vulgaris reveals a blister within the epidermis, the base of which is one or two cells above the basal layer. The underlying pathologic process is the loss of cohesion between epidermal cells, termed *acantholysis*. There is relatively little inflammatory infiltrate; acantholytic cells can be seen within the blister cavity. Direct immunofluorescence shows IgG and complement in the intercellular spaces of the epidermis. Indirect immunofluorescence testing is also positive for a specific intercellular substance–reactive antibody.

Figure 511

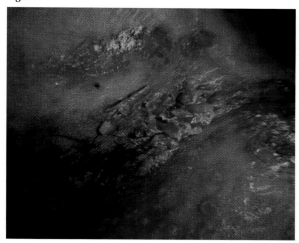

Figure 512

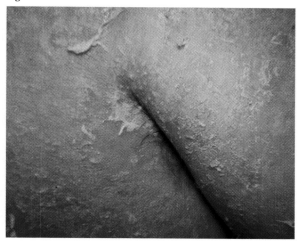

Pemphigus vegetans When the cutaneous changes of pemphigus take place in intertriginous spaces, clear blistering is not evident. Rather, one sees boggy inflammation and tumid granulation. The essential histologic process is again epidermal acantholysis, but blister roofs part almost at once and secondary infection is inevitable. This figure is a good representation of the kind of clinical appearance that develops in pemphigus vegetans. Lesions on other parts of the body take the form of pemphigus vulgaris.

Pemphigus foliaceus This figure illustrates the type of scaling that accompanies pemphigus foliaceus. What one sees is largely exfoliating stratum corneum, not blisters. On biopsy analysis, one finds acantholysis occurring high in the epidermis, usually in the granular layer. There may be a subcorneal cleft, but the rest of the epidermis remains attached. The autoantibodies that are seen by immunofluorescence are identical to those in pemphigus vulgaris.

Figure 513

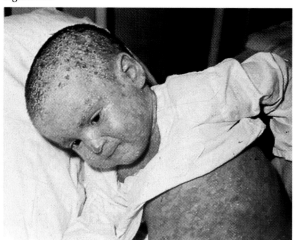

Figure 514

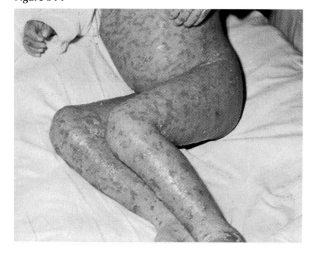

Pemphigus foliaceus This form of pemphigus is less severe than pemphigus vulgaris, because blister formation occurs higher in the epidermis. As a result, there is less compromise of vital cutaneous functions. In most areas of the world, pemphigus foliaceus is extremely unusual in children. In Brazil, there is an endemic form of pemphigus foliaceus, termed *fogo selvagem,* which affects individuals of all ages. Pictured here

are the typical lesions of pemphigus foliaceus. The disease often begins in the scalp with areas of erythema and scaling. As it progresses to involve the trunk and extremities, there evolve numerous crusting and erythematous plaques. Severe scaling is common, but there is usually no blister formation and no involvement of the oral cavity. Treatment consists of topical or systemic steroids, depending on the severity of the disease.

Figure 515

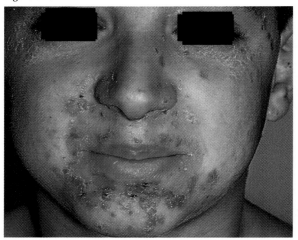

Figure 516

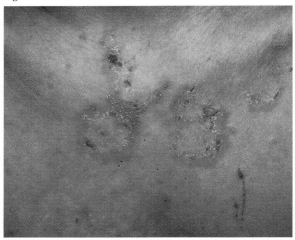

Pemphigus foliaceus (cont.)   Lesions in the perioral area, as seen in this figure, are quite common. Oral mucosal involvement is less common, in contrast to pemphigus vulgaris. Often, patients with pemphigus foliaceus are initially thought to have recurrent impetigo, although the infection does not totally clear with appropriate antibiotics. It is important to realize that secondary infection often occurs in these patients, and this should be considered when patients have flare-ups or the disease is difficult to control.

Pemphigus foliaceus   This figure shows annular lesions that are seen in childhood forms of pemphigus foliaceus. Direct immunofluorescence is important in making the diagnosis. In addition, antibodies to desmoglein, an epidermal desmosomal component, have been found. Treatment consists of topical or systemic steroids, depending on the severity of the disease.

Figure 517

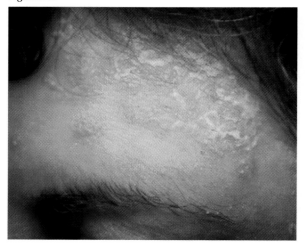

Figure 518

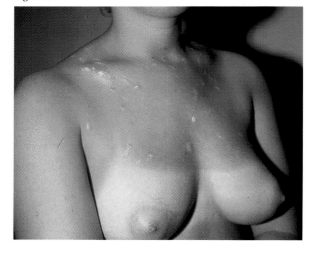

Pemphigus erythematosus   This is the least serious form of the pemphigus group of diseases and is probably best considered as a localized form of pemphigus foliaceus. It is unusual in children but does occasionally occur. Typically, there is scaling and crusting in a "butterfly distribution" on the face, as well as involvement of the chest, back, and scalp. The disease may be mistaken for severe seborrheic dermatitis or systemic lupus

erythematosus. Biopsy analysis of a lesion of pemphigus erythematosus reveals an intraepidermal bulla in the upper layers of the epidermis. As in all forms of pemphigus, IgG antibody to intercellular substance is present in the serum. Pemphigus erythematosus tends not to be a severe disease; most cases can be controlled with topical steroids alone.

Figure 519

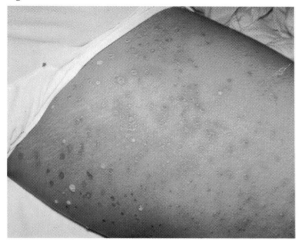

Figure 520

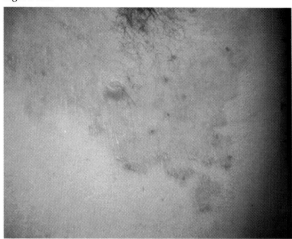

Subcorneal pustulosis (Sneddon-Wilkinson disease) This condition is most common during adulthood, but it does occur in children. Characteristically, crops of vesicles and pustules (Fig. 519) spring up and evolve into areas of superficial crusts and scales. As the lesions coalesce, they form the type of arcuate plaque that is illustrated in Fig. 520. The most common locations are the axillae, groin, and flexures of the upper and lower ex-

tremities. The lesions are often pruritic, and, especially in childhood, there may be fever and an elevated white blood count. The etiology of this condition is completely unknown. Diagnosis is best confirmed by classic histologic appearance, which consists of collections of neutrophils just beneath the stratum corneum. The disease process is essentially benign, but dapsone is an effective therapy for the patient with frequent or severe recurrences.

Figure 521

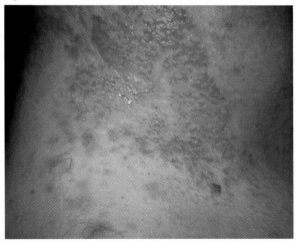

Figure 522

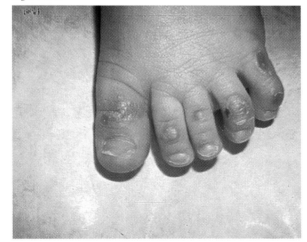

Familial benign chronic pemphigus (Hailey-Hailey disease) This blistering disease is inherited in autosomal dominant fashion. Onset tends to occur during late adolescence. Patients with this disorder have a pruritic vesicular eruption in intertriginous areas that is worse during the summer months. Intact bullae may be absent, and there is often only an erosive and crusted intertrigo in the axillae, in the groin, and on the neck. Control of this condition is best achieved by the avoidance of the causative factor, such as heat or friction, and the treatment of superinfection when it occurs.

Epidermolysis bullosa simplex This autosomal dominant condition is among the mildest of the diseases that are termed *epidermolysis bullosa*. The exact deficit is not known but is postulated to be an abnormal structural protein or a cytolytic enzyme. Epidermolysis bullosa simplex begins at birth or in early infancy, and throughout life the site of blistering corresponds to areas of friction or other trauma. During infancy, blisters occur on the neck, lower extremities, and hands and feet. In the child who is old enough to wear shoes, the dorsa of the toes are a common site of bulla formation.

Figure 523

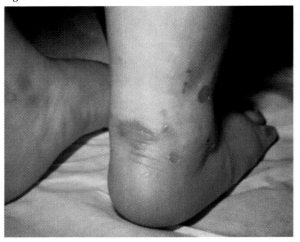

Epidermolysis bullosa simplex (cont.) In this condition, cleavage occurs through the basal cell layer of the epidermis, and the dermoepidermal junction is otherwise undisturbed. The result is that the lesions are superficial in appearance, and cutaneous function is well preserved. The lesions of epidermolysis bullosa simplex heal without scarring. In children with this disorder, mucous membrane involvement is minimal and usually does not produce serious difficulty. There may be some nail dystrophy, but this also heals with the cutaneous process.

Figure 524

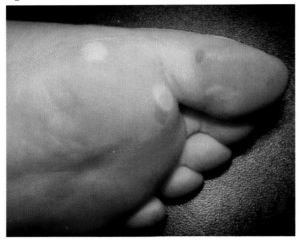

Recurrent epidermolysis bullosa of the hands and feet (Weber-Cockayne type) This particular variant of epidermolysis bullosa involves only the hands and feet; the cleavage plane is above the basal layer. The lesions tend to appear first during late childhood and adolescence. Pictured here are blisters on and near the great toe; the appearance of the bullae is modified by the thickness of the stratum corneum in this area. Patients with this disease tend also to suffer from hyperhidrosis. Minimizing trauma to the hands and feet and the use of antiperspirants help to prevent blister formation.

Figure 525

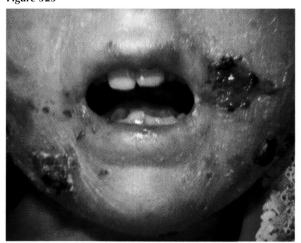

Epidermolysis bullosa dystrophica The autosomal recessive, dystrophic form of epidermolysis bullosa is a multisystem disease that is characterized by chronic and recurrent subepidermal blistering. The disorder often leads to severe disability, interfering with the normal processes of growth and development. Blister formation usually begins at or shortly after birth, and intraoral involvement may lead to early feeding difficulties. Normal handling of the infant with this disease results in the formation of tense bullae, which quickly evolve into ulcerations. The typical blisters, crusts,

Figure 526

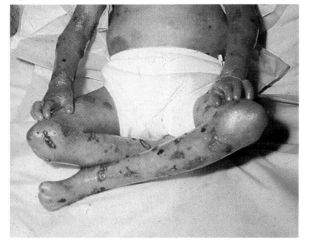

and erosions of dystrophic epidermolysis bullosa are seen in Fig. 525. The most serious sequelae of this disorder are due to the fact that the blisters heal with scarring. The recurrent episodes of bulla formation and healing on the hands and feet may result in an acquired syndactyly, as illustrated in Fig. 526. In the esophagus, the same process eventuates in mechanical obstruction. The strictures that form lead to nutritional difficulties and even perforation or squamous cell carcinoma of the esophagus. Eye involvement, with ulcers, keratitis, and opacities, is an additional problem.

Figure 527

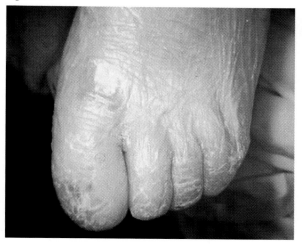

Epidermolysis bullosa dystrophica This figure shows a foot with complete destruction of the toenails, induced syndactyly of the fourth and fifth toes, and typical wrinkled scarring of the skin surface. Appropriate care for the child with epidermolysis bullosa must begin in the nursery and involves the use of topical dressings to protect eroded skin and the careful handling of the infant to avoid new blister formation. Subsequent management includes efforts to minimize skin trauma, good dental and ophthalmic care, and careful attention to diet and nutrition.

Figure 528

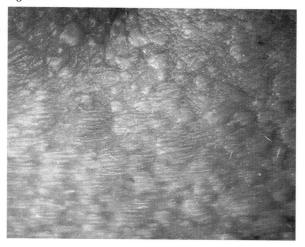

Epidermolysis bullosa (albopapuloid of Pasini) This is a dystrophic form of epidermolysis bullosa that is inherited in autosomal dominant fashion. Widespread blistering may be present at birth. During puberty, patients with this disorder develop distinctive ivory-white follicular papules on the chest and lower back. The albopapuloid form of epidermolysis bullosa has been associated with a defect in anchoring fibrils. The prognosis tends to be good.

Figure 529

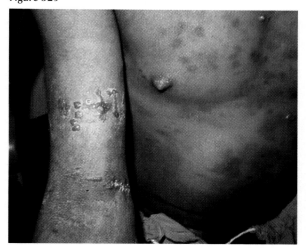

Epidermolysis bullosa dystrophica (dominant) This figure illustrates another patient with a dominant form of scarring epidermolysis bullosa. The Cockayne-Touraine form tends to begin during infancy and is associated with widespread blistering and milia formation. Shown here are a number of tense bullae on the flexor surface of the arm. Mouth involvement and nail dystrophy may also occur.

Figure 530

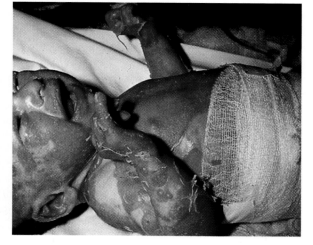

Epidermolysis bullosa atrophicans gravis This disorder, also known as *epidermolysis bullosa letalis,* is a severe variant. The bullae are junctional, and the disease is inherited in autosomal recessive fashion. Extensive cutaneous involvement is often present from birth. Severe erosions of the oral mucous membranes are commonplace and lead to early feeding difficulties. Gastrointestinal involvement leads to severe dysphagia, pyloric stenosis, or chronic malabsorption. Lesions in the genitourinary and respiratory systems are additional problems. Most patients do not survive into adulthood.

Figure 531

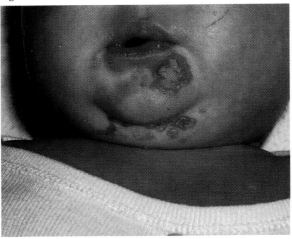

Figure 532

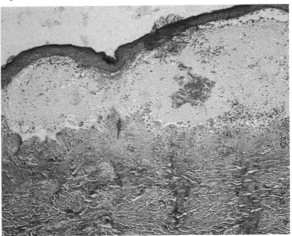

Epidermolysis bullosa simplex, Dowling-Meara type This form of epidermolysis bullosa is characterized by grouped, herpetiform blistering that generally occurs on the trunk but is also seen on the face and extremities. Blistering in infancy is often severe and extensive. After a few months, infants develop frequent blistering of the palms and soles. This disorder is associated with a defect in keratin 5 genes that causes clumping of tonofilaments in epidermal basal cells.

Histopathology of epidermolysis bullosa Random biopsy of a vesicle of epidermolysis bullosa is generally of no help in distinguishing types of the disease. All show the nonspecific picture of a subepidermal blister. A biopsy specimen taken from a newly formed, preferably induced, vesicle is helpful if the subepidermal basement membrane is stained with periodic acid–Schiff stain. Then the bulla may be seen formed through the basal cells, just above or just beneath the basement membrane. Electron microscopy is of particular value in establishing an exact diagnosis.

Figure 533

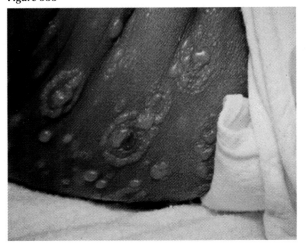

Figure 534

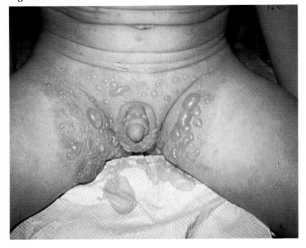

Chronic bullous dermatosis of childhood This is a distinct blistering disease that occurs exclusively during childhood, most commonly during the first 5 years of life. The disorder is characterized by large, tense bullae that tend to occur in the genital area, lower abdomen and back, and lower extremities. The degree of pruritus is variable. Figure 533 illustrates the particular fashion in which the blisters tend to cluster. Note the circular or oval configuration of blisters. As an early lesion heals with crusting and hyperpigmentation, new lesions arise in a string-of-pearls or rosette-like pattern along the periphery. The blisters themselves may be elongated or sausage-shaped. Figure 534 shows the clustering of tense blisters on the inner thighs. This is probably the most common location for chronic bullous dermatosis of childhood.

Figure 535

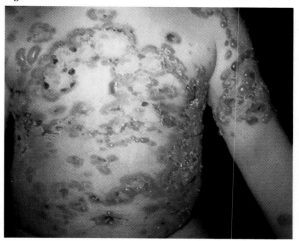

Figure 536

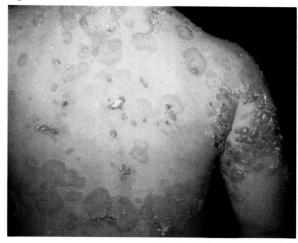

Chronic bullous dermatosis of childhood These two figures show the annular and polycyclic clustering of blisters that is so typical of this disorder. Biopsy of a lesion reveals a sub-epidermal blister with an infiltrate of neutrophils and/or eosinophils. Immunofluorescence is more distinctive and usually shows a linear deposit of IgA along the basement membrane (in the lamina lucida). In most patients, there are also circulating IgA antibodies directed against the basement membrane. For most affected children this is a self-limited disease, and it resolves spontaneously over a period of several years. Sulfapyridine and dapsone are the most effective therapies. These drugs have hemolytic activity, and the patients must be monitored for induced anemia and methemoglobinemia. A test for adequate glucose-6-phosphate dehydrogenase should be done before initiation of therapy, and hemoglobin determinations should be made subsequently until stabilization occurs.

Figure 537

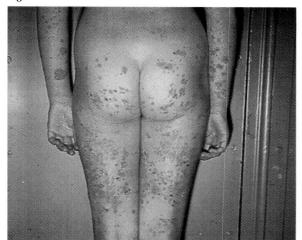

Figure 538

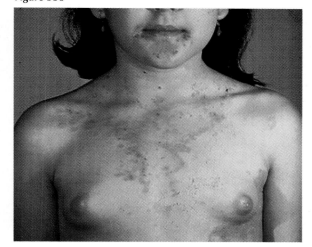

Dermatitis herpetiformis This intensely pruritic papulovesicular eruption is fairly unusual during childhood. Figure 537 shows the symmetrical distribution of the grouped, excoriated lesions on the extensor extremities and buttocks. Additional papules and vesicles on the upper chest and face are seen in Fig. 538. Dermatitis herpetiformis is a disease that affects both the skin and the gastrointestinal tract. The majority of children with this disorder have a gluten-sensitive enteropathy. This may lead to diarrhea and malabsorption, or it may be evidenced only by villous atrophy on jejunal biopsy analysis. The approaches to treatment of this disease include sulfapyridine or dapsone and a gluten-free diet. As mentioned above, children treated with dapsone or sulfapyridine must be carefully monitored for the development of hemolytic anemia. Adherence to a diet that contains no gluten is extremely difficult but, if accomplished, will often lead to prolonged remission.

Figure 539

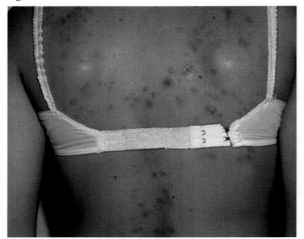

Dermatitis herpetiformis (cont.)   This picture of lesions of dermatitis herpetiformis shows them in a highly characteristic distribution on the back. Because of the intense pruritus, excoriations tend to outnumber the primary papulovesicles. Direct immunofluorescence of perilesional skin is an effective means of confirming the diagnosis of dermatitis herpetiformis. Typically, there are granular deposits of IgA at the tips of the dermal papillae.

Figure 540

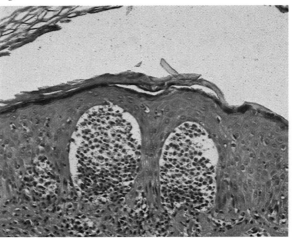

Histopathology of dermatitis herpetiformis   Biopsy analysis of erythematous and edematous skin around a blister is helpful in establishing the diagnosis of dermatitis herpetiformis. Such a specimen tends to show the unique histologic features, namely the formation of neutrophilic microabscesses in papillary bodies. The individual papillae show crescentic empty spaces between the epidermis and the cellular infiltrate.

15

Cutaneous Manifestations of Systemic Disease

Figure 541

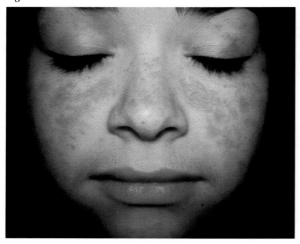

Figure 542

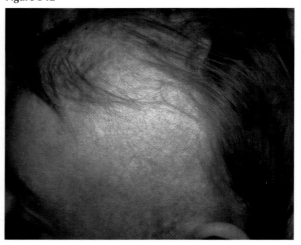

Cutaneous expressions of systemic lupus erythematosus
Figure 541 illustrates cutaneous involvement of systemic lupus erythematosus (SLE) in the classic butterfly pattern on the face. This macular and intensely erythematous eruption is frequently aggravated by sun exposure and may flare with other symptoms of systemic disease. Figure 542 shows the temporary alopecia that is also a hallmark of SLE. This autoimmune disease of un-

known etiology affects almost every organ system. The most common findings in the child with SLE are fever, arthralgias, and arthritis. In addition, pleuritis, pericarditis, and central nervous system involvement are frequently seen in children with SLE. Lupus nephritis develops in the vast majority of affected children and may eventually cause renal failure.

Figure 543

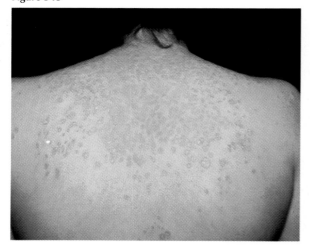

Figure 544

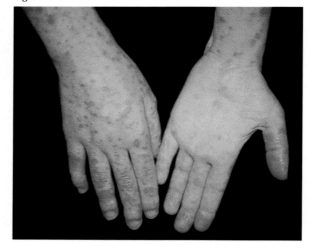

Cutaneous expressions of systemic lupus erythematosus
These photographs illustrate additional cutaneous features of SLE. The lesions on the back (Fig. 543) and the hands (Fig. 544) are intensely erythematous macules and slightly edematous papules and plaques. Childhood SLE occurs most frequently during adolescence and is more common among African-Americans and among girls. The diagnosis is established when four of eleven clinical and laboratory criteria are

met. Clinical criteria include rash (either malar or discoid), photosensitivity, oral ulcers, and disease of the joints, lungs, kidneys, and central nervous system. The single most reliable laboratory test is antinuclear antibody, which will be positive in almost every case of childhood SLE. Other laboratory criteria include leukopenia, thrombocytopenia, and the presence of anti–native DNA antibodies. Corticosteroids remain the mainstay of therapy for SLE.

Figure 545

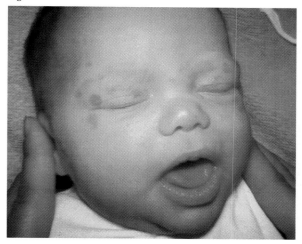

Figure 546

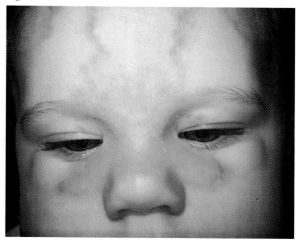

Neonatal lupus erythematosus   This condition is due to the transplacental passage mainly of anti-Ro (anti–SS-A) antibodies from mother to infant. However, anti-La (anti–SS-B) and anti-RNP antibodies may be implicated. The mother may suffer from a form of connective tissue disease or may be completely asymptomatic. The infants pictured in Figs. 545 and 546 were born with these atrophic and telangiectatic plaques on the face. The lesions may also resemble those of subacute cutaneous lupus in the older

patient. The skin lesions, which are more common in girls, tend to resolve without scarring. Nonfluorinated topical steroids and avoidance of the sun are the only treatments that may be required. A frequent complication of neonatal lupus is congenital heart block. This situation is potentially life threatening and may sometimes require implantation of a pacemaker. Although neonatal lupus is self-limited, there are reports of affected infants going on to develop connective tissue disease during adolescence.

Figure 547

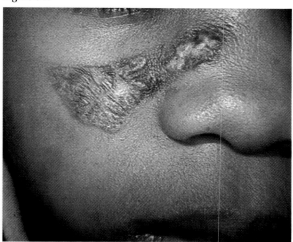

Figure 548

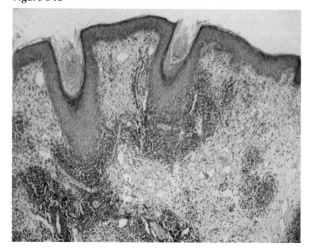

Discoid lupus erythematosus   Illustrated here is the characteristic plaque of a discoid lesion of lupus erythematosus. There is a violaceous hue at the border and central atrophy with scarring. Similar involvement in the scalp can cause permanent alopecia. Discoid lesions may be a cutaneous manifestation of systemic lupus erythematosus or the sole physical finding in a disease that does not go on to affect any other organ system. Treatment consists of avoidance of the sun or the use of sunscreens, antimalarial agents, and topical or intralesional corticosteroids.

Histopathology of lupus erythematosus   The diagnosis of discoid lupus erythematosus is based on clinical and histologic morphology. The histologic features are keratotic follicular plugs, vascular dilatation beneath the epidermis, damage to the dermoepidermal interface, patchy collections of lymphocytes, and loss of pilosebaceous units.

Figure 549

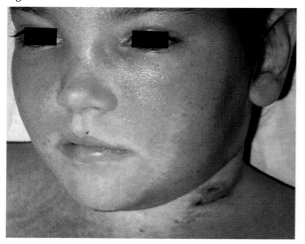

Figure 550

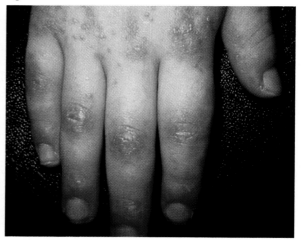

Dermatomyositis   This collagen vascular disease is characterized by a combination of symmetrical proximal upper and lower extremity muscle weakness and cutaneous disease. Early symptoms of muscle involvement include general malaise, difficulty in playing or climbing stairs, myalgias, and muscle tenderness. These illustrations are highly characteristic of the cutaneous part of the syndrome. Figure 549 shows symmetrical, intense erythema and edema of the face. The violaceous color of the periorbital rash is sometimes described as heliotrope in hue; the edema is so intense that it makes the face look puffy.

Erythematous and edematous papules and plaques may also be present on the dorsum of the hand (Fig. 550) and on the elbows and knees. The lesions that occur over the distal interphalangeal joints are referred to as Gottron's papules. An additional cutaneous finding, which is particularly characteristic of childhood dermatomyositis, is calcinosis cutis. This may present as firm, superficial nodules or plaques or as painful deposits of calcium in muscle or fascia. A psoriasiform dermatitis of the scalp may also occur.

Figure 551

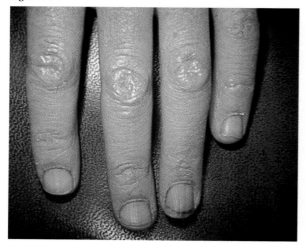

Figure 552

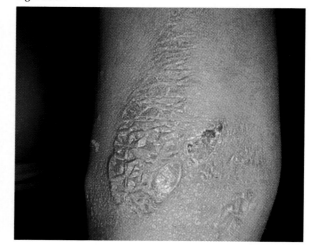

Dermatomyositis   These illustrations show more of the cutaneous manifestations of dermatomyositis. Figure 551 again shows the classic Gottron's papules, and in Fig. 552 there is a nearly identical process on and around the elbow. In both these pictures, the cutaneous disease has advanced to wrinkling and atrophy. The diagnosis of dermatomyositis is usually made on the basis of elevated muscle enzymes (especially creatinine

phosphokinase and aldolase), electromyography, and muscle biopsy. Skin biopsy tends not to be helpful in differentiating dermatomyositis from other collagen vascular disease. Early therapy with systemic corticosteroids is vital in the treatment of both muscular and cutaneous disease and in the prevention of calcinosis. In contrast to the adult form of the disease, childhood dermatomyositis is not associated with malignancy.

Figure 553

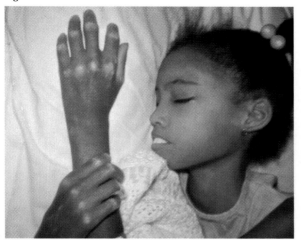

Figure 554

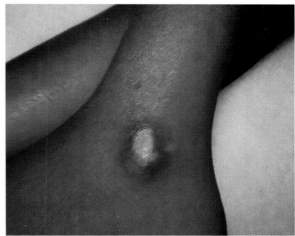

Scleroderma (progressive systemic sclerosis) This is a multisystem connective tissue disease that is relatively rare in childhood. Patients may suffer from arthritis and muscle weakness and from the results of pulmonary, esophageal, cardiac, and renal involvement. The condition of the skin on the face and hands is shown in Fig. 553. The induration and hidebound quality are hard to capture in photography, but they can be imagined from the fixed expression in the face, from the exposure of the teeth by the indurated lips, and, on the hands, from the pallor of the knuckles and seeming inflexibility of the fingers. The chest may appear hidebound from the outline of the ribs and its general shape. Figure 554 shows scleroderma on a leg and a foot, the latter also scarred from ulceration. Again, photography cannot bring out the hardness of the skin as palpation can.

Figure 555

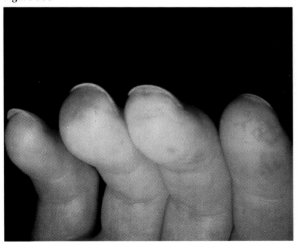

Figure 556

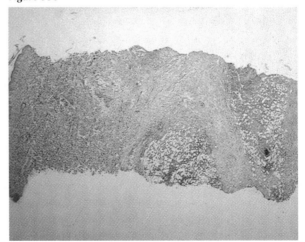

Scleroderma (progressive systemic sclerosis) This photograph of fingertips shows the pallor of Raynaud's phenomenon and telangiectasia. The patient also has scleroderma of the hands, forearms, and face. If calcinosis cutis were present or supervened, this type of case would be designated as the CRST syndrome, that is, marked by calcinosis, Raynaud's phenomenon, sclerodactyly, and telangiectasia. Such a combination is the most severe of the cutaneous possibilities of progressive systemic sclerosis.

Histopathology of scleroderma The biopsy specimen, oriented here with the surface to the left, shows nothing abnormal in the epidermis or dermis. The essential changes are in the subcutis on the right and consist of increased cellularity and replacement of fat cells by newly formed abnormal connective tissue. Fibrosis and sclerosis of the underlying fascia may also be present.

Figure 557

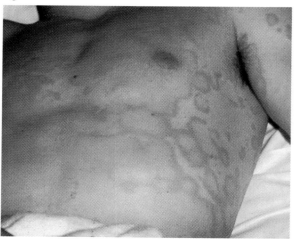

Figure 558

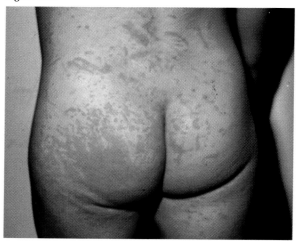

Cutaneous expressions of rheumatic fever and rheumatoid arthritis *Erythema marginatum* is a specific cutaneous expression of rheumatic fever. An unusually good representation of erythema marginatum at a static moment is shown in Fig. 557. As the term indicates, the condition is redness in the form of margination. What is not told is that the red margination is around normal-appearing skin and that it is transient and re-

current over days and weeks and may precede cardiac or joint symptoms or signs. Rheumatoid arthritis sometimes has a cutaneous expression that is of the nature of urticarial dermographism or edematous erythema provoked by scratching, especially during a febrile period of the illness. Figure 558 provides an illustration of this, showing persistent and transient stripes of erythema and edema on the back and buttocks.

Figure 559

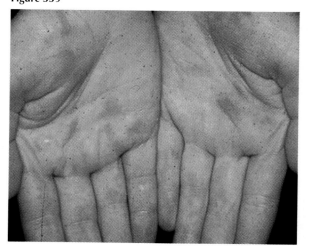

Figure 560

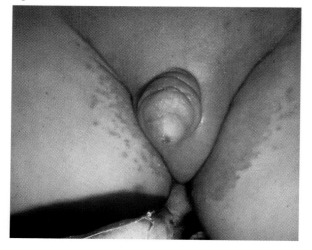

Cutaneous expressions of polyarteritis nodosa This multisystem disease is a form of necrotizing vasculitis that affects small and medium-sized arteries. Frequent areas of systemic involvement are the gastrointestinal tract and kidneys. Palpable purpuras are the most common cutaneous manifestation of this disease. In addition, there may be necrotic ulcers and distal gangrene. Tender cutaneous nodules are occasionally seen, but these are more characteristic of benign cutaneous periarteritis nodosa, which has no systemic manifestations.

Cutaneous expressions of chronic granulomatous disease This X-linked recessive inherited disorder is characterized by recurrent granulomatous infections of multiple organ systems. The underlying defect is in the neutrophils' inability to produce hydrogen peroxide and to kill bacteria; this abnormality can be verified by the nitroblue tetrazolium slide test. Pneumonia, meningitis, and septicemia are among the most serious complications of this disease. An intertriginous eczematous eruption and granulomatous nodules and plaques are among the cutaneous manifestations.

Figure 561

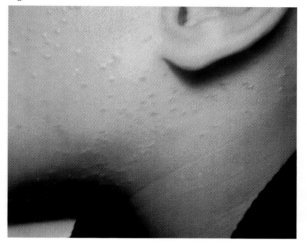

Figure 562

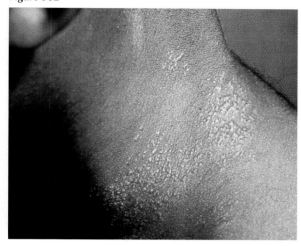

Sarcoidosis This is a disease of unknown etiology that is characterized by the formation of noncaseating granulomas in many different organ systems. Sarcoidosis is more common among African-Americans. It is unusual in children, but it does occur. During childhood, the most common presenting signs and symptoms are lymphadenopathy, uveitis, and cutaneous disease. In very young children, arthritis, eye disease, and skin disease

tend to predominate. Children with sarcoidosis may also have weight loss, fever, and respiratory involvement. Disorders of calcium metabolism are evidenced by hypercalcemia and hypercalcuria. These photographs illustrate the erythematous and flesh-colored papules that may be the sole cutaneous manifestation of sarcoidosis. Systemic steroids remain the treatment of choice in this disease.

Figure 563

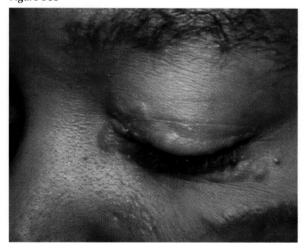

Figure 564

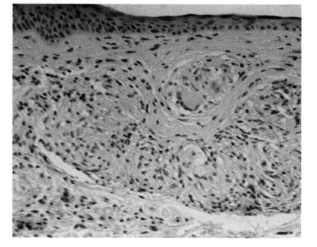

Sarcoidosis Here illustrated are highly characteristic papules of sarcoidosis on and around the eyelids. Similar lesions are common around the nose and mouth. Sarcoidosis such as this may be cutaneous only, or, more likely, may involve other organs. Investigation for systemic disease should include x-rays of the lungs and pulmonary function tests. The eyes should be examined for uveitis and lacrimal gland enlargement.

Histopathology of sarcoidosis Sarcoidosis, whatever may be its single or multitudinous causes, shows a consistently uniform histologic picture. That picture in skin or any other organ is a "naked" tubercle consisting of epithelioid and giant cells with few or no lymphocytes and no necrosis. These collections or granulomas in the skin may be small or large, discrete or confluent, and situated superficially or deeply in the dermis. In this photomicrograph, the so-called naked tubercles are seen superficially placed.

Figure 565

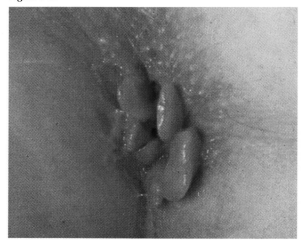

Figure 566

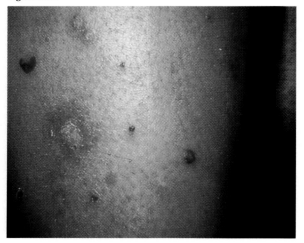

Cutaneous manifestations of Crohn's disease   This chronic inflammatory bowel disease has several cutaneous manifestations. Most common are perianal fissures, fistulas, and granulomatous nodules. The exophytic lesions pictured here could easily be confused with condylomata acuminata. Metastatic Crohn's disease may present with ulcerations in intertriginous folds. Children with Crohn's disease may also suffer from erythema nodosum and aphthous ulcers.

Cutaneous manifestations of thalassemia major   The homozygous form of thalassemia (thalassemia major, Cooley's anemia) presents with a severe hemolytic anemia during infancy or early childhood. Affected children are usually small for their age and have distinctive frontal bossing, along with jaundice and hepatosplenomegaly. Illustrated here are the chronic leg ulcers that are fairly common in this hematologic disorder.

Figure 567

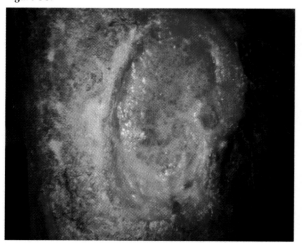

Figure 568

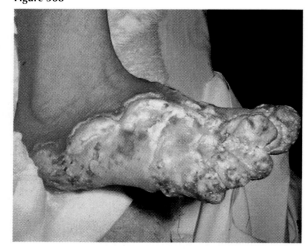

Cutaneous manifestations of sickle cell anemia   Leg ulcers, commonly around the malleoli, are a frequent manifestation of sickle cell anemia. In size, shape, and appearance they are very similar to stasis ulcers. The occurrence of leg ulcers in sickle cell anemia is attributed to sludging of the sickled cells, local ischemia, and stasis. Treatment consists of bed rest, occlusive or semi-occlusive dressings, and the use of topical and oral antibiotics when superinfection is present. Oral zinc therapy may be of value.

Pyoderma gangrenosum   This form of gradually enlarging necrotic ulceration usually involves the distal lower extremity. Typical characteristics include a purulent base and a purplish undermined border. Etiologies include inflammatory bowel disease, chronic active hepatitis, and Behçet's syndrome. Arthritis may be an associated finding. Treatment consists of bed rest, local care, and the injection of intralesional steroids along the border of the lesion. Dapsone, sulfapyridine, and oral corticosteroids are additional therapies.

Figure 569

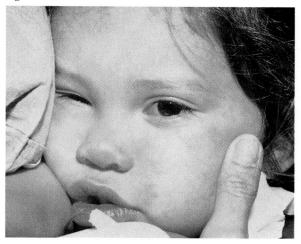

Figure 570

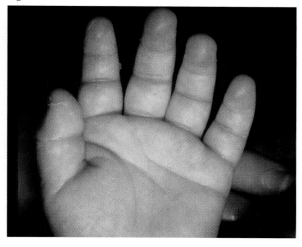

Kawasaki's disease   This childhood disease of unknown etiology is officially diagnosed by the presence of high fever lasting 5 or more days, and four of the following criteria: con-
junctival injection (Fig. 569), mucous membrane changes,
erythema or edema of the palms and soles (Fig. 570), rash (Fig.

571), and cervical lymphadenopathy. A common cutaneous
finding during the second week of the illness is desquamation
of the palms and soles and, very frequently, of the perineum
(Fig. 572). Systemic aspects of Kawasaki's disease include
arthritis, aseptic meningitis, and hydrops of the gallbladder.

Figure 571

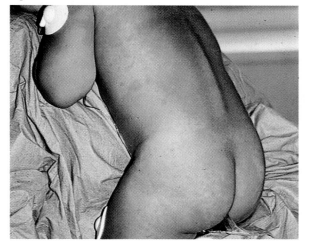

Figure 572

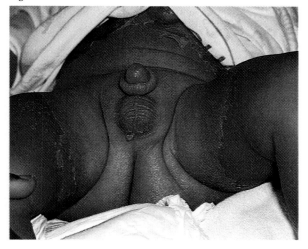

Kawasaki's disease   Coronary artery aneurysms develop in 20
percent of patients who are not treated, and some children go
on to develop myocardial infarction. Current therapy, consisting of aspirin and intravenous gamma globulin, seems to reduce
the incidence of cardiac disease. Children who do not meet the

strict diagnostic criteria for Kawasaki's disease should be treated
as if they did, if there is a strong clinical suspicion. All children
with Kawasaki's disease should be followed with serial two-
dimensional echocardiography.

Figure 573

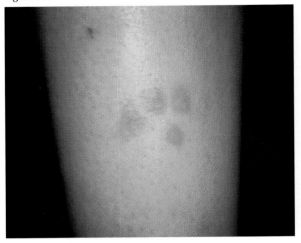

Figure 574

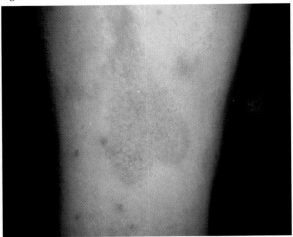

Necrobiosis lipoidica   This condition has some resemblance to granuloma annulare, more histopathological than clinical, but the two conditions are far from being the same. For one thing, the lesions of necrobiosis lipoidica are generally much larger than those of granuloma annulare. (The lesions in Fig. 573 are exceptional, probably because the disease is in early development; Fig. 574 is more typical for size.) The border is not ringed with papules, and the center, unlike that in granuloma annulare, is eventually atrophied or scarred. Ulceration may occur. Necrobiosis lipoidica does not abate spontaneously or with reasonable treatment to the point of *restitutio ad integrum* as granuloma annulare does. The condition is common in diabetes mellitus, in which case it is distinguished by addition of the term *diabeticorum*. Occasionally it is seen in patients who themselves do not have diabetes, but often those patients have familial histories of consanguineous relatives with diabetes mellitus.

Figure 575

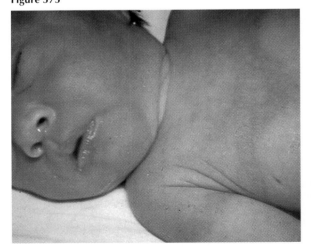

Figure 576

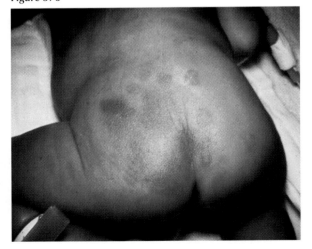

Cutaneous effects of *Pseudomonas* sepsis   Sepsis caused by *Pseudomonas aeruginosa* occurs most commonly in the child with an underlying illness. It is seen in children with immune deficiency due to cancer chemotherapy, in those with malnutrition, and in those with extensive burns. Some of the less specific cutaneous manifestations, specifically erythematous macules and petechiae, are pictured in Figs. 575 and 576. *Pseudomonas* sepsis may also present with discrete small nodules and bullae. The classic skin lesion of *Pseudomonas* sepsis is termed *ecthyma gangrenosum*. This form characteristically progresses quickly from a well-circumscribed area of edema, to a centrally located blister, to a gangrenous ulcer with a gray eschar. Multiple lesions in different stages of evolution may be present, and the lesions may appear on any body surface. Gram's stain and culture of tissue scraped from the base of a blister will be positive for *Pseudomonas*.

Figure 577

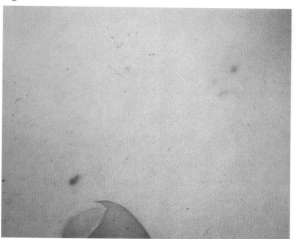

Figure 578

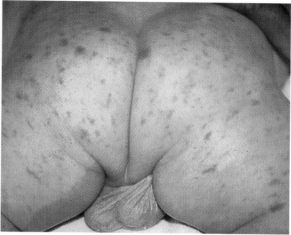

Cutaneous effects of meningococcemia The early treatment of meningococcemia with appropriate parenteral antibiotics can often be lifesaving. Cutaneous manifestations of this disease may provide the single most important diagnostic clue in the acutely ill child. The most common findings on the skin are petechiae and purpuras. The small petechial lesion pictured in Fig. 577 develops early in the course of the disease, and a scraping yields gram-negative diplococci on both Gram's stain and culture. Subsequently, the lesions arise in additional crops,

enlarge, and coalesce. The numerous ecchymoses pictured in Fig. 578 are the result of this rapidly ongoing process. These areas may become necrotic and develop eschars. Other cutaneous manifestations, occurring subsequently, include peripheral gangrene and purpura fulminans, with confluent areas of necrosis of the skin. These are the result of vasospasm, shock, and a consumption coagulopathy. A deficiency in protein C may play a particular role in this process.

Figure 579

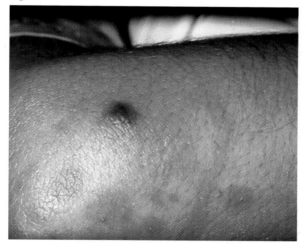

Figure 580

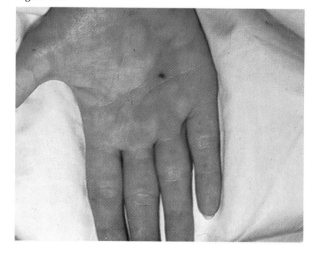

Cutaneous effects of gonococcemia Infection with *Neisseria gonorrhoeae* may manifest as a purulent conjunctivitis in the newborn or as a genital discharge in the sexually abused child or sexually active adolescent. Disseminated gonococcal infection, as illustrated here, is quite rare. Gonococcemia presents with a migratory polyarthralgia or septic arthritis and fever. The skin lesions are few, are often located on extremities,

and may overlie the involved joints. Initially, there are small erythematous macules that progress to papules. These tender lesions may develop a small vesicle and then a gray, umbilicated center. Rarely, bullae, petechiae, and larger hemorrhagic lesions are also seen. The two photographs show the macules and necrotic papules that are typical of disseminated gonococcal infection.

Figure 581

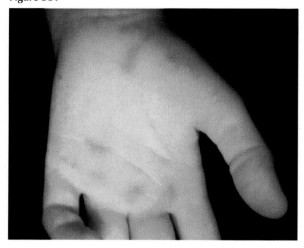

Cutaneous effects of endocarditis (Janeway lesions) Mucocutaneous lesions are common in subacute bacterial endocarditis. The erythematous and hemorrhagic macules shown here are termed *Janeway lesions.* They may occur on the distal finger pads, palms, or soles. Other manifestations of this disease include petechiae on the oral mucosa and skin and splinter hemorrhage under the nails. Large, painful nodules or areas of gangrene involving the fingers or toes are signs of embolus formation.

Figure 582

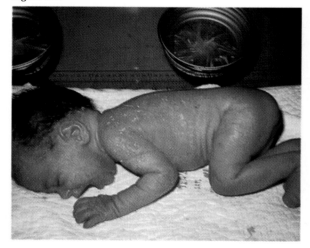

Figure 583

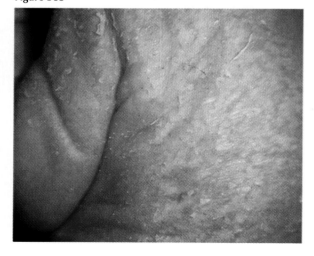

Erythroderma with immunodeficiency The infant pictured here has a severe generalized erythroderma with diffuse scaling. In the past, the term "Leiner's disease" was used to describe children with severe and widespread seborrheic dermatitis–like eruptions, diarrhea, failure to thrive, and recurrent infections. The clinical presentation, which includes erythroderma, diarrhea, and growth failure, may result from a variety of immunologic abnormalities. A complete workup is mandatory in patients with this constellation of symptoms.

16

Cutaneous Manifestations of HIV Infection

Figure 584

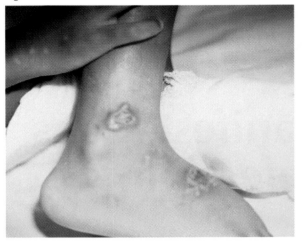

Cutaneous manifestations of HIV infection (chronic vari-cella zoster infection)   This figure illustrates a form of infection with varicella zoster virus that is unique to patients with immune suppression from HIV. The 6-year-old child pictured here developed recurrent vesicular and ulcerative lesions of the trunk and extremities following an episode of chickenpox. The lesions contain numerous multinucleated giant cells and are culture-positive for varicella zoster virus. This form of infection responds to treatment with intravenous acyclovir but tends to recur when therapy is discontinued.

Figure 585

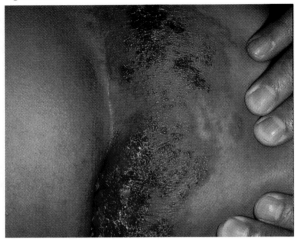

Cutaneous manifestations of HIV infection (herpes zoster infection)   In addition to chronic infections with varicella zoster, many patients develop unusual forms of herpes zoster infection. These patients also develop prolonged episodes of shingles that do not respond quickly to appropriate antiviral agents; they may also develop generalized herpes zoster infections. In addition, these patients are at risk for the development of herpes simplex infections that are resistant to the more commonly used antiviral agents.

Figure 586

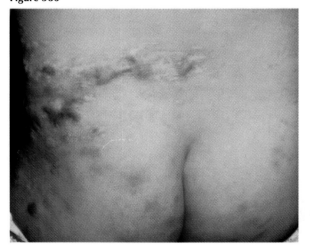

Cutaneous manifestations of HIV infection (scarring from herpes zoster)   This 3-year-old girl developed herpes zoster as an early manifestation of her immune deficiency. Despite therapy with intravenous acyclovir, severe scarring resulted. Herpes zoster occurs more frequently in children who have had chickenpox very early in life. Although herpes zoster is certainly seen in the healthy child, its occurrence in a child who is at risk for HIV infection should signal concern.

Figure 587

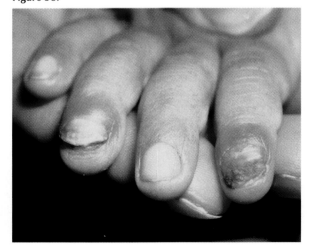

Cutaneous manifestations of HIV infection (candidal paronychias and nail dystrophy)   Candidiasis is the most common mucocutaneous manifestation of pediatric HIV infection. Children with AIDS or lesser forms of HIV-related disease frequently develop oral thrush, which recurs or persists despite topical antifungal therapy. Recalcitrant infections of the diaper area and neck folds are also common. Illustrated here are chronic paronychias with a resultant nail dystrophy.

Figure 588

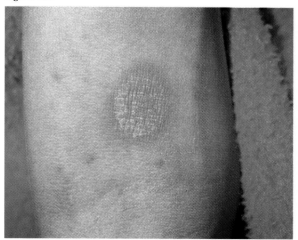

Cutaneous manifestations of HIV infection (drug eruption)
Drug eruptions, usually due to therapy with trimethoprim-sulfa-methoxazole, are particularly common among children with HIV infection. This young girl developed a rash subsequent to treatment with that drug combination for *Pneumocystis carinii* pneumonia. Biopsy analysis of the skin lesion illustrated here revealed an interface dermatitis. A generalized blanchable erythema and true Stevens-Johnson syndrome may also be seen. The frequency of drug eruptions in children with AIDS illustrates the complex effect of HIV on the immune system.

Figure 589

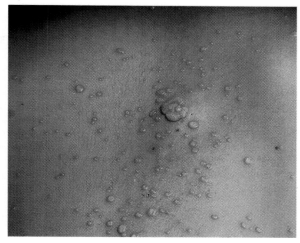

Cutaneous manifestations of HIV infection (molluscum contagiosum) Children in general are more prone to infection with the virus causing molluscum contagiosum. Children infected with the human immunodeficiency virus are more likely to develop persistent, widespread eruptions due to molluscum contagiosum.

Figure 590

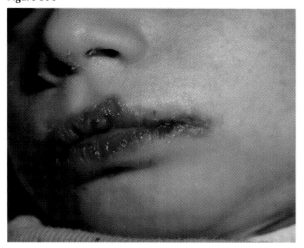

Cutaneous manifestations of HIV infection (chronic herpetic gingivostomatitis) Children with AIDS frequently suffer from persistent herpetic infections of the mucous membranes or skin. The gingivostomatitis shown here would be typical of primary infection in a healthy child. One would then expect recurrences to be considerably milder. By contrast, the child with HIV infection may have recurrent episodes of gingivostomatitis or may develop infection that does not respond at all to acyclovir.

Figure 591

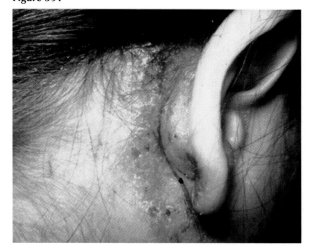

Cutaneous manifestations of HIV infection (seborrheic dermatitis) Seborrheic dermatitis occurs with particular severity in individuals who are infected with HIV. The infantile form consists of severe scaling and erythema of the scalp and flexural areas, and sometimes of the entire skin surface. The latter resembles the clinical appearance of the child with Leiner's disease. Illustrated here is an older child with recalcitrant inflammation in the skin folds behind the ears. She also had severe crusting and scaling of the entire scalp.

Figure 592

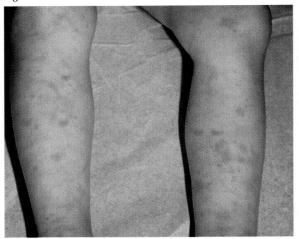

Cutaneous manifestations of HIV infection (leukocyto-clastic vasculitis)   Occasionally, chronic leukocytoclastic vasculitis occurs in children who are infected with HIV. It is not certain whether this is the direct result of this virus or of some other, concurrent infection. The palpable purpuras seen here on the lower extremities are indistinguishable from those observed in Henoch-Schönlein purpura. The chronicity of this patient's eruption, however, was atypical, and pointed to the possibility of HIV-related disease.

Figure 593

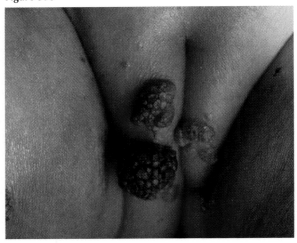

Cutaneous manifestations of HIV infection (condylomata acuminata)   Children who are infected with the human immunodeficiency virus are prone to a wide variety of viral infections. Lesions caused by human papillomavirus may be unusually widespread and persistent. A case of condylomata acuminata in a 1-year-old girl is illustrated here. Extensive flat warts or periungual warts may also be seen.

17

Disorders of the Dermis (Infiltrates, Atrophies, and Nodules)

Figure 594

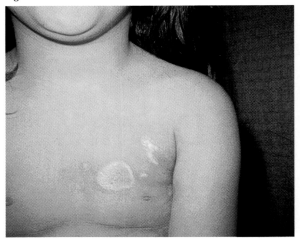

Morphea There are conditions that take the title scleroderma but are not related to progressive systemic sclerosis. They are marked by areas of hardened skin, small or large, scattered or localized, single or multiple, and of variable shape. Here illustrated is morphea in the form of several discrete lesions of different shapes, all confined to the skin on the left side of the chest. The lesions are firm and atrophic.

Figure 595

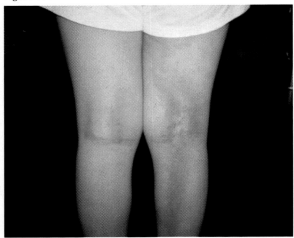

Morphea (linear, en bande) Illustrated is a type of morphea that is linear in shape and situated on the flexor aspect of a leg, extending from the medial aspect of the thigh through the popliteal space to near the Achilles tendon. Again the affected skin is hard, slightly depressed, and dyschromic. Extensive areas of linear morphea are the most difficult to treat. There is a tendency toward permanent deformity, in the form of atrophy or contractures.

Figure 596

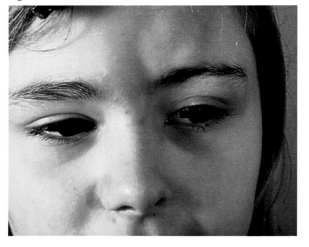

Morphea (en coup de sabre) Here is another kind of hardened skin in the form of a depression, as though the result of a blow from a blunt instrument or a weapon like a saber. Location on one side of the brow is highly characteristic. Such lesions are seen with no other associated anomaly or as part of hemiatrophies. Atrophy or absence of subcutaneous fat is also part of such a process.

Figure 597

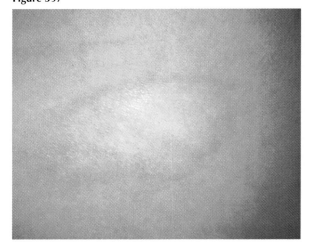

Morphea This kind of morphea is highly characteristic. The solitary or individual lesion of the condition is a circle or oval of firm skin that is whitish, slightly depressed, and surrounded by a different color that is lilac or purple. There may be only one such lesion of moderate size or many of about the same size or very large ones covering large areas of skin. The course of the condition is variable too. Spontaneous recovery in children is common.

Figure 598

Figure 599

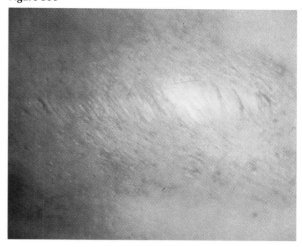

Morphea　Illustrated here is a lesion of morphea resolving. From an appearance like that in Fig. 597, the lesion has become reddish, has risen to the level of the surrounding skin, and will eventually leave nearly completely or with minor dyschromia. The cause of circumscribed scleroderma of any form is unknown.

Atrophoderma (Pasini-Pierini)　This condition is most common in adolescent girls, and its etiology is completely unknown. Characteristically, there develop single or multiple well-circumscribed, slightly hyperpigmented areas of cutaneous atrophy, with a sharp "cliff-drop" border. The lesions tend to enlarge slowly, and then persist. Some believe that this form of atrophoderma represents a variant of morphea, in which atrophy is more evident than is sclerosis.

Figure 600

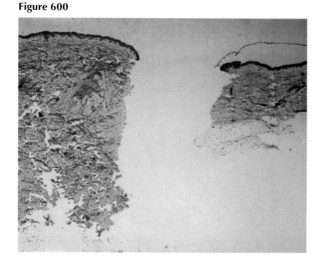

Figure 601

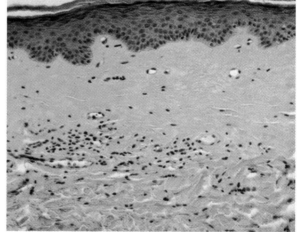

Histopathology of atrophoderma (Pasini-Pierini)　Atrophy of the skin may involve epidermis, its appendages, dermal collagen and elastic tissue, adipose tissue, or combinations thereof. In atrophoderma of Pasini and Pierini, the atrophic process is limited strictly to the dermal collagen. The two specimens shown here represent markedly atrophic skin on the right and comparable uninvolved skin from the same patient on the left.

Histopathology of lichen sclerosus et atrophicus　The most constant histologic feature of this condition, well illustrated here, is a zone directly beneath the epithelium that is sparse of cells, pale, and almost "sclerotic." Separating this abnormal zone from the deeper, uninvolved corium is a horizontal patchy band of mononuclear inflammatory cells. The epithelium may show hyperkeratosis, atrophy, and liquefaction degeneration of the stratum malpighii, features that do not appear in this photomicrograph.

Figure 602

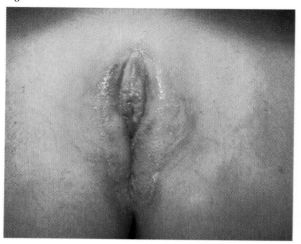

Figure 603

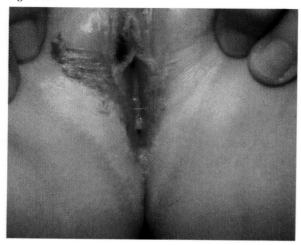

Lichen sclerosus et atrophicus   These two figures illustrate lichen sclerosus et atrophicus in its most typical location. This cutaneous disorder is more common in girls and is usually confined to the skin surrounding the anogenital region. The onset of the disease may be accompanied by pruritus, burning, or vaginal discharge, or it may be completely asymptomatic. Porcelain-colored or slightly erythematous macules gradually co-alesce to form plaques. The end result is an area of induration and shiny atrophy in an hourglass shape around the rectum and vagina. Childhood lichen sclerosus et atrophicus tends to be a self-limited disease, with improvement occurring at the time of puberty. The use of topical corticosteroids provides some symptomatic relief and may hasten the resolution of the process.

Figure 604

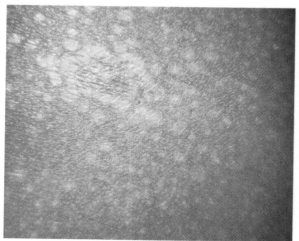

Figure 605

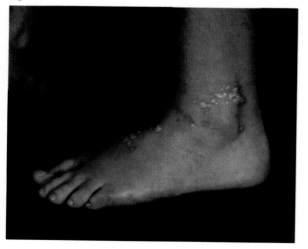

Lichen sclerosus et atrophicus   In Fig. 604, discrete and confluent ivory-colored macules are shown on an area of skin that might be of the trunk, arms, or thighs. Extragenital lesions tend to be asymptomatic. Figure 605 illustrates lichen sclerosus et atrophicus involving the ankle, which is not an unusual location. Another common site is the male genitalia, especially the foreskin and glans penis. The result may be a nonretractable foreskin, or stenosis of the urethral meatus. It appears that lichen sclerosus et atrophicus may be a common cause of phimosis in young boys.

Figure 606

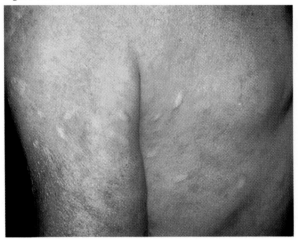

Figure 607

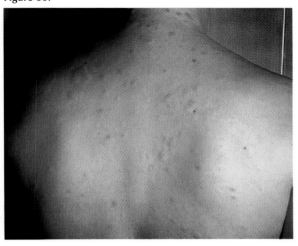

Anetoderma (macular atrophy) The term *anetoderma,* meaning slack skin, is most often used to describe a form of cutaneous atrophy that has no clear preceding cause. Anetoderma is divided into two clinical types. The Jadassohn form of anetoderma, most common among girls, is characterized by the eruption of round, slightly erythematous macules over large ar-

eas of the trunk and proximal extremities. The lesions quickly evolve into small areas of atrophy, each with an outpouching of shiny white skin (Fig. 606). The second form of anetoderma bears the eponym Schweninger-Buzzi. This form, illustrated in Fig. 607, is distinguished by the slow evolution of lesions that arise without any preceding inflammation.

Figure 608

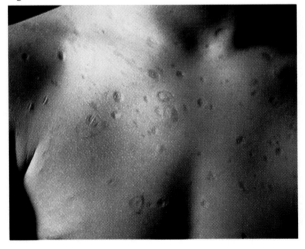

Figure 609

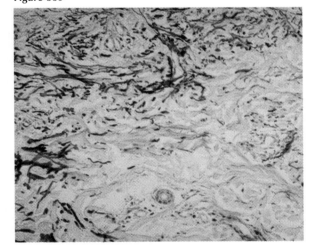

Anetoderma (macular atrophy) Here is another illustration of idiopathic macular atrophy. In this patient the lesions arose with no evidence of prior inflammation. Occasionally, skin changes that are similar to the primary anetodermas can be seen as a sequela of sarcoidosis, granuloma annulare, Hansen's disease, secondary syphilis, or penicillamine therapy. In either situation, the biopsy analysis reveals the localized loss of elastic tissue.

Histopathology of anetoderma Anetoderma (macular atrophy), whether primary or secondary to some other dermatosis, shows a stereotypic histopathologic picture. The atrophy affects dermal elastica, and a special elastic tissue stain is required for its demonstration. The destruction of elastic tissue usually involves a spherical or ellipsoidal mass. In this photomicrograph, elastic tissue is absent in the right lower half of the field and is present adjacent to it.

Figure 610

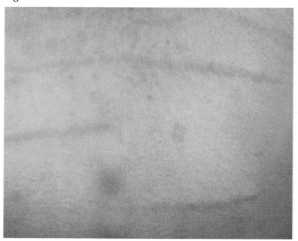

Figure 611

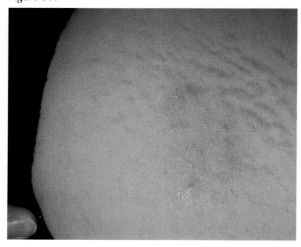

Striae distensae   Ruptures within the dermis in the lines of cleavage of the skin that are not associated with obvious external trauma are common in pregnancy and obesity. In pregnancy, mechanical stretching of the skin by the developing fetus and its housing and, in obesity, extreme storage of fat can be taken to be cause enough for dermal ruptures; but a factor of endocrinopathy or idiopathic response to hormone balance also seems to be operative. Athletes, particularly weight lifters, sometimes show striae distensae, and again, mechanical stretching and idiopathic hormonal influence may be adduced in explanation, since the phenomenon is not universal. In Fig. 610 one sees striae on a back that may well be of a weight lifter. Figure 611 shows striae and telangiectasia in a patient who is and has long been on topical corticosteroids for good reason. The hormonal influence in the latter case is indubitable.

Figure 612

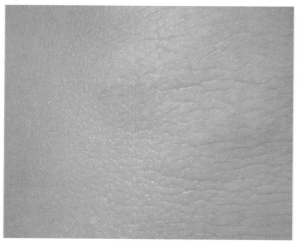

Figure 613

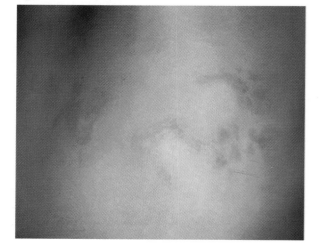

Connective tissue nevus   This group of hamartomas may be composed of the various elements of the extracellular connective tissue: collagen, elastic fibers, and glycosaminoglycans. One example of the collagen variety is the shagreen patch, a cutaneous manifestation of tuberous sclerosis. These yellow or orange plaques of coalescent papules are often seen in the lumbosacral area. Other varieties of connective tissue nevus are not associated with tuberous sclerosis. Particularly, collagenomas may be seen in solitary, eruptive, and multiple forms. The last of these is a familial disorder. Elastic fibers are found in isolated elastomas and in the small yellowish papules of the autosomal dominant Buschke-Ollendorf syndrome. The latter is also characterized by asymptomatic sclerotic densities of the bones.

Figure 614

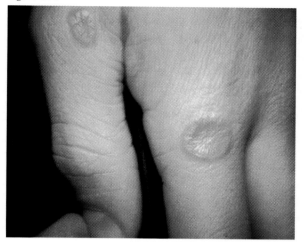

Figure 615

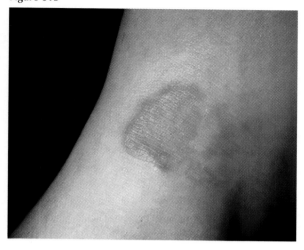

Granuloma annulare This benign condition is characterized by one or more circular plaques, consisting of rings of papules around a depressed center. Figure 614 is most typical; Fig. 615 is somewhat variant. The hands and feet are the commonest sites for the lesions of granuloma annulare. One or two lesions are the usual number. Occasionally, eruptive and widespread lesions are seen. For the most part, granuloma annulare is not associ-

ated with any other disease, nor is there any known cause. The condition is symptomless. It has been known to vanish spontaneously after a procedure such as a biopsy of part of it. Topical or intralesional corticosteroids are a standard therapy. Parent and child should be warned that the lesions may persist for months or years before response to therapy or spontaneous resolution. Lesions may also recur.

Figure 616

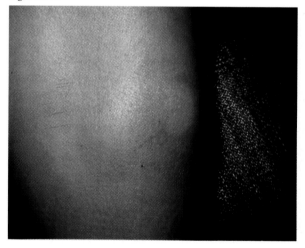

Figure 617

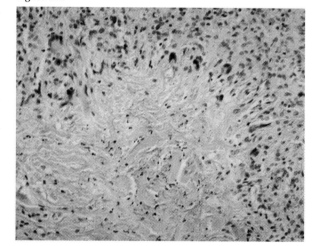

Subcutaneous granuloma annulare (pseudorheumatoid nodule) There is a form of granuloma annulare that presents with deep nodules. A more typical annular lesion may overlie the nodule or may be present at another anatomic site. These lesions are most frequently localized to the digits, scalp, dorsa of the feet, or anterior tibial region.

Histopathology of granuloma annulare Granuloma annulare is a granuloma of a group that includes necrobiosis lipoidica and the nodule of rheumatoid arthritis and rheumatic fever. All have similar histopathologic pictures that cannot always be distinguished from one another without clinical correlation. Here, in a typical example of granuloma annulare, one sees a central zone sparse of cells, surrounded by mononuclear and multinucleated cells in palisade pattern.

Figure 618

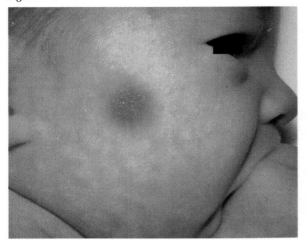

Figure 619

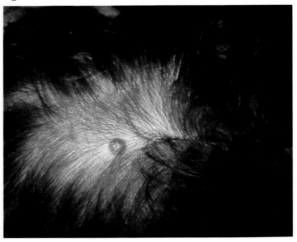

Juvenile xanthogranuloma This is a common and completely benign cutaneous nodule. Typically, a juvenile xanthogranuloma is firm and dome-shaped. The lesion is reddish at first, as in Fig. 618, but develops a fairly typical orange-brown hue over time (Fig. 619). Most juvenile xanthogranulomas are located on the head or neck, as pictured in these two infants, but the lesions sometimes occur on the trunk or extremities. They may be present at birth, but most develop during the first year of life. Juvenile xanthogranuloma is not associated with abnormalities in serum cholesterol or triglycerides, and the individual lesions undergo spontaneous involution, usually over a period of 1 to 2 years. A diagnostic biopsy analysis is sometimes needed, but surgical intervention beyond this is certainly not required. A juvenile xanthogranuloma on the skin may be accompanied by intraocular lesions. For this reason, the physician must pay careful attention to the examination of the eyes. An abnormality in the color of the iris or an enlargement of the globe should trigger a prompt ophthalmologic referral.

Figure 620

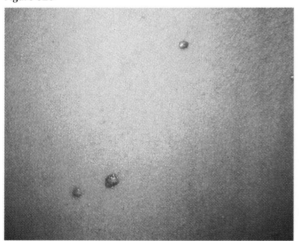

Figure 621

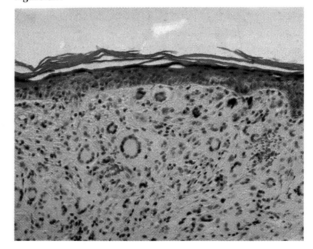

Juvenile xanthogranuloma This photograph shows four lesions. It is somewhat more common to see multiple juvenile xanthogranulomas than a solitary lesion. Rarely, they may number in the hundreds. As mentioned, xanthogranuloma of the eye is the most common complication of this generally benign and self-limited condition. Multiple small juvenile xanthogranulomas seem to be slightly more common in children with neurofibromatosis, and these patients have an additional tendency toward juvenile chronic myelocytic leukemia.

Histopathology of juvenile xanthogranuloma This lesion, also designated *nevoxanthoendothelioma,* is a benign, localized histiocytoma. Because lipid is often present in such lesions, they qualify histologically as xanthomas. In addition to mononuclear, lipid-filled histiocytes, one finds multinucleated giant cells of a distinctive type (Touton) that have a ring of nuclei set in cytoplasm that is foamy at the periphery only. Touton giant cells are almost never seen in the xanthomas of systemic dyslipidoses.

Figure 622

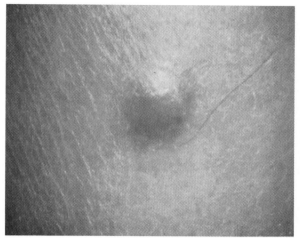

Figure 623

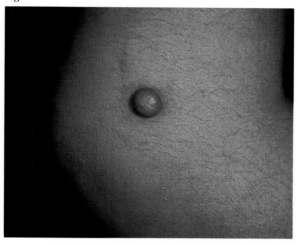

Dermatofibroma   These are benign dermal nodules that represent a focal proliferation of fibroblasts; the overlying epidermis is slightly thickened. Their occurrence is not unusual in children and adolescents. Dermatofibromas are firm and may be black, red, brown, or flesh-colored. Their diameter generally ranges from 0.5 to l.5 cm, although they may occasionally be larger. Dermatofibromas may be solitary or multiple, and they develop either spontaneously or after minor trauma to the skin, such as an insect bite. Most are asymptomatic. A very useful diagnostic maneuver is executed by exerting lateral pressure on the lesion. The skin overlying a dermatofibroma will frequently dimple. Dermatofibromas require surgical treatment only when they are of cosmetic concern to the patient. However, biopsy analysis is occasionally required in order to confirm the diagnosis and to differentiate it from more serious disorders.

Figure 624

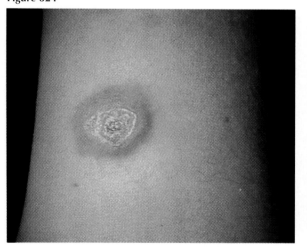

Figure 625

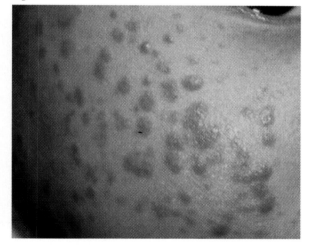

Granular cell tumor   These are unusual nodular lesions that vary from 0.5 to 3.0 cm in diameter. They may be single or multiple and are firm, elevated, and circumscribed. The tongue is a common site. The lesion pictured here is fairly typical of the cutaneous variety. The original name *granular cell myoblastoma* derived from an early theory that these tumors arise from immature striated muscle cells. In fact, Schwann cells are a more likely origin. The condition is benign and lends itself to any form of extirpation.

Benign cephalic histiocytosis   This very distinctive eruption consists of numerous brownish-yellow macules and papules involving the head and neck. The mucous membranes are spared. Benign cephalic histiocytosis usually begins during the first 3 years of life, and the lesions continue to evolve for several years. The condition then resolves spontaneously during childhood but may leave small atrophic or pigmented scars. These children do not develop systemic disease and are not at risk for histiocytosis X. Electron microscopy of the histiocytic infiltrate reveals comma-shaped bodies in the cytoplasm.

Figure 626

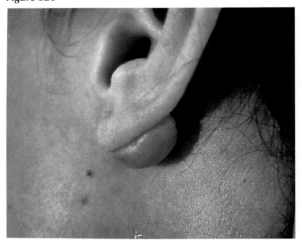

Figure 627

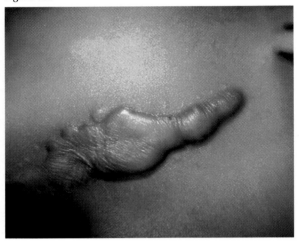

Keloids   The lesions pictured here are typical of the disfiguring changes that sometimes occur after trauma to the skin. In children, a laceration, a surgical procedure, or a bout of chicken pox may be the inciting event for keloid formation. Figure 626 shows a keloid that was caused by ear-piercing. Keloid formation is more common in African-American children, is very rare in infants, and becomes somewhat more frequent with increasing age. Keloids begin as firm, telangiectatic plaques confined to the site of the initial wound. Over time, they become less erythematous and extend beyond the site of injury. Pruritus,

burning, and hyperesthesia are frequent complaints. In contrast to hypertrophic scars, keloids do not resolve spontaneously. In fact, they may continue to grow over a period of years. The monthly intralesional injection of corticosteroids is currently the preferred treatment for most keloids. This modality is most successful in the newly forming keloid, which is softer and smaller than the well-established one. Surgical excision will almost always result in recurrence but is somewhat more successful when accompanied by the injection of corticosteroids.

Figure 628

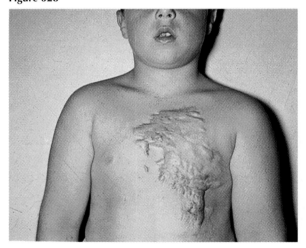

Figure 629

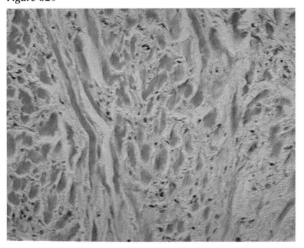

Keloids   The keloid pictured here is a common variety that develops after a thermal burn. The irregular contour and crab-like projections are characteristic and illustrate the root of the word *keloid:* from the Greek word *chele,* meaning crab's claw. The size and thickness of lesions of this type make treatment difficult. The chest and back are also common sites for keloids of another cause, namely, inflammatory acne. In that situation, repeated injections of intralesional corticosteroids are often of cosmetic benefit.

Histopathology of keloids   In many instances it is impossible clinically to distinguish a keloid from a hypertrophic scar. Histologically, however, distinction can almost always be made. Both lesions show proliferation of fibroblasts and collagen, but in keloids one finds in addition broad bands of hyalinized collagen separated by pale-staining areas. This particular histopathologic pattern is not seen in hypertrophic scars. Keloids, unlike hypertrophic scars, persist indefinitely.

Figure 630

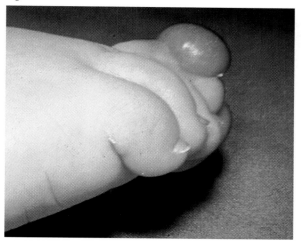

Figure 631

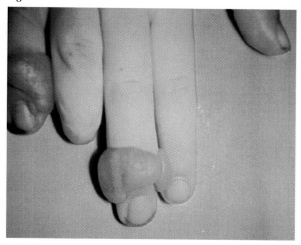

Digital fibrous tumor of childhood   This is a rare fibromatosis that starts in infants either as a single nodule or, less commonly, as several nodules. Parents may be alarmed by the rapid growth of the lesions. Digital fibrous tumors usually occur on the dorsal and sometimes the lateral aspects of the distal phalanges of fingers and toes. They may be globular, red, and smooth, as illustrated in Fig. 630, or reddish-brown and convoluted, especially when they wrap around digits, as illustrated in Fig. 631. Deformity of the adjacent nail plate may occur. The lesions are benign and have never been known to become malignant and metastasize. Recurrence is a common event after surgical excision, but many such tumors will involute without treatment over a period of several years. In most cases, the best treatment is simple observation.

Figure 632

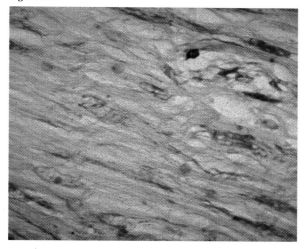

Histopathology of digital fibrous tumor of childhood   Fibromatoses are localized overgrowths of mature fibrocellular and collagenous connective tissue. Dupuytren's contracture, Peyronie's disease, and the desmoid tumor of the rectus sheath are examples. Such processes have the ability to invade contiguous structures. Infantile digital fibromatosis is unique in that the fibroblasts contain round intracytoplasmic bodies, here distinctively stained red, whose presence permits precise diagnosis.

Figure 633

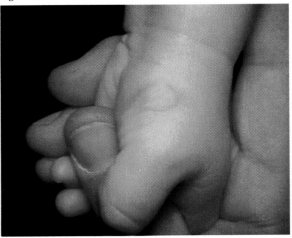

Figure 634

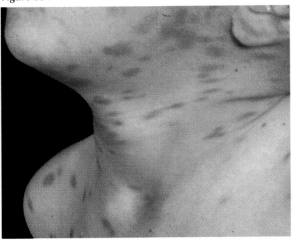

Mastocytosis   This is a set of disorders that are characterized by the accumulation of mast cells in the skin and sometimes in other organs. There is a wide clinical variety. The plaque shown in Fig. 633 represents a solitary mastocytoma, which occurs almost exclusively during infancy. This is most often a reddish-brown or orange nodule or plaque that is rubbery in consistency. There is occasionally a history of repeated blister formation on the surface. Figure 634 shows the numerous macules and papules of reddish or brownish hue that are typical of urticaria pigmentosa. This generalized form is the most common type of mastocytosis, and it also usually develops during early childhood. The whealing of lesions when they are rubbed (Darier's sign) is virtually pathognomonic for this disorder. Mechanical trauma is thought to degranulate mast cells and cause a local release of histamine. Dermographism in uninvolved skin is not uncommon.

Figure 635

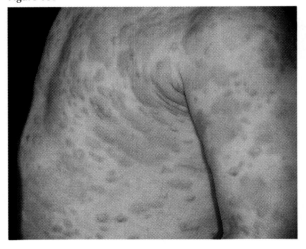

Figure 636

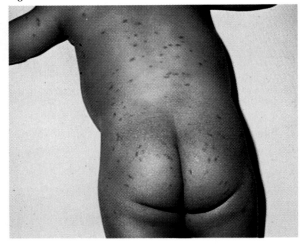

Mastocytosis   Figure 635 is another good representation of the typical lesions of the skin, this time involving papules in great abundance and of red-brown hue. Figure 636 shows the same process in an African-American infant who, incidentally, has a large mongolian spot on the lower part of the back above the buttocks. Patients who develop urticaria pigmentosa during early childhood tend to have only cutaneous involvement, and their disease will almost always involute over a period of years. No treatment is necessary, but it is important to provide the parents with a list of medications that might cause the sudden and potentially life-threatening release of histamine. These include aspirin, codeine, morphine, polymyxin B, aminoglycosides, and nonsteroidal anti-inflammatory drugs. Immersion in a very hot bath may have the same effect.

Figure 637

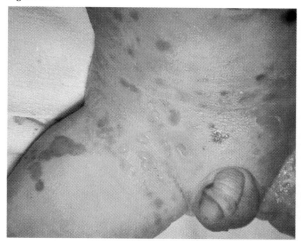

Figure 638

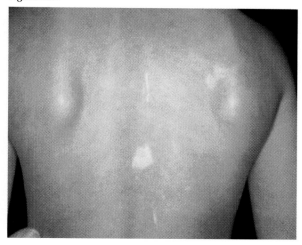

Mastocytosis Figure 637 illustrates the blister formation that may occur in infants with urticaria pigmentosa. Mast cells may sometimes be detected by staining the material from a scraped blister with Giemsa stain and examining it microscopically. Occasionally, a biopsy is necessary in order to differentiate bullous mastocytosis from other blistering diseases of infancy. Figure 638 is a photograph of the same patient in later life; he has gone on to develop diffuse infiltrative mastocytosis of the entire skin surface. The prognosis in this rare form of the disease,

and in individuals who first develop mastocytosis later in life, is not as good. Particularly common is involvement of the gastrointestinal and skeletal systems with the infiltrative process. Elevated urinary histamines or histamine metabolites are indicative of such widespread disease. Patients with this type of systemic mastocytosis are prone to attacks of pruritus, flushing, and hypotension. The massive release of mast cell products is sometimes fatal.

Figure 639

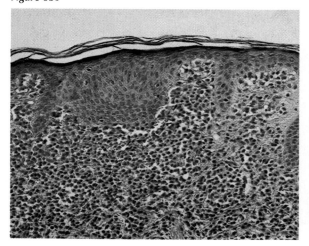

Figure 640

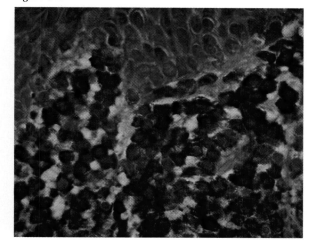

Histopathology of mastocytosis Mastocytosis most often involves the skin, producing the clinical picture known as urticaria pigmentosa. Histologic confirmation of the diagnosis depends on the demonstration of an excessive number of mast cells within the dermis. The biopsy specimen should not be taken from a lesion that has been rubbed, because rubbing causes degranulation of the cells. In the lesions of children with the condition, mast cells are generally present in large numbers,

but when they are only slightly increased in number, a special stain is necessary to establish the diagnosis with certainty. In Fig. 639, one sees sheets of uniform mononuclear cells beneath the epidermis that are suggestive of the diagnosis. By use of a metachromatic stain, which specifically colors the heparin-containing cytoplasmic granules a violet or reddish color and other structures blue (Fig. 640), the diagnosis is confirmable.

Figure 641

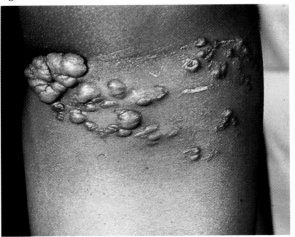

Figure 642

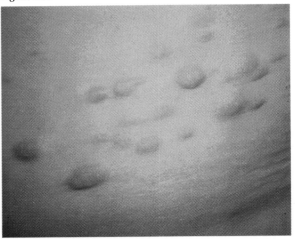

Nevus lipomatosus superficialis   Fat tissue is no more exempt from nevoid anomaly than is any other tissue. Here illustrated is a condition in which fat tissue is redundant and situated high in the dermis, well above its normal position in the hypoderm. The result is papillomatosis of yellowish hue and variable shape. There are no great consequences from the condition beyond the cosmetic, which may be remedied by plastic surgery in cases like the one pictured.

Leiomyoma   There are several neoplasms of the skin that are notably tender or painful. Leiomyoma is of this class. The intense pain associated with it takes the form of unprovoked paroxysms that reach a crescendo of torture before subsidence. The lesions are fleshy papules or nodules of no great morphologic distinctiveness. They have no malignant potential. Surgical ablation is curative and simple enough for solitary lesions but may be more complicated for numerous and widely spaced lesions such as those illustrated.

Figure 643

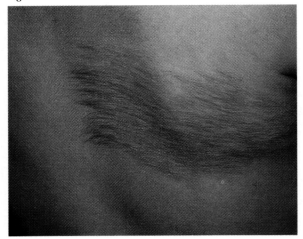

Smooth muscle and pilar hamartoma   This lesion typically presents as a solitary firm plaque, most often located on the trunk and proximal limbs and noted at birth or within the first few weeks of life. The lesions are flesh-colored to slightly erythematous initially but then tend to develop a light brown color. There is usually increased hair growth within the lesion. Histologically, the lesion is characterized by the presence of well-defined bundles of smooth muscle. Firm stroking may elicit fasciculations.

18

Drug Eruptions

Figure 644

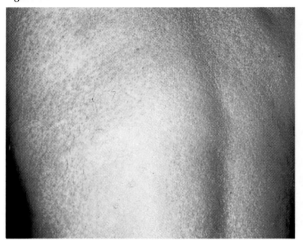

Figure 645

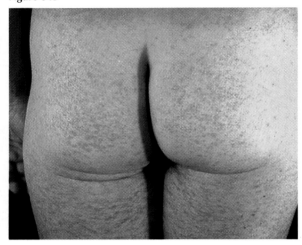

Drug eruptions (dermatitis medicamentosa) Diagnosing drug eruptions has become a common experience to practitioners in all branches of modern medicine. The profusion of drugs now available, the continuous influx of new drugs, and the capability of drugs to cause actions different from or in addition to their pharmacologically desirable actions make adverse cutaneous reactions an inevitable fact of modern medical practice. The kinds of cutaneous reactions are varied. Exanthems (ery-

thematous, morbilliform, or maculopapular), urticaria, fixed drug eruptions, and erythema multiforme are the most common. Both illustrations here are of the morbilliform type of reaction. Figure 644 resulted from novobiocin and Fig. 645 from ampicillin. Constitutional symptoms of low-grade fever and malaise may be associated with such drug eruptions. Morbilliform eruptions from ampicillin are more frequently seen in children with infectious mononucleosis.

Figure 646

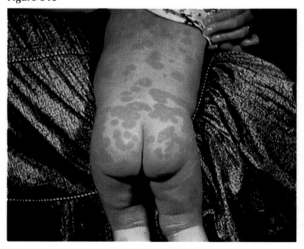

Figure 647

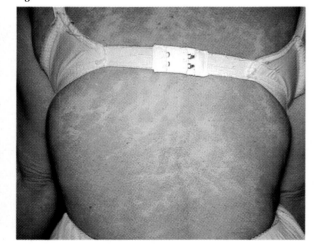

Drug eruptions (dermatitis medicamentosa) Drug eruptions may mimic nearly the entire range of dermatoses of other causes. One of the commonest forms is the exanthematic, whose lesions are usually erythematous and edematous. Common causes of drug eruptions include ampicillin, cephalosporins, semi-synthetic penicillins, and barbiturates. We have just illustrated cases that were morbilliform. Illustrated here are cases clinically resembling erythema multi-

forme. Figure 646 resulted from a sulfonamide and Fig. 647 from a chloroquine (Plaquenil). Note again the tendency to universality and symmetry. Drug eruptions of the types so far illustrated may be uncomfortably pruritic and attended at their onset by prodromal malaise, but they are rarely serious and usually subside fairly quickly upon elimination of the causative drug and, on occasion, even in the face of continued administration of an absolutely required drug.

Figure 648

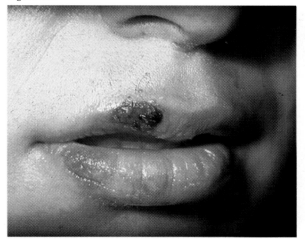

Figure 649

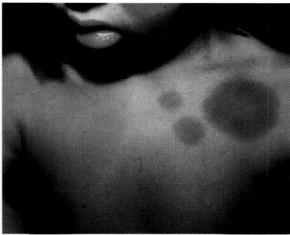

Fixed drug eruption   Another common type of adverse reaction to drugs is the so-called fixed drug eruption. The term *fixed* is intended to suggest that the cutaneous change, occurring for the first time in given sites (anywhere), recurs in those same sites upon subsequent and repeated administration. Upon subsequent provocation, new reactions in new sites may occur, but original sites always flare again. There are several drugs that are well known for their propensity to cause fixed drug eruptions, namely, phenolphthalein, salicylates, phenacetin, barbiturates, antipyrine, arsenicals, and gold salts. The clinical morphology of a fixed drug eruption is usually a roundish plaque that is palpably edematous and purplish. Sometimes fixed drug eruptions are bullous. Both illustrations here are of fixed drug eruptions caused by phenolphthalein.

Figure 650

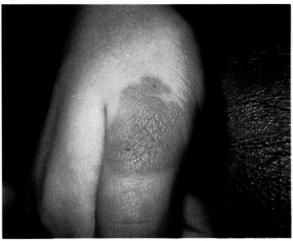

Figure 651

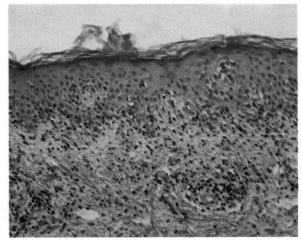

Fixed drug eruption   This cutaneous change appeared after institution of treatment of an unrelated condition with an antihistamine. The proof of a drug as cause of an eruption is sometimes certain, on the basis of repeated experience, but often conjectural or circumstantial, especially in the case of newly introduced drugs. Proof by withdrawing a suspected drug and observing subsidence of the eruption and then reappearance upon resumption of the drug is usually not wise or safe practice.

Histopathology of fixed drug eruption   Fixed drug eruptions are acute inflammatory plaques that tend to leave post-inflammatory hyperpigmentation upon resolution and to recur in the same sites upon readministration of the causative drug. During the inflammatory stage, the histopathologic changes are similar to those of erythema multiforme (Fig. 484). The changes are damage to the lower level of the epidermis and appearance of eosinophilic prickle cells and a mononuclear infiltrate. Often there is melanin within macrophages in the upper dermis.

Figure 652

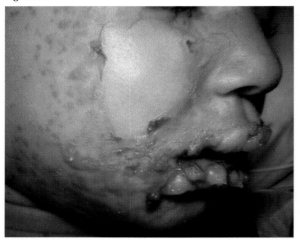

Figure 653

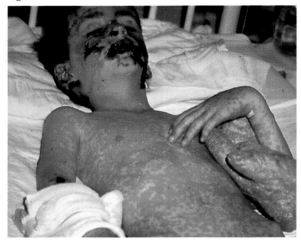

Toxic epidermal necrolysis This is a severe generalized eruption that is almost always the result of a reaction to a medication. The most common agents are sulfonamides, anticonvulsants, and nonsteroidal anti-inflammatory drugs. Combinations of bullae and erosions are seen; the bullae occur especially on or around the lips, in the mouth, and on other mucous surfaces. Frozen section processing of a biopsy specimen of toxic epidermal necrolysis allows for rapid diagnosis. In patients with

erosions and blisters, one sees necrotic keratinocytes, severe degeneration of the basal layer, and a subepidermal separation. The mortality rate in this disease is significant; most deaths are related to superinfection and sepsis. Patients with toxic epidermal necrolysis benefit enormously from intensive medical care, in a burn unit when possible. The role of systemic steroids in this disease remains extremely controversial.

Figure 654

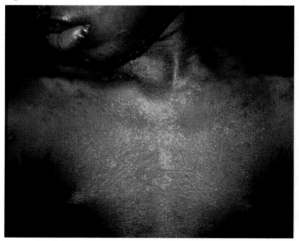

Figure 655

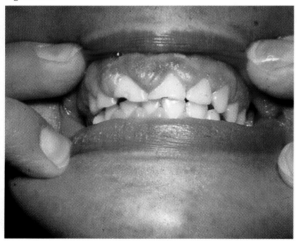

Acute exanthem syndrome Each of the anticonvulsant medications phenytoin (Dilantin), phenobarbital, and carbamazepine (Tegretol) may cause this severe form of drug reaction. The mucocutaneous manifestations are strawberry tongue and a generalized scarlatiniform eruption that is followed by desquamation. The rash may also be purpuric. The presence of high fever, lymphadenopathy, and hepatosplenomegaly may give the false impression of an infectious disease. Elevations in blood urea nitrogen, liver enzymes, and peripheral eosinophil count may also be present.

Gingival hyperplasia from phenytoin The mechanisms of adverse reactions to drugs vary. Some, like the urticarial or eczematous, are clearly based on an allergic or immunologic mechanism; others are utterly obscure in mechanism. Such is the gingival hyperplasia caused by phenytoin. Since it occurs in almost all patients receiving the drug, all one can say is that the effect probably is within the normal pharmacologic action of the drug.

Figure 656

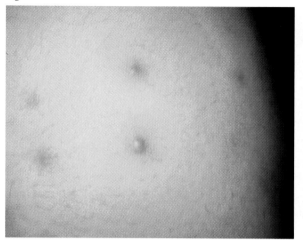

Figure 657

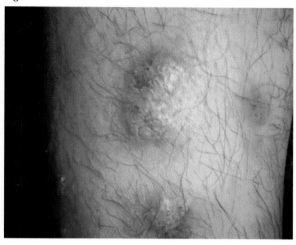

Iododerma and bromoderma Iodides and bromides are drugs that can cause severe adverse cutaneous reactions, and of these, the worst are acneiform, furuncular, carbuncular, chancriform, pyodermatous, or granulomatous. Iodides and bromides are widely distributed, not only in foods and in the environment but also in proprietary and formally prescribed medicaments. These photographs are of still relatively minor consequences of adverse reactions from the two halides, of which bromides are usually worse than iodides. Lesions like those of acne or folliculitis caused by an iodide are shown in Fig. 656. Figure 657 is a granulomatous reaction caused by a bromide. Another baleful characteristic of drug eruptions from halides is persistence and extension of reaction once it occurs. The reason for such persistence or extension, even when a known source of the offending drug is removed, is the wide dispersion of occult iodine or bromine salts in foods, in the environment, and indeed in the body's own chemistry. Iodine, for example, is a constituent of thyroid hormone.

Figure 658

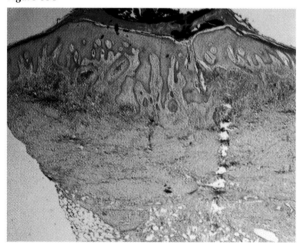

Histopathology of bromoderma The halides (bromine and iodine salts) may, in certain individuals, induce a variable combination of acute inflammatory and hyperplastic changes in the epidermis, which clinically may range from pustules to large, destructive, chancriform lesions. In this illustration, one sees surface crust, pseudocarcinomatous hyperplasia of the epidermis, and intense inflammation, mainly in the superficial dermis and subcutaneous fat. Eosinophils are often numerous in the cellular infiltrate.

19

Panniculopathies

Figure 659

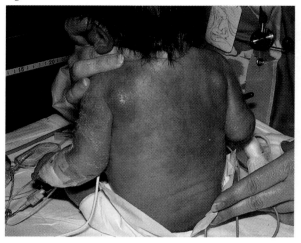

Figure 660

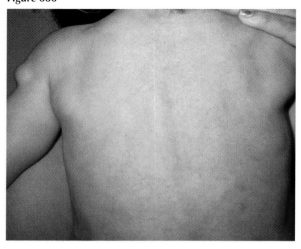

Subcutaneous fat necrosis of the newborn   This is a self-resolving and benign condition that is seen in healthy newborns. The infants develop single or multiple firm red-purple nodules or plaques that are asymptomatic. Cheeks, back, buttocks, and thighs are the most common locations. Lesions may be present at birth, or they may develop during the first month of life. Most lesions resolve spontaneously over a period of 2–4 weeks, but

some last significantly longer. There is usually no residual atrophy or scarring. It is difficult to capture the quality of panniculitis in photography, but a sense of it can be appreciated on the buttock of the patient pictured in Fig. 659. The etiology of this disorder is probably ischemic injury to subcutaneous fat. Lesions often develop at sites of pressure. Subcutaneous fat necrosis is occasionally associated with hypercalcemia.

Figure 661

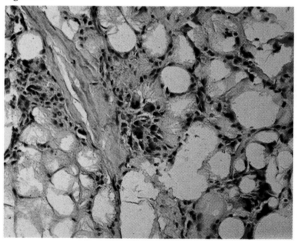

Figure 662

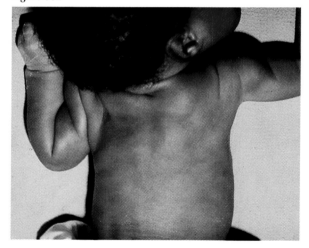

Histopathology of subcutaneous fat necrosis of the newborn   In this clinically dramatic but essentially benign condition, needle-shaped triglyceride crystals form and incite a foreign-body reaction characterized by giant cells. In tissue routinely processed, as here, the lipid has been dissolved by solvents, but one can still see thin protoplasmic strands that had separated the acicular crystals. Upon resolution, normal structure reappears.

Sclerema neonatorum   Unlike the condition just described, sclerema neonatorum presents itself as symmetrical areas of induration on cheeks, shoulders, buttocks, and calves. The skin over involved subcutaneous fat is uniformly board-like, cold, and livid in color, as though frozen. Infants so affected appear rigid because mobility is interfered with by the sclerema, and they are severely ill. Mortality is high. The condition is more common in premature infants and in those with severe underlying disease, such as sepsis or dehydration.

Figure 663

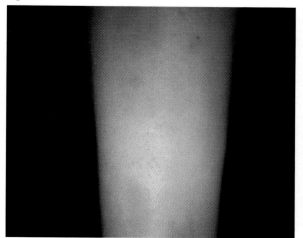

Figure 664

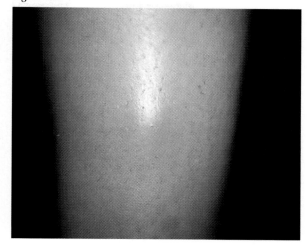

Erythema nodosum Red, tender, subcutaneous nodules on the extensor aspects of the legs between knees and ankles are a common condition of many causes, some clear, some likely, and many obscure. The most important conditions that are heralded or attended by erythema nodosum are such infections as streptococcal upper-respiratory infections, ulcerative colitis, histoplasmosis, coccidioidomycosis, tuberculosis, syphilis, and leprosy. Another condition that is sometimes revealed by investigation of erythema nodosum is sarcoidosis. Drugs appear to be the cause of particular cases of erythema nodosum. In many cases, however, no clear cause can be found.

Figure 665

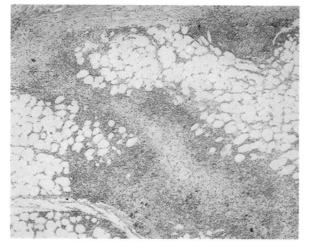

Figure 666

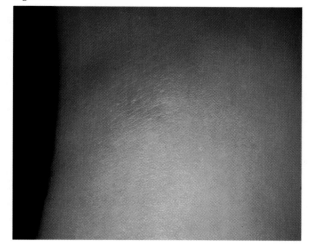

Histopathology of erythema nodosum Erythema nodosum is a panniculitis. The panniculitises in general are difficult to distinguish clinically and microscopically, but of them, erythema nodosum is easiest to so distinguish. The inflammatory process affects chiefly the fibrous septa; the fat lobules are less involved. Here one sees pronounced inflammation of a septum diagonally cut and some involvement of the adjacent fat lobules. Scattered multinucleated giant cells are present.

Relapsing, febrile, nodular, nonsuppurative panniculitis (Weber-Christian) This is a rare panniculitis in children that is characterized by recurrent crops of tender subcutaneous plaques and nodules in association with fever. The lower extremities are primarily involved, although the upper extremities, trunk, and face may also be involved. Myalgias and arthralgias may also occur. The etiology of Weber-Christian syndrome is unknown.

Figure 667

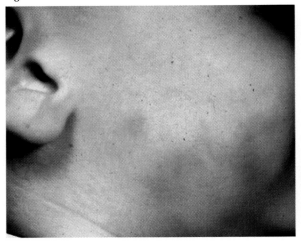

Panniculitis from cold   Local exposure to cold leads to the formation of ice crystals within cells. Injury to cell contents occurs during both cooling and thawing. Cold panniculitis may occur in a child whose glove or boot has filled with snow. It is also seen in the youngster who has been sucking on a frozen dessert product—called Popsicle panniculitis. The self-limited injury sustained in that condition is illustrated in Fig. 667.

Figure 668

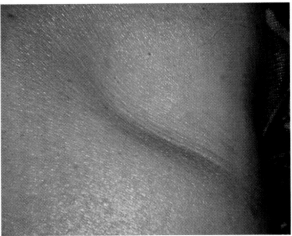

Lipoatrophy (lipodystrophy)   The localized lipoatrophy illustrated here resulted from the injection of insulin. This side effect can sometimes be avoided by use of a single-peak insulin preparation. Atrophy of tissue may follow injection into it of many materials. For example, deposition of corticosteroids often causes temporary atrophy. Localized lipoatrophy may sometimes occur in patients with a number of different autoimmune diseases, and it occurs very rarely as an isolated finding in the otherwise healthy child.

Figure 669

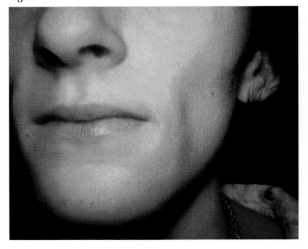

Lipoatrophy (lipodystrophy)   Progressive lipoatrophy is characterized by the loss of all adipose tissue in the upper portion of the body. Patients characteristically have the emaciated "sunken cheek" appearance that is seen in Fig. 669. A frequent complication of progressive lipoatrophy is membranoproliferative glomerulonephritis, associated with decreased levels of the third component of complement. The majority of patients are female.

Figure 670

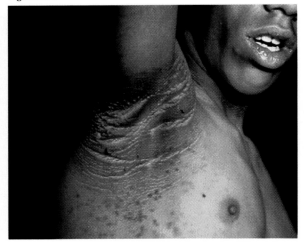

Acanthosis nigricans and lipoatrophy   Patients with either partial lipodystrophy or congenital total lipodystrophy may develop severe acanthosis nigricans. Note the severity of acanthosis nigricans in this young patient. The congenital form of lipodystrophy evolves during the first 2 years of life and is inherited in autosomal recessive fashion. Other features include insulin-resistant diabetes mellitus and accelerated growth. This combination may be referred to as the Lawrence-Seip-Beradinelli syndrome.

20

Vascular and Lymphatic Dysplasias

Figure 671

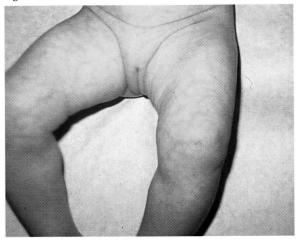

Cutis marmorata This term means "marbled skin" and is intended to describe the appearance of skin in which the terminal vessels are so superficial and dilated that they are constantly visible in patterns that vaguely suggest veined marble. This condition is physiologic in the newborn and represents a vasomotor response to lowering of the environmental temperature. Persistent cutis marmorata is seen in Down syndrome and in trisomy 18.

Figure 672

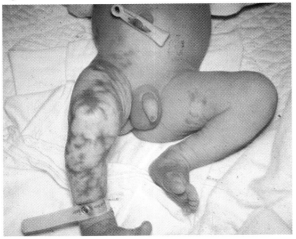

Cutis marmorata telangiectatica congenita (phlebectasia congenita) This condition is present at birth and consists of accentuated vascular markings (cutis marmorata), along with areas of telangiectasia, ulceration, and atrophy. The lesions may be localized or generalized. A minority of children with this condition have other abnormalities, among them mental retardation and hemiatrophy or hemihypertrophy. The mottling resolves gradually with age in most patients.

Figure 673

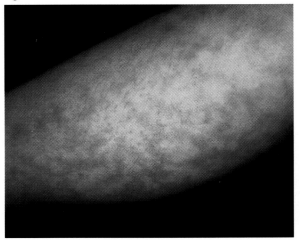

Livedo reticularis *Livedo* means a slate-gray blueness. *Reticularis* means "like a net." The term describes a network of grayblueness that is generally seen on the lower extremities. The idiopathic form of this disorder, most common in young women, carries a good prognosis. However, livedo reticularis is also seen in association with polyarteritis nodosa, systemic lupus erythematosus, and cryoglobulinemia.

Figure 674

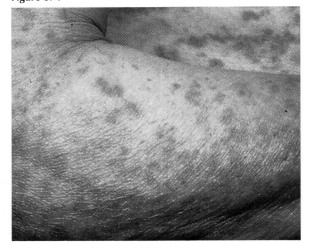

Angioma serpiginosum This rare vascular disorder is most commonly seen in girls and tends to favor the extremities. The patient shown here has numerous areas of vascular ectasia in a gyrate pattern. As one observes the condition over long periods of time, one sees resolution of old lesions and development of new ones at the periphery. Though the condition tends to abate, it never quite leaves.

Figure 675

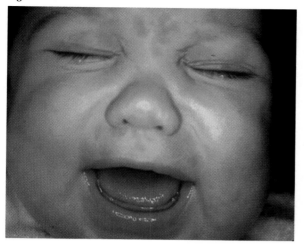

Figure 676

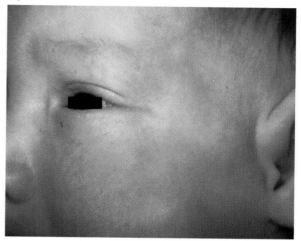

Salmon patch The salmon patch is by far the most common vascular lesion in the newborn. This midline or symmetrical pink macular lesion is most commonly seen on the eyelids, the nape of the neck, and the glabella. The last two are commonly described as "stork bite" and "angel's kiss," respectively. The glabellar lesion in Fig. 675 can be expected to resolve spontaneously, as do lesions on the eyelids. Rarely, a salmon patch on the neck may persist into adult life.

Port-wine stain This unilateral vascular malformation has a markedly different histology, significance, and natural history from that of the salmon patch. The port-wine stain is made up of capillary ectasias that may be present throughout the dermis and that gradually increase with age. The color changes from pink to purple as the patient grows, and the lesions may become nodular during adult life. Because port-wine stains show no tendency to involute, they may represent a significant, lifelong cosmetic problem.

Figure 677

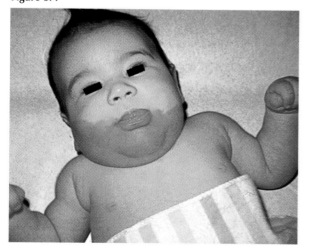

Figure 678

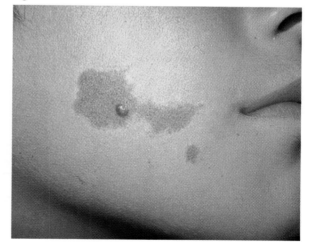

Port-wine stain In Fig. 677 we see the kind of port-wine stain that is a serious cosmetic hardship. Previous therapeutic approaches, including surgery, dermabrasion, tattooing, and use of the argon laser, have met with poor to variable results. The tunable pulsed dye laser is a considerably more successful modality in the treatment of disfiguring port-wine stains. Success is related to the fact that hemoglobin preferentially absorbs

laser energy at the 577 nm wavelength. The very brief pulse duration prevents the heat from spreading from the blood vessels into the surrounding connective tissue, and the danger of scarring is thus minimized. Shown in Fig. 678 is a relatively small port-wine stain that has a small papule of angiomatosis on it. Both of these patients would be excellent candidates for treatment with the pulsed dye laser.

Figure 679

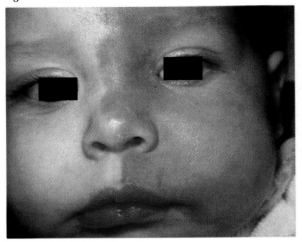

Sturge-Weber syndrome This is one of the most serious of the angiopathies because more than merely skin is involved with the excess of blood vessels. In the case shown here, deep structures (namely, the eye and the meninges) have extensive vascular reduplication. The result here is glaucoma and a seizure disorder. The association between port-wine stain, seizures, and glaucoma only occurs when skin involvement includes the forehead and upper eyelid (ophthalmic or V1 trigeminal area).

Figure 680

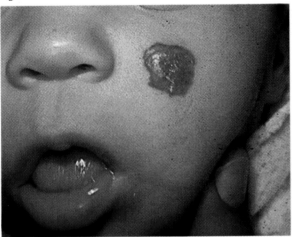

Hemangioma Hemangiomas occur in a variety of sizes, locations, and degrees of combination of capillaries, larger vessels, and venous lakes. The hemangioma pictured here is of the simplest sort. It is limited, superficial, and largely capillary. Lesions of this sort tend to increase in size for a period of time and then to involute partially or totally. Most often, the best cosmetic result is achieved by allowing this spontaneous process to run its course.

Figure 681

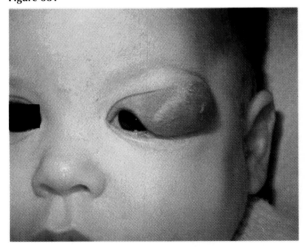

Hemangioma The hemangioma illustrated here is not serious in itself; it will eventually resolve spontaneously. There is, however, a danger in so young a child if the lesion should grow and mechanically close the eye. There may then be a failure of development of the cerebral area that receives visual stimuli for interpretation. This could result in amblyopia ex anopsia, a blindness from disuse. Treatment with a course of oral prednisone is indicated in such a case. The use of intralesional steroids has been advocated by some.

Figure 682

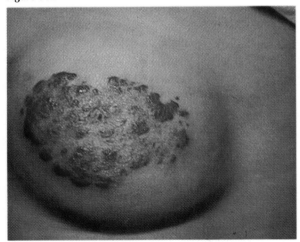

Hemangioma This picture is a good illustration of how a hemangioma resolves spontaneously. After a year or so of development, most hemangiomas begin to thrombose, and some ulcerate. Repeated events of this sort diminish the vascular bulk until nothing more than some telangiectasia, atrophy, or redundancy of overlying skin remains. Frequently no additional treatment is needed, but if necessary, minor plastic surgery is all that is required for an acceptable cosmetic result.

Figure 683

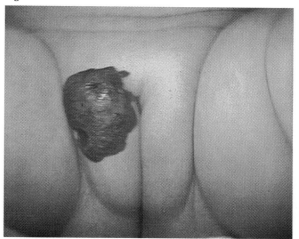

Figure 684

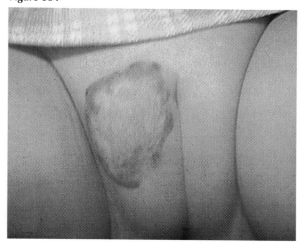

Hemangioma These are illustrations of a hemangioma at the height of its development on a labium majus and in almost complete spontaneous resolution. No treatment has been applied. If one could have followed the events of such a case from recognizable beginnings to end points, one would have seen originally a bit of redness, then a flowering of the lesion to the extent pictured in Fig. 683 about 1 or 1½ years later, and finally, in the course of 2, 3, or 4 more years, the condition shown in Fig. 684. Perhaps at the very end, nothing more than some macular telangiectasia or some redundancy of skin would remain. In a site like this, whatever remains could be left alone. Serial photographs of this sort may be reassuring to the parents of a child with a hemangioma.

Figure 685

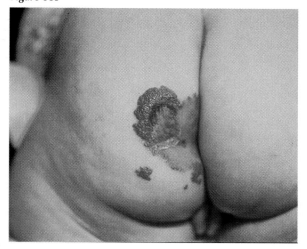

Figure 686

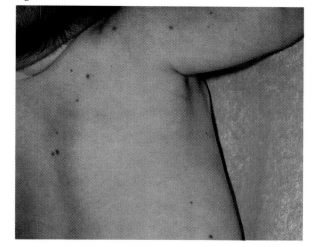

Hemangioma (ulcerated) During the growth phase of hemangiomas, especially in the groin area, ulceration may develop. Ulcerations are prone to secondary bacterial infection and can be very tender. These lesions result in scars upon healing. Treatment is aimed at treating secondary infection. Recently, pulsed dye lasers have been used in an attempt to expedite healing and decrease pain.

Disseminated hemangiomatosis Pictured here is a neonate with multiple small hemangiomas. Children with this degree of cutaneous involvement may suffer from visceral hemangiomatosis. Liver, spleen, lungs, and the gastrointestinal and central nervous systems may be involved. Risks include high-output congestive heart failure, thrombocytopenia, and neurologic complications. If a complete workup establishes the presence of extensive visceral disease, early corticosteroid therapy is advisable.

Figure 687

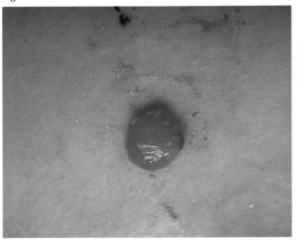

Pyogenic granuloma   This is a common acquired lesion that develops at the site of an obvious or unnoticed trauma. It is the result of a local vascular proliferation. Typically, a pyogenic granuloma grows rapidly, and there is often a history of spontaneous bleeding.

Figure 688

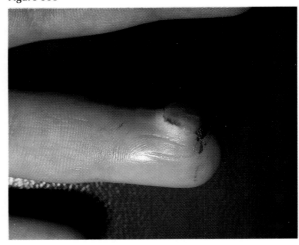

Pyogenic granuloma   The lesion is usually a red papule or nodule the size of a small nut, and it can be located anywhere on the body. The surface is usually friable, with a collarette of epidermis at the base. Treatment consists of thorough electrodesiccation and curettage.

Figure 689

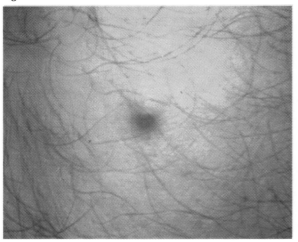

Figure 690

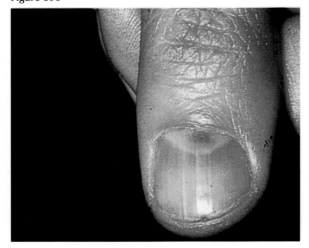

Glomus tumor   Vascular shunts are special structures abundant in acral parts of the body that have a large area and a relatively small volume, such as the fingertips, the nose, and the pinnae of the ears. They are much sparser elsewhere. Their function is to alter circulation under the stimulus of cold in such a manner as to conserve heat by turning off much of the arterial circulation. Their structure is of a myoepithelium, i.e., a conglomeration of epithelial cells that have contractile ability. Such tissue sometimes becomes benignly hyperplastic and somewhat bulky. The purplish nodule in Fig. 689 is typical of the glomus tumor. Solitary glomus tumors are often located in the nail bed, as in Fig. 690, and may give rise to severe episodes of paroxysmal pain. The subungual lesions seem to be more common in females. Excision of painful lesions is the treatment of choice. In addition, a rare syndrome of multiple glomus tumors exists. These lesions tend to be asymptomatic, and the condition is inherited in autosomal dominant fashion.

Figure 691

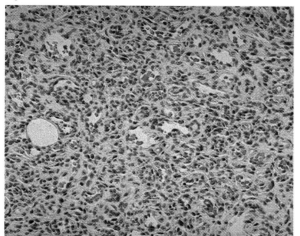

Histopathology of superficial and deep hemangiomas
These vascular hamartomas are cellular angiomas in which one finds almost confluent sheets of proliferating endothelial cells; small, well-formed vascular channels (illustrated here); and at times somewhat larger (cavernous) vessels. Whatever the clinical and histologic pictures, they are all the same in their embryonic dysgenesis and in their strong tendency to eventual spontaneous resolution.

Figure 692

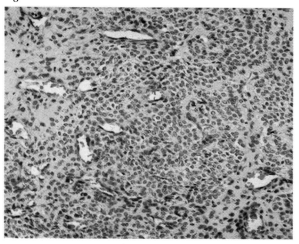

Histopathology of glomus tumors Glomangiomas are uncommon vascular tumors, usually acral, solitary, and tender, but at times multiple, asymptomatic, and scattered. The solitary ones tend to be highly cellular; the multiple tend to be cavernous. In addition to the endothelial-lined vessels, there is a proliferation in the form of sheets of cells that are contractile like smooth muscle cells. They have round nuclei and resemble epithelial cells. Tenderness is probably produced by contraction of these cells and stimulation of nerve fibers.

Figure 693

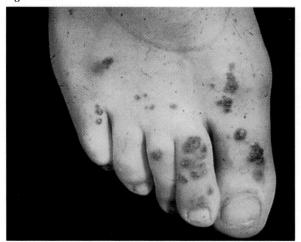

Angiokeratoma (angiokeratoma of Mibelli) There are many forms of angiogenesis that are benign. Pyogenic granuloma, nevus araneus, and ruby spots are examples. Angiokeratoma of Mibelli is another type and is distinguished by the development of hyperkeratosis on small papular angiomas. The feet and lower extremities are common sites for this condition.

Figure 694

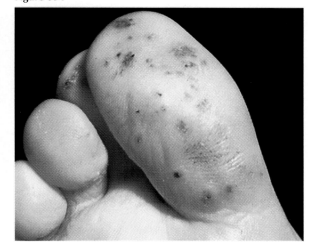

These lesions arise during adolescence and may be associated with cold intolerance. Papular lesions of the same sort are common on the scrotum, where hyperkeratosis does not develop. These are sometimes labeled *angiokeratoma of Fordyce*. At first glance, one might think the condition as illustrated might be verruca vulgaris. Biopsy distinguishes with certainty.

Figure 695

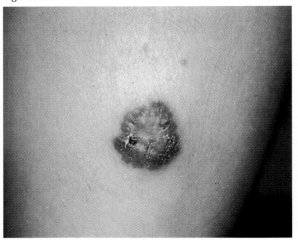

Solitary angiokeratoma This lesion usually develops on the lower extremities, sometimes in response to trauma. The lesion pictured here could easily be mistaken for a melanoma or a pigmented basal cell carcinoma. Biopsy is indicated, and the combination of dilated blood vessels, hyperkeratosis, and acanthosis enables the dermatopathologist to make the correct diagnosis. When lesions of this type enlarge to the size of a plaque, the term *angiokeratoma circumscriptum* is used.

Figure 696

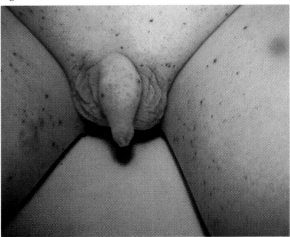

Fabry's disease (angiokeratoma corporis diffusum) This condition is serious because it is a sphingolipidosis associated with an enzyme anomaly that leads to the deposition of a ceramide trihexoside in the smooth muscle of blood vessels. The cutaneous lesions are tiny papules that are angiomatous. When this happens in the blood vessels of the heart, kidneys, eyes, and nervous system, symptoms of functional disturbance and failure appear. Fucosidosis and sialidosis may cause a similar clinical appearance.

Figure 697

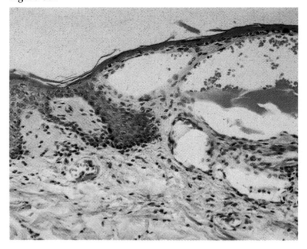

Histopathology of Fabry's disease Fabry's disease (angiokeratoma corporis diffusum) is histologically classed among the angiokeratomas, i.e., hemangiomas that show a variable degree of surface hyperkeratosis. It is known to be caused by an inborn error of metabolism (a specific, heritable enzyme defect). Microscopically, one sees cavernous, endothelium-lined blood vessels directly beneath a thinned epidermis. There is no hyperkeratosis visible in this figure. The microscopic picture is typical, but not unique.

Figure 698

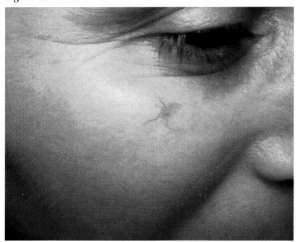

Spider angioma (nevus araneus) This is a trivial and common childhood angioma, highly characteristic in its central vascular punctum, from which radiate fine vessels that give the entire lesion the fanciful appearance of a spider in its web. Such lesions are usually solitary, and the face is a common site for them. The dorsa of the hands are another common site. Persistent lesions are easily extirpated by skillful electrodesiccation or by the use of the tunable pulsed dye laser.

Figure 699

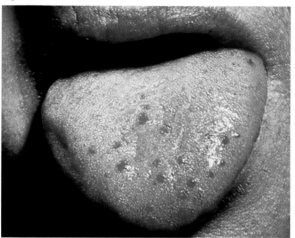

Figure 700

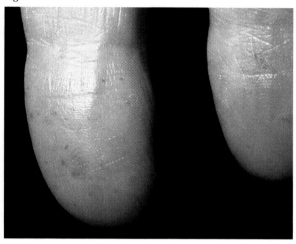

Hereditary hemorrhagic telangiectasia (Osler-Rendu-Weber syndrome) This is an autosomal dominant syndrome with both cutaneous and visceral involvement. In most children with the disease, the presenting symptom is recurrent epistaxis. Patients go on to develop vascular papules that stud the lips, tongue, palate, and nasal mucosa. The ears, palms, soles, digital tips, and nail beds are other common sites for lesions. As the disease progresses, melena and hematemesis may develop as a result of gastrointestinal involvement. A significant number of patients with this syndrome have hepatic and pulmonary arteriovenous fistulas. The latter may lead to cyanosis, shortness of breath, polycythemia, and digital clubbing. Patients must be monitored carefully for hemorrhage in the liver, brain, urinary bladder, and retina and for the development of a secondary anemia.

Figure 701

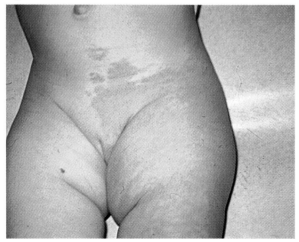

Figure 702

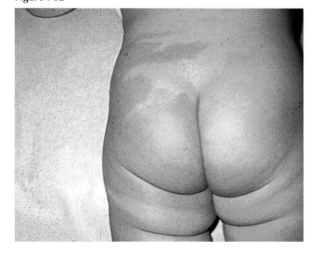

Klippel-Trénaunay-Weber syndrome This is a condition in which hemangiomas, varicosities, and phlebectasia cover an entire limb or other body area. There may be associated skeletal abnormalities, including macrodactyly and syndactyly. A combination of port-wine stain and hemangiomas may be present from birth. The osteohypertrophy develops during the first several years of life. These photographs are front and back views of an infant who has the beginning of the angiomatous process. At this stage, the condition appears almost like a nevus flammeus. Over time, more massive vascularization and enlargement of the limb will develop.

Figure 703

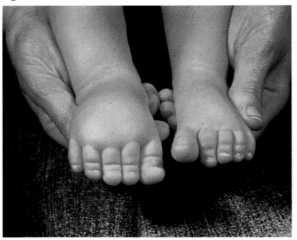

Milroy's disease This term refers to a form of primary lymph-edema that is inherited in autosomal dominant fashion. The swelling of the feet and legs is either unilateral or bilateral. The edema is pitting at first, but fibrosis of the lower extremities gradually leads to a firmer and more persistent enlargement. Over time, the overlying epidermis may become verrucous and hyperkeratotic.

Figure 704

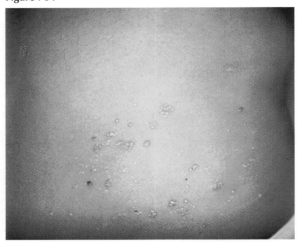

Lymphangioma The proliferation of lymphatic channels in the skin or subcutaneous tissue may give rise to lesions with a variety of clinical appearance. Most lymphangiomas develop during the first 2 years of life, and some are present at birth. The cluster of clear vesicles pictured here is termed *lymph-angioma circumscriptum*. The lesions are benign but may be distressing because of their tendency to increase in size and number over time and occasionally to become irritated or superinfected.

Figure 705

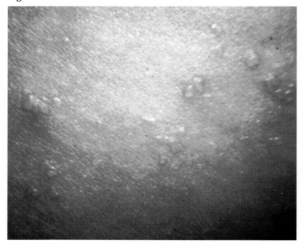

Lymphangioma Illustrated in these two photographs are additional examples of lymphangioma circumscriptum. Figure 705 shows why the appearance of these glistening papules is sometimes compared to frog spawn. Figure 706 is a mixed hamartoma composed of both lymphatic channels and blood vessels.

Figure 706

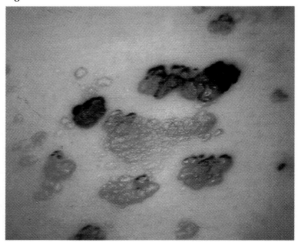

The surgical treatment of lymphangioma circumscriptum is complicated by the fact that the associated lymphatic channels may be deeper than can be clinically appreciated. The result is a high rate of recurrence. Laser surgery may be a reasonable approach for some of these lesions.

Figure 707

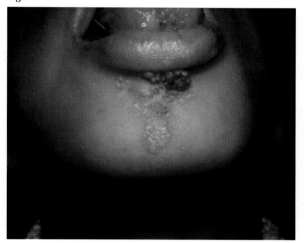

Figure 708

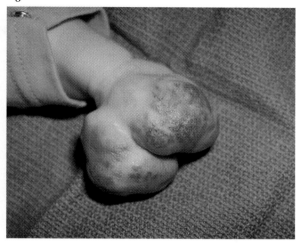

Lymphangioma Lymphangioma circumscriptum is usually localized to the neck, proximal extremities, abdomen, tongue, and mucous membranes. The lesion pictured here is in an unusual location. The surface is hyperkeratotic, and one can imagine confusing this lymphangioma with a large verruca. Plastic surgery would possibly yield a good result in a localized, easily accessible lesion like this one.

Vascular malformations These are congenital malformations that consist of capillary, venous, arterial or lymphatic abnormalities. There are often combined malformations that are comprised of different types of vessels. Examples of vascular malformations include port wine stains (capillary malformation), cystic hygroma (lymphatic malformation), and venous malformations. Vascular malformations are present at birth and grow proportionately with the child. Some vascular malformations may not manifest themselves until adolescence or adulthood.

21

Neoplastic Diseases

Figure 709

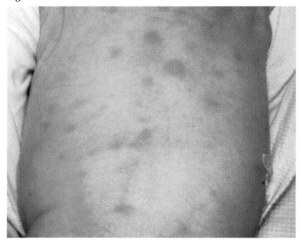

Figure 710

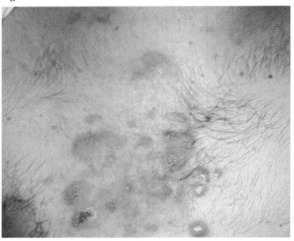

Leukemia cutis   A dermal infiltrate of leukemic cells results in the papulonodular lesions, or plaques, that are illustrated here. Such primary involvement of the skin is relatively rare in childhood leukemia. The wide variety of secondary manifestations of leukemia includes petechiae and ecchymoses and pyoderma gangrenosum. A polymorphonuclear dermal infiltrate termed *Sweet's syndrome* (see Fig. 489) may be associated with leukemia. In addition, children receiving chemotherapy are prone to bacterial and fungal infections of the skin, severe varicella, and ulcerative or chronic herpes simplex.

Hodgkin's disease   Like other lymphoproliferative disorders, Hodgkin's disease may have both specific and nonspecific cutaneous manifestations. Figure 710 illustrates a relatively rare event in children with Hodgkin's disease: the direct infiltration of malignant cells into the skin. A biopsy analysis of these brownish papules, nodules, and plaques reveals a histology similar to that of affected lymph nodes. These lesions may occasionally ulcerate, and pruritus is a distressing symptom.

Figure 711

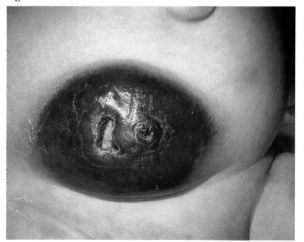

Chloroma   Also known as granulocytic sarcomas, these lesions may be seen in acute and chronic myelocytic leukemias. The lesions, which are infiltrates of masses of leukemic cells, occasionally present with a green color due to myeloperoxidase activity.

Figure 712

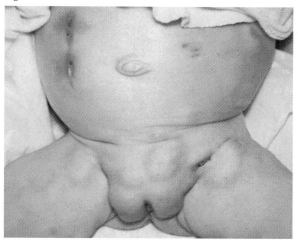

Neuroblastoma, metastatic This malignant tumor of the autonomic nervous system occurs most frequently in young children. Metastatic disease is often present at the time of diagnosis. Cutaneous metastases appear as bluish papules or nodules involving the trunk or extremities.

Figure 713

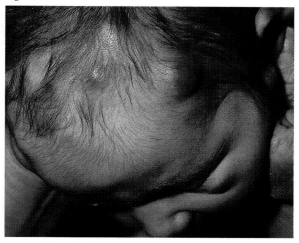

Neuroblastoma, metastatic The lesions are sometimes noted to blanch upon stroking and may sometimes exhibit increased sweating. Children who are under 1 year of age at the time of diagnosis, as was the case in the patient in this figure, may experience spontaneous regression of their illness. The prognosis in older children and in those with very widespread disease tends to be poor.

Figure 714

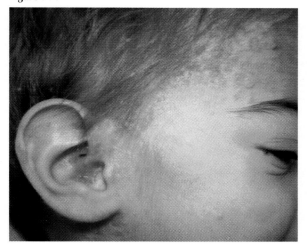

Figure 715

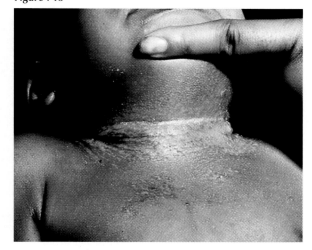

Histiocytosis X (Langerhans' cell histiocytosis) This is a spectrum of disease that encompasses Letterer-Siwe disease, Hand-Schüller-Christian disease, and eosinophilic granuloma. The disorder is characterized by the proliferation of Langerhans' histiocytes in the skin and other organ systems. Figure 714 shows the characteristic seborrheic-like, scaly, erythematous eruption on the scalp, face, and ears. A similar eruption, accompanied by erosive and granulomatous changes, may be seen in the neck folds, as in Fig. 715, or in the axillae and diaper area. In general, an unusual or recalcitrant diaper rash of this general appearance should alert the physician to consider the diagnosis. The presence of petechiae is a particularly helpful sign. Diagnosis is confirmed by skin biopsy and electron microscopy. More rapid confirmation is sometimes possible if one observes the presence of histiocytes in a lesion that has been scraped onto a microscopic slide and stained. Histiocytosis X may be accompanied by hepatosplenomegaly, lymphadenopathy, anemia, and thrombocytopenia.

Figure 716

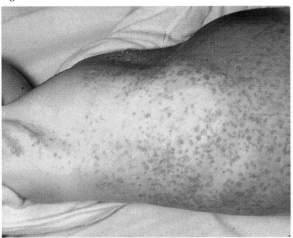

Histiocytosis X (Langerhans' cell histiocytosis) (cont.) The child shown here is covered with numerous red-brown crusted papules, which may become hemorrhagic. Rarely, this clinical picture is present at birth. The prognosis of children with histiocytosis X is extremely variable but is certainly worse in patients who de-velop organ dysfunction from their disease. The decision to initiate chemotherapy should be based on the clinical course of the individual patient.

Figure 717

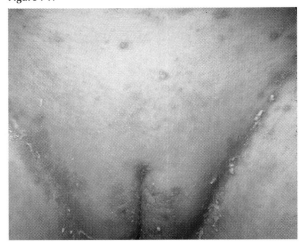

Histiocytosis X (Langerhans' cell histiocytosis) The diaper area may occasionally be the first area of involvement for infants. The inguinal creases appear erythematous, with scaling, fissuring, and a white mucoid material that may be the result of a secondary candidal infection. The presence of individual erythematous papular and petechial lesions will aid in the diagnosis.

Figure 718

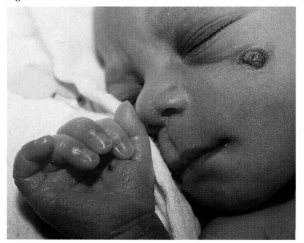

Congenital self-healing reticulohistiocytosis This is a rare condition that may present as a nodular form, solitary (Fig. 718) or multiple, or a generalized form with vesicles, papules, pustules, and crusts (Fig. 719). Mucous membranes are spared. Lesions are almost always present at birth, but new lesions may

Figure 719

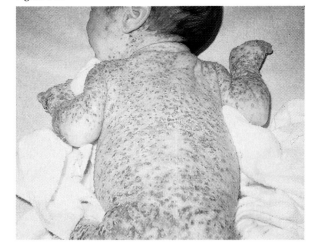

erupt in the early neonatal period. Most cases have only cutaneous involvement, but all patients should be evaluated for other organ involvement. The lesions typically resolve without any treatment within a few months. Ongoing monitoring is essential even after apparent clinical resolution.

22

Adnexal Dysplasias

Figure 720

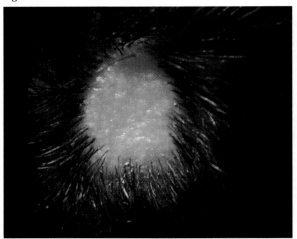

Figure 721

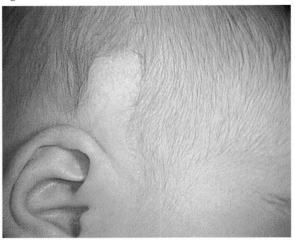

Nevus sebaceus This congenital lesion is composed of hamartomatous sebaceous glands and abortive hair follicles. It usually presents at birth as a yellow nodule or pebbled, hairless plaque on the scalp, forehead, or neck. Figure 720 shows the color and shape of the congenital lesion. With the loss of the effect of maternal hormones during the first few months of life, the lesion may quickly flatten and lose its distinctive color. During puberty, the nevus sebaceus again becomes raised, yellow,

and verrucous. After this change, and usually during adulthood, nevus sebaceus may give rise to a wide variety of benign and malignant neoplasms. These include basal cell hamartomas, keratoacanthomas, syringocystadenoma papilliferum, basal cell epitheliomas, and, rarely, squamous cell carcinomas. Figure 721 shows a basal cell carcinoma that has developed on a plaque of nevus sebaceus.

Figure 722

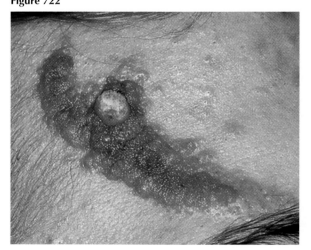

Figure 723

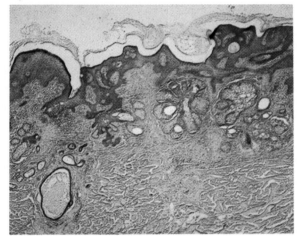

Nevus sebaceus Here pictured is another nevus sebaceus on which basal cell carcinoma has developed. In this case the color appears more brown and blackish in the main lesion, but the yellow color can still be appreciated in the small outlying papules. The nodule near the center represents the malignant change. Because neoplasms eventually occur in about one-third of patients with nevus sebaceus, it is considered advisable to arrange for the excision of all such lesions before puberty.

Histopathology of nevus sebaceus This is a localized cutaneous dysplasia in which disordered structure involves the epidermis, cutaneous appendages, and dermis. In the illustration one sees a rugose, hyperplastic epidermis; sebaceous glands without hair follicles; and cystic sweat gland elements (presumably apocrine) on the left. The impression conveyed is of a flawed attempt to form normal structures. Basal-cell epithelioma and a variety of adnexal neoplasms develop in a nevus sebaceus.

Figure 724

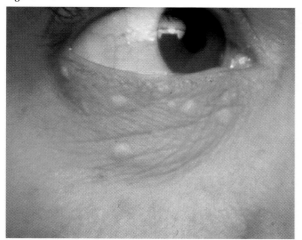

Figure 725

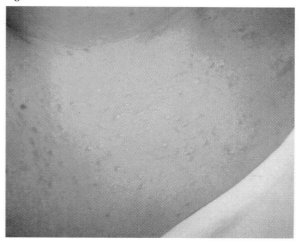

Syringoma These very small papules are adenomas of intraepidermal eccrine ducts. Most commonly, syringomas develop on the eyelids of women during adolescence or early adult life. Figure 724 is a good example of the fine papules that occur on the lower eyelids. They have no malignant potential, but the lesions are usually multiple and therefore the cause of cosmetic concern. Syringomas of this type may be delicately re-

moved by electrodesiccation and curettage. Figure 725 is a representation of even smaller lesions, this time on the upper part of the chest. Rarely, a child or adolescent will develop successive crops of syringomas on the skin of the anterior neck, antecubital fossa, axilla, and groin. This condition, termed eruptive syringoma, is sometimes inherited in autosomal dominant fashion.

Figure 726

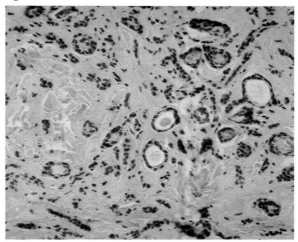

Figure 727

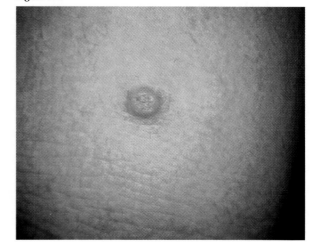

Histopathology of syringomas Syringomas are the most common malformations of cutaneous appendages. The microscopic picture is essentially the same in the common periorbital and the rare disseminated variety. One sees numerous epithelial elements in the form of solid cords and tubules containing pink secretory material situated in dense, relatively acellular stroma.

Clear cell hidradenoma This benign eccrine sweat gland tumor occurs as a solitary lesion in most cases. Most commonly, the growth appears as a small intraepidermal nodule. Ulceration or discharge of serous material rarely occurs. The lesion is harmless and may be extirpated by shaving it off level with the surrounding skin and electrodesiccating the base.

Figure 728

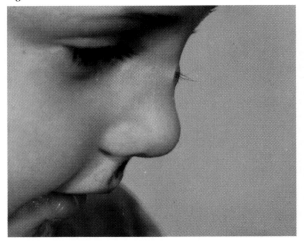

Figure 729

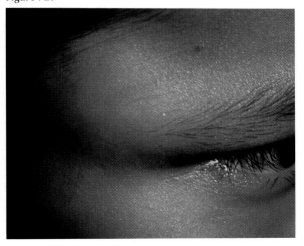

Dermoid cyst   These lesions present in the newborn as soft, round, subcutaneous tumors that are freely movable beneath the overlying epidermis. They represent ectodermal hamartomas and occur at the site of closure of embryonic clefts. The vast majority of dermoid cysts are found near the lateral eyebrow or on the forehead. The neck is the second most common location. The lesion pictured in Fig. 728 has protruding hairs and was

present at birth. In Fig. 729 there is a typical mass just lateral to the eyebrow. Histologic examination of these lesions reveals combinations of epidermis, dermis, sweat glands, sebaceous glands, and hair. Surgical excision is required when the dermoid cyst interferes with closure of the eyelid and is sometimes desirable for cosmetic reasons.

Figure 730

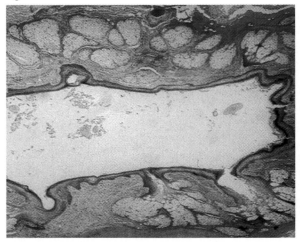

Figure 731

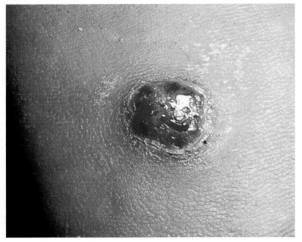

Histopathology of dermoid cysts   Dermoid cysts probably result from defective fusion of embryonic structures, most commonly on the face. When in the midline of the nose, a tuft of hairs commonly emerges from a sinus. The cyst itself is lined with stratified squamous epithelium, usually with sebaceous glands and hair follicles in continuity, opening into a cyst lumen, as seen here. Sweat ducts are present less commonly; abundant smooth muscle is sometimes found.

Eccrine poroma   This is a solitary benign tumor that is most common in adults but is occasionally seen in adolescents. Eccrine poromas are usually located on the sole of the foot, although they may rarely occur in a variety of other areas. The vascular appearance of the lesion, as shown in the illustration, could lead to confusion with pyogenic granuloma. Treatment consists of complete surgical excision.

Figure 732

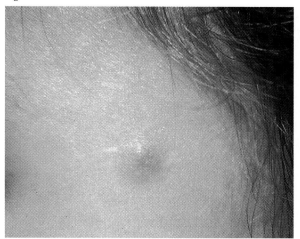

Pilomatricoma (benign calcifying epithelioma of Malherbe) This solitary benign tumor arises most commonly during childhood, usually on the face or upper extremities. Pilomatricomas range in size from 0.5 to 3.0 cm, although they are occasionally even larger. They appear as hard, freely movable dermal nodules. The skin overlying the lesion is usually normal but is sometimes erythematous or bluish. The overlying surface may feel irregular and exhibit a "tent sign." Multiple pilomatricomas are occasionally associated with myotonic muscular dystrophy.

Figure 733

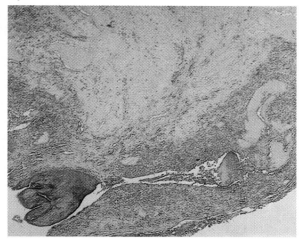

Histopathology of pilomatricoma This lesion is a solid tumor that clinically simulates an epidermoid cyst. Histologically, it shows differentiation like that of the matrix of a hair bulb and hence is called *pilomatricoma*. At the lower left of this photomicrograph one sees some undifferentiated basaloid cells, but most of the tumor is composed of sheets of what are called ghost or shadow cells. Calcification, usually present, is not seen here; even ossification occasionally occurs.

Figure 734

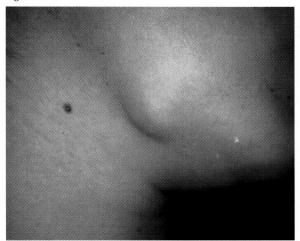

Figure 735

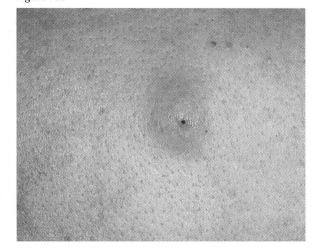

Epidermal cyst The lesions that were long termed *sebaceous cysts* are now renamed *epidermal cysts*, because their points of origin are not the sebaceous glands, and their content is not purely sebum. Epidermal cysts are exceedingly common lesions on the face and trunk. They consist of an epithelium-lined cavity that is filled with a caseous mixture of lipid and proteinaceous matter. They may have no apparent opening onto the surface of the skin, as in Fig. 734, or they may have a small aperture, as in Fig. 735. They may be as small as large seeds or as large as good-sized nuts. Uncomplicated epidermal cysts may be surgically removed in toto by clean dissection. They frequently become secondarily infected, and then incision and repeated drainage are required for their cure. They have no malignant potential, but sooner or later require attention because of size, location, or secondary infection.

Figure 736

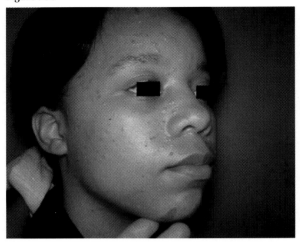

Figure 737

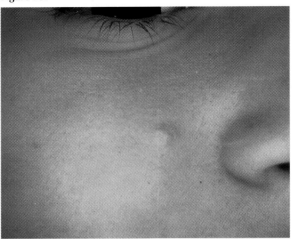

Trichoepithelioma　Trichoepithelioma is a benign neoplasm that differentiates toward hair structures. Lesions of this type may be multiple or solitary. Figure 736 illustrates a patient with multiple trichoepitheliomas. Individuals with this condition have numerous firm, rounded, skin-colored papules that are located mainly near the nasolabial folds. In more extensive cases, the rest of the face may become involved. The lesions usually begin to emerge during puberty, and the tendency for them to develop is inherited in autosomal dominant fashion. Figure 737 shows a solitary trichoepithelioma. These single flesh-colored papules develop on the face during childhood or adolescence. Solitary trichoepitheliomas are usually not hereditary.

Figure 738

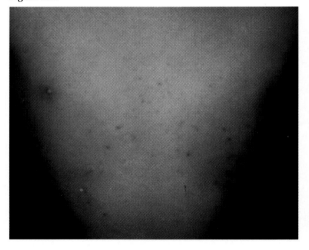

Figure 739

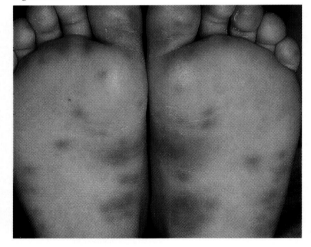

Eruptive vellus hair cysts　This condition is characterized by the rapid appearance of numerous small pigmented and flesh-colored papules. The tiny, dome-shaped lesions are usually clustered on the chest but may also involve the proximal extremities, buttocks, and back. The onset of this asymptomatic condition usually occurs during mid-childhood. Biopsy analysis of a lesion reveals a mid-dermal cyst containing laminated keratinous material. Autosomal dominant inheritance of this condition is sometimes observed. Spontaneous resolution frequently occurs.

Palmoplantar eccrine hidradenitis　This entity is characterized by the acute onset of painful erythematous papules and nodules located on the palms and/or soles in otherwise healthy children. Histopathology is remarkable for a neutrophilic infiltrate involving eccrine structures. The changes are similar to those seen in a condition known as neutrophilic eccrine hidradenitis, an eruption sometimes seen in oncology patients, especially myelogenous leukemia, receiving chemotherapy. The cause is unknown and the condition is self-limited.

23

Benign and Malignant Pigmented Lesions

Figure 740

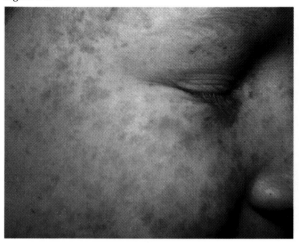

Figure 741

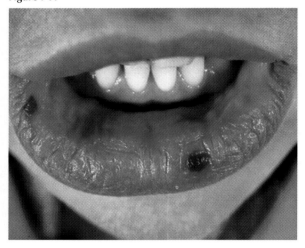

Ephelis This is the learned word for a freckle. The plural is ephelides (pronounced ĕf-ĕl´ĭ-dēz). These small, brown macules that are exceedingly common on the face in some children. They appear after exposure to sunlight and are more common in children with very fair skin or red hair. They tend to disappear in adult life. Histologically, these lesions show increased amounts of epidermal melanin but no abundance of melanocytes.

Lentigo This tan-to-brown to almost brown-black macular lesion may be found on any area of the body surface, which includes mucous membranes. There is no relation to ultraviolet light exposure. The illustration here is of lentigines on the lip. Lentigines may be present at birth and tend to increase in number during childhood and adult life. Histologically, there is a proliferation of melanocytes and elongation of the rete ridges. Lesions of this sort show no tendency to resolve spontaneously.

Figure 742

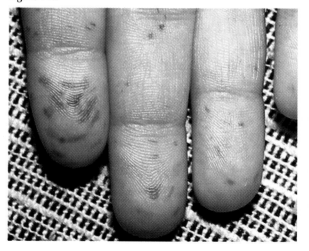

Figure 743

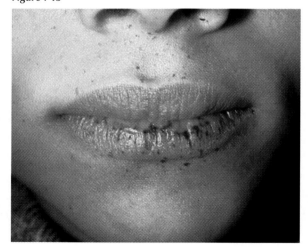

Peutz-Jeghers syndrome This autosomal dominant syndrome is notable for highly characteristic lentigines seen on the vermilion of the lips and adjacent skin, on the buccal mucosa, and on the palmar aspect of the fingertips. The pictures here are good representations of the lentigines in a typical case. Patients with this syndrome may also have gastrointestinal polyps

throughout the GI tract but most frequently in the jejunum. These benign hamartomas have very little malignant potential but may be the cause of obstruction, diarrhea, bleeding, or intussusception. Unlike common lentigines, the cutaneous lesions in these patients tend to fade during adult life. Mucous membrane lesions persist.

Figure 744

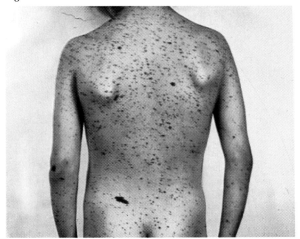

Multiple lentigines syndrome This autosomal dominant syndrome features numerous small lentigines, which are present at or soon after birth and cover the entire cutaneous surface. The possibilities of organ involvement are summed up in the mnemonic word *leopard*, in which *l* stands for lentigines, *e* for electrocardiographic conduction defects, *o* for ocular hypertelorism, *p* for pulmonary stenosis, *a* for abnormalities of genitalia, *r* for retardation of growth, and *d* for deafness.

Figure 745

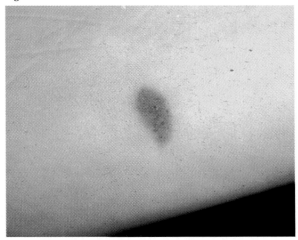

Nevocytic nevus (junction type) The macule of hyperpigmentation here pictured is the most common form of nevocytic nevus in childhood. The so-called junction nevus is a benign lesion that is composed of melanocytic nevus cells along the dermoepidermal junction. Lesions of this sort may arise in crops after the first year of life. As nevus cells migrate into the dermis, the typical junction nevus becomes a compound nevus. This process usually occurs during adolescence and early adulthood.

Figure 746

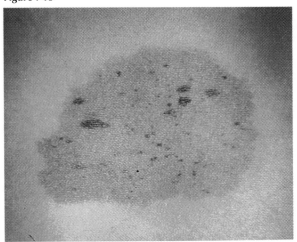

Nevus spilus This is a solitary flat area of light-brown pigmentation that may vary in size from 2 to 25 cm. Illustrated here is the tendency for numerous brown or black freckles of pigmentation to develop on top of the larger and lighter-colored macule. Nevus spilus should not be confused with either a congenital melanocytic nevus or a café-au-lait spot. The nevi within carry no more malignant potential than any other acquired nevus, and no treatment is required.

Figure 747

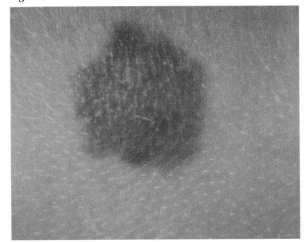

Atypical nevus Nevi that show an irregular mixture of tan, black, brown, and pink and feature an uneven border are termed *atypical nevi*. The central portion may be darker and slightly elevated. The premalignant potential of a solitary atypical-appearing nevus is controversial. However, it is widely recognized that patients with a family history of melanoma and those who have numerous atypical nevi should be observed carefully. Individuals with the so-called atypical mole syndrome are at higher risk for developing melanoma.

Figure 748

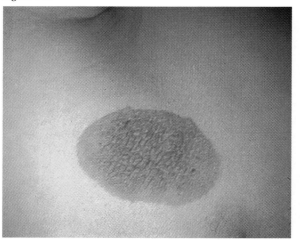

Figure 749

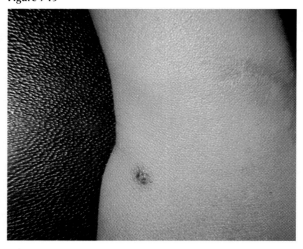

Compound nevus The ordinary mole has great variety in intensity of brown color, size, shape, and location. Those termed *compound nevi* are composed of melanocytes that are gathered into thèques or nests at the dermoepidermal junction and in larger, less compact collections deeper in the dermis. Shown in Fig. 748 is a plaque that is light brown and of fairly large size as compound nevi go. Figure 749 shows a papule that is reddish-brown and of a more usual size. Such lesions are thought to start out as junction nevi, which then go on to more

melanocytic proliferation; melanocytes continue to drop off and down, becoming collections in the dermis. At any time in the development of compound nevi, melanocytes are found both at the dermoepidermal junction and in the dermis. Generally speaking, these lesions are benign and remain so. If cosmetically objectionable, they may be excised in toto or shaved off. Histologic examination of all surgically removed pigmented lesions is advisable.

Figure 750

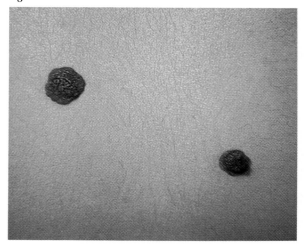

Figure 751

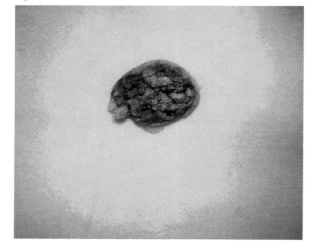

Intradermal nevus The illustrations here are of common moles in which the collections of melanocytes are entirely intradermal. Such lesions do not show any thèques or nests of melanocytes at the dermoepidermal junction. They too come in a great variety of colors, shapes, sizes, and sites. Intradermal nevi are the end stage of development of junction and com-

pound nevi. As with junction and compound nevi, they are extremely common and benign. Like compound nevi, they may be ablated by shaving or elliptical excision. Treatment by these methods does not increase the possibility of malignant transformation.

Figure 752

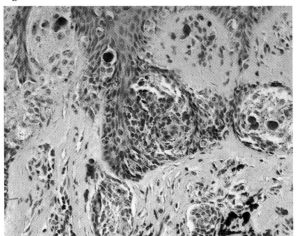

Figure 753

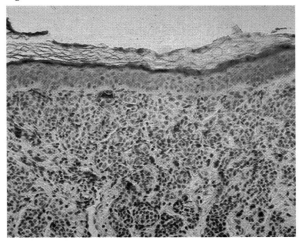

Histopathology of compound and intradermal nevi The precursors of the pigment-producing cells (melanocytes) migrate early in fetal development from the neural crest through the mesenchyme to the epidermis, where they normally remain in the basal (germinative) layer in functional harmony with the more numerous keratinocytes. About every sixth cell in the basal layer is a melanocyte. The melanin that melanocytes produce is transferred by dendrites to nearby keratinocytes. Should melanocytes proliferate but remain with the epidermis, a junction (intraepidermal) nevus forms. The proliferating cells generally gather into nests (thèques) at the tips of rete ridges. If some of these cells "drop" into the dermis, a compound nevus (illustrated on the left) develops. When intraepidermal proliferation of melanocytes ceases and all of them come to be in the corium (illustrated on the right), the nevus is designated *intradermal.*

Figure 754

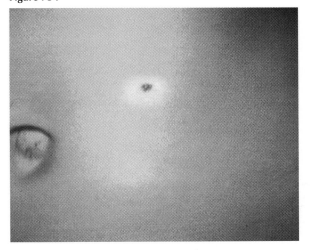

Figure 755

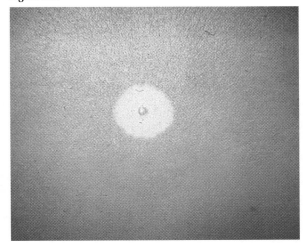

Halo nevus This is a relatively common condition in which an area of depigmentation develops around an existing melanocytic nevus. Lesions of this type, also termed *leukoderma acquisitum centrifugum,* are not unusual during childhood. They may be single or multiple. Figure 754 shows a small halo around a typical compound nevus. Over time, the nevus itself may depigment (Fig. 755) and disappear, and the skin color of the entire area may return to normal. The development of a halo around a nevus is probably due to an immune response to the melanocytes of the original lesion. Halo nevi are more common in children with vitiligo and have been very rarely seen in association with malignant melanoma at another site. For most halo nevi, no treatment is required. When biopsy analysis is performed, there is a dense lymphohistiocytic infiltrate around the central pigmented lesion.

Figure 756

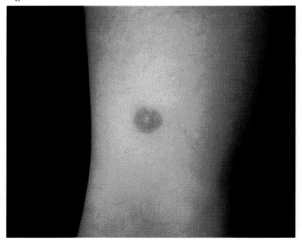

Figure 757

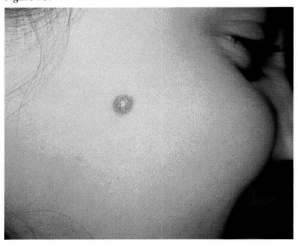

Spitz nevus   This completely benign melanocytic lesion most often occurs during childhood. Spitz nevi are usually solitary, dome-shaped papules or nodules. They frequently arise on the face and extremities. The red-to-red-brown color of the papular lesions in these illustrations is fairly typical. Occasionally, they may be flesh-colored or brown-black. There is often a his-

tory of rapid growth. There are little data on the natural history of these lesions, but the customary treatment consists of a conservative complete excision. Rarely, patients may develop multiple Spitz nevi. These multiple and agminated Spitz nevi may occur over a large café-au-lait spot.

Figure 758

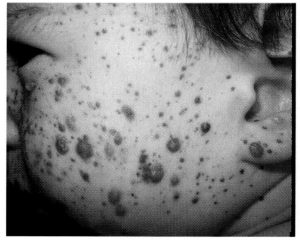

Figure 759

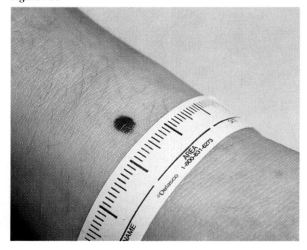

Multiple and agminated Spitz nevi   Rarely, a patient may present with multiple Spitz nevi on an underlying light tan macular base. These patients must be closely observed for the possible development of malignant melanoma.

Pigmented spindle cell nevus   This lesion, first described by Reed, is a variant of a Spitz nevus that is heavily pigmented. Although this lesion is benign, clinically it may mimic a malignant melanoma. Biopsy of such a lesion is advised.

Figure 760

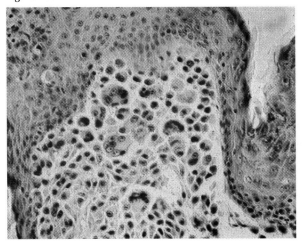

Figure 761

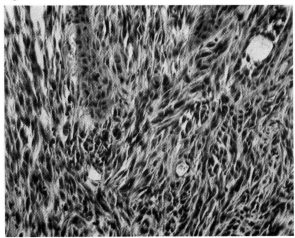

Histopathology of Spitz nevus   Spitz nevus, formerly termed *benign juvenile melanoma,* is felt by most dermatopathologists to be a form of compound nevus. The presence of pleomorphism, numerous mitotic figures, and a dense inflammatory cell infiltrate may at times suggest the diagnosis of nodular malignant melanoma. Before the historic work of the late Dr. Sophie Spitz, many such lesions were in fact misdiagnosed as mela-

noma. Dr. Spitz defined a typical architecture and cell morphology that are associated with a good prognosis. Pictured in Fig. 760 is the nest of large, epithelioid cells, which are typical of this lesion. Spindle cells, the other cell population in Spitz nevus, are shown in Fig. 761. Such lesions have also been termed *spindle-* and *epithelioid-cell nevi.*

Figure 762

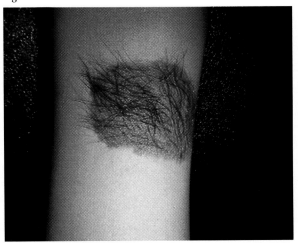

Figure 763

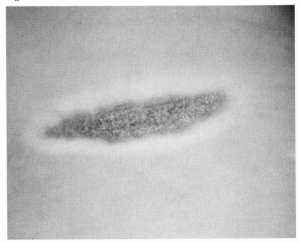

Congenital melanocytic nevus   This pigmented lesion is present at birth in about 1 percent of all infants. The typical appearance is a flat, tan or brown macule of irregular shape. The lesion may be studded with fine papules or may even be nodular. As illustrated here, a congenital melanocytic nevus may develop numerous coarse hairs. Biopsy of a lesion reveals nevus cells in the deep dermis between collagen bundles and adjacent to adnexa. Because the true incidence of malignant melanoma arising in small congenital melanocytic nevi is uncertain, management remains controversial.

Congenital melanocytic nevus   The lesion shown here is surrounded by a border of depigmentation. The occurrence of a halo congenital melanocytic nevus is fairly unusual. The spontaneous regression of a portion of a pigmented lesion is probably due to a host antibody response to a subset of melanocytes. This phenomenon is sometimes associated with the development of melanoma. However, in most cases, the formation of such a halo is a benign event. Complete and spontaneous resolution of even very large congenital melanocytic nevi may occur.

Figure 764

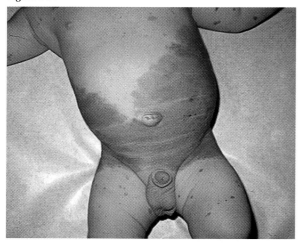

Figure 765

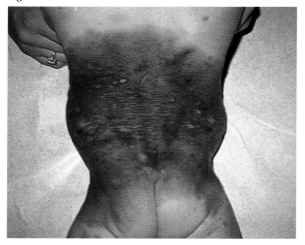

Congenital melanocytic nevus   A congenital melanocytic nevus may cover large parts of the cutaneous surface. A lesion in the distribution illustrated here is sometimes referred to as a bathing trunk nevus. The possibility of malignant melanoma developing within such a large congenital melanocytic nevus represents a significant problem. Varying studies estimate the incidence of this occurrence somewhere between 6 and 36 percent.

Therefore, the excision of giant congenital melanocytic nevi is recommended whenever feasible. The use of inflatable tissue expanders enables the surgeon to remove large portions of lesions like this one without skin grafting. Patients with congenital melanocytic nevi on the scalp or midback must also be investigated for the possibility of leptomeningeal melanocytosis or other neurologic defects.

Figure 766

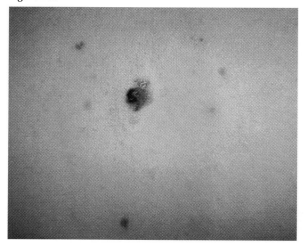

Figure 767

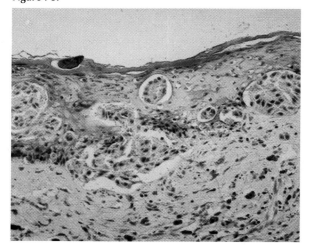

Malignant melanoma   Less than 2 percent of all melanomas occur during childhood. Nonetheless, attention must be paid to signs and symptoms suggestive of this potentially fatal disease. Variegations of color are of particular concern. Irregular or notched borders, bleeding, and ulceration are other signs of malignant change. The patient may give a history of itching, and the parents may have noted rapid growth of the lesion. Because the prognosis of a melanoma is most closely related to the thickness of the lesion at the time of treatment, emphasis should be on early diagnosis.

Histopathology of malignant melanoma   Three types of melanoma may occur in children: superficial spreading, nodular, and acral lentiginous. The commonest is the superficial spreading variety, pictured here. The photomicrograph shows nests of atypical melanocytes lying at all levels of the epidermis. These tumors may have a long phase of radial growth in the epidermis and at the dermoepidermal junction. Eventually, penetration into the dermis occurs, with a rapid worsening of prognosis. Measurements of tumor depth are used to establish prognosis and appropriate therapy.

Figure 768

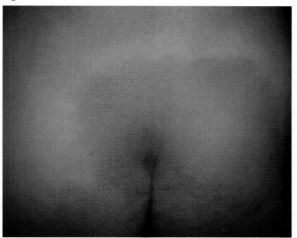

Dermal melanocytosis (mongolian spot) This very common cutaneous lesion is caused by a collection of melanocytes scattered through the deep dermis. The sacral location shown here is by far the most frequent, but dermal melanosis may be present in other areas as well. Mongolian spots are found in many African-American and Asian newborns and are significantly less common among white infants. The areas of blue-gray pigmentation are usually present at birth and almost always fade during the first years of life.

Figure 769

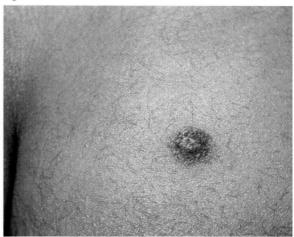

Blue nevus Collections of melanocytes deep in the dermis produce a blue macule or papule such as that illustrated. The physics of color in the skin is such that melanin high in the dermis makes for black coloration, and lower in the dermis, blue. Blue nevi are small, dome-shaped nodules that are often located on the dorsa of the hands or feet. They frequently arise during childhood. The common blue nevus has little or no potential for malignancy. Malignant degeneration of a cellular blue nevus occurs rarely.

Figure 770

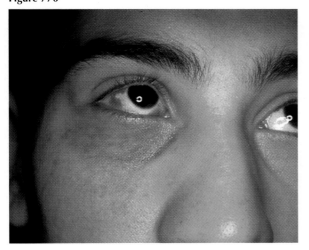

Nevus of Ota This rare dyschromia is characterized by a persistent bluish-gray discoloration of the skin around the eye. The proliferation of melanocytes in the upper dermis may extend to the forehead, malar area, and nose. Ocular involvement always includes the sclera, as in this patient, and sometimes the iris, conjunctiva, and optic nerve. Nevus of Ota is considered a benign dermatosis, but melanoma on the ipsilateral side has been known to occur.

Figure 771

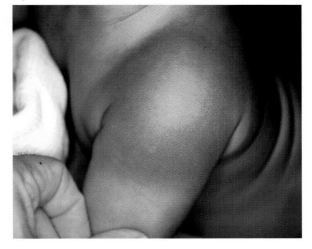

Nevus of Ito The occurrence of a pathological process identical to nevus of Ota but occurring on the skin of the deltoid, scapular, and clavicular regions is termed *nevus of Ito*. The color tends to be somewhat browner than the mongolian spot, because of the distribution of melanocytes higher in the dermis. In contrast to the mongolian spot, these lesions tend to persist through adult life.

Figure 772

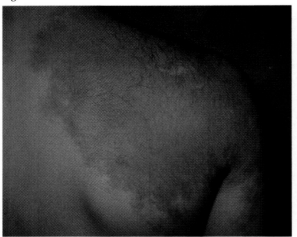

Figure 773

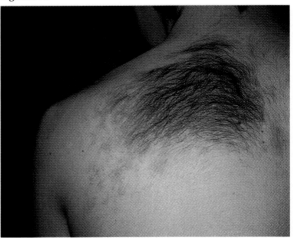

Becker's nevus This lesion is an irregular, pigmented macule that most commonly arises in males at puberty, although it may be seen in females. The light-brown area of pigmentation, which may be quite large, eventually develops thick hairs. The most typical location for Becker's nevus is on the shoulder or upper back. Less commonly, lesions arise on the forearm, upper chest, abdomen, and rarely, the lower extremity. Becker's nevus has no malignant potential, and therefore surgical removal is not necessary. The pigmentation and hypertrichosis both tend to persist into adult life.

24

Miscellaneous Pigmentary Disorders

Figure 774

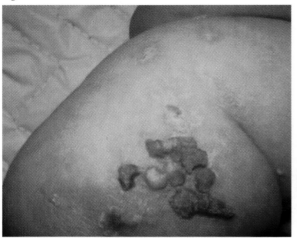

Figure 775

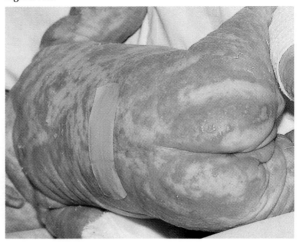

Incontinentia pigmenti This rare condition is characterized by linear and whorled lesions and a wide variety of systemic manifestations. Incontinentia pigmenti is inherited as an X-linked dominant trait and is seen almost exclusively in girls. The cutaneous eruption is usually present at birth and evolves

through three stages. Lesions typical of the first two stages, vesicular and verrucous, are seen in these figures. The vesicular phase of incontinentia pigmenti can be quite extensive and lasts for about 2 weeks. The verrucous phase lasts for about 6 weeks, although it may go on for many months.

Figure 776

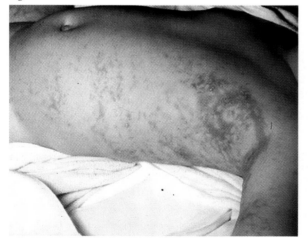

Figure 777

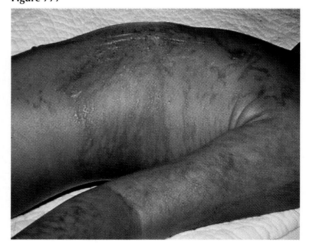

Incontinentia pigmenti Over several months the raised areas flatten, and the patients develops whorled, or "marble-cake," hyperpigmentation, as pictured here. In turn, the lesions of this third, hyperpigmented stage fade over a period of several years. A fourth, hypopigmented stage can develop in the second and third decade. The disorder may also result in scarring alopecia of the scalp, dystrophic nails, and abnormalities of the teeth.

Incontinentia pigmenti This illustration is a good representation of how extensive and bizarre the dyschromia of incontinentia pigmenti can be. Central nervous system and ocular abnormalities are the most serious aspects of this disease. One-third of patients will develop seizures, mental retardation, or spastic paralysis. Eye involvement may include the presence of a retrolental mass, retinal detachment, cataracts, and optic atrophy. Skeletal anomalies are sometimes seen.

Figure 778

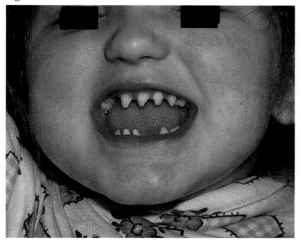

Figure 779

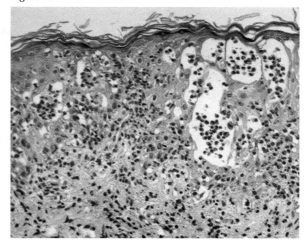

Incontinentia pigmenti   The most common extracutaneous abnormality in incontinentia pigmenti involves teeth and occurs in about two-thirds of patients. There may be a marked delay in the eruption of deciduous teeth. Dental defects such as partial or complete absence of teeth as well as conical teeth may be seen.

Histopathology of incontinentia pigmenti   The three classic stages of incontinentia pigmenti differ histologically and clinically. The third stage, from which the condition derives its name, is microscopically the least specific. In the early vesicular stage, illustrated here, one sees intraepidermal spongiotic blisters containing mainly eosinophils. Both this stage and the second, verrucous, stage display keratinized, eosinophilic malpighian cells, one of which is seen on the left.

Figure 780

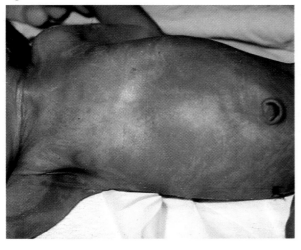

Figure 781

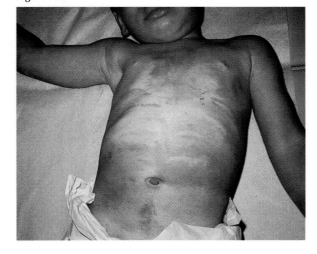

Hypomelanosis of Ito   This condition is characterized by whorled areas of hypopigmentation following lines of Blaschko that are present from birth or evolve during early childhood. The lesions may be generalized, with individual areas of hypopigmentation assuming whorled or streaked patterns. A num-

ber of patients with this pigmentary disorder have central nervous system disease, usually manifest as seizures or mental retardation. Other reported abnormalities include skeletal and ocular defects.

Figure 782

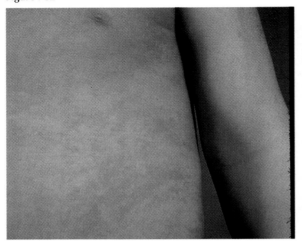

Linear and whorled nevoid hypermelanosis This is a congenital condition characterized by hyperpigmenation that follows lines of Blaschko in a linear pattern on the extremities and a whorled pattern on the trunk. The hyperpigmentation may be present at birth or develops shortly thereafter, spreading during the first two years of life, at which time it stabilizes.

Figure 783

Nevus depigmentosus (achromicus) These are localized areas of hypopigmentation that are usually present at birth. The lesions may be irregular in size and shape and occasionally follow a linear or segmental pattern. Electron microscopic study of these areas suggests that melanosomes are not being transferred from melanocytes into surrounding keratinocytes. There are no associated abnormalities.

Figure 784

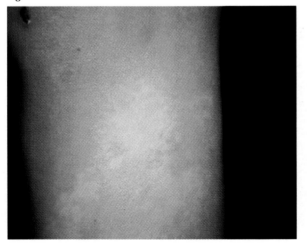

Nevus anemicus This circumscribed area of macular hypopigmentation is due to a localized vascular abnormality. Chest and back are the most common locations. In contrast to nevus depigmentosus, erythema does not develop in response to stroking or the application of ice or warm water. Hypersensitivity of the involved vessels to catecholamines has been postulated as a cause.

Figure 785

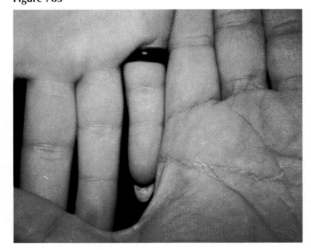

Carotenemia The vegetable pigment carotene is widely distributed in carrots, lettuce, squash, and many other vegetables and fruits. A diet that is very rich in these foods results in a yellowish-orange discoloration of the skin. This appearance is usually localized to the palms and soles (note the hand on the left) but may also involve the skin of the face. The presence of normal sclerae distinguishes the clinical appearance of this condition from that of jaundice. Return to normal skin color follows a reduction in dietary intake of carotene.

Figure 786

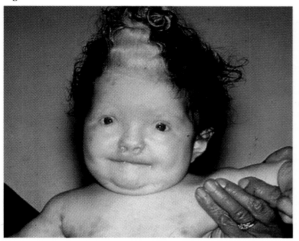

Figure 787

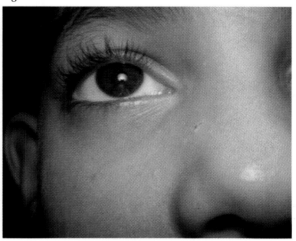

Waardenburg's syndrome　This genetic disorder is transmitted as an autosomal dominant, with variable penetrance. It is characterized grossly by partial albinism in the form of a white forelock (Fig. 786), broad nasal root (Figs. 786 and 787), hypertrichosis of the inner portions of the eyebrows, lateral displacement of the medial canthi (Figs. 786 and 787), partial or complete heterochromia of the irides (Fig. 787), and complete or unilateral deafness. In African-Americans, blue irides, vitiligo, and pigmentary changes in the fundi may be seen. There are no other constitutional symptoms, but the hearing loss and unusual appearance may pose handicaps.

Figure 788

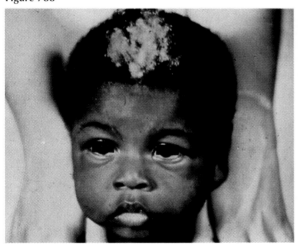

Figure 789

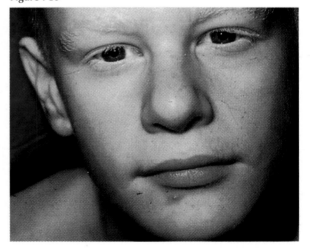

Piebaldism　Patients with this autosomal dominant condition have congenital patches of depigmentation. Most have a white forelock, with involvement of adjoining scalp and forehead in a triangular pattern. There may be other areas of involvement on the trunk and extremities. Electron microscopic examination of affected areas reveals a complete absence of melanocytes. Management must include the appropriate use of sunscreen lotions on depigmented skin.

Albinism　This condition is characterized by congenital hypopigmentation of the skin, hair, and eyes. Almost all of the many varieties are inherited in autosomal recessive fashion. Photophobia is a significant problem for most patients. The lack of protective melanin leads to extreme sun sensitivity and results in a high incidence of actinic keratoses, basal cell carcinomas, and squamous cell carcinomas. The avoidance of sun exposure through the use of protective clothing and sunscreen preparations is critical.

Figure 790

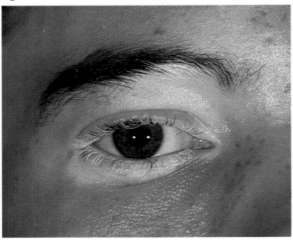

Figure 791

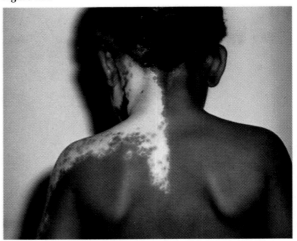

Vitiligo About one-half of patients with vitiligo have onset of their disease during childhood or adolescence. Patients may present with hypopigmented and depigmented macules of various sizes and shapes. The area of involvement surrounding the eye in Fig. 790 represents one fairly typical distribution. Note the associated depigmentation of eyebrows and eyelashes. Periorificial vitiligo may also involve the skin around the mouth, rectum, and genitalia. Vitiligo may occur only on the distal ex-

tremities or may be unilateral and segmental, as in Fig. 791. Vitiligo may be associated with uveitis and peripheral retinal scarring, but these changes rarely affect vision. The frequent presence of antibodies to melanocytes in individuals with vitiligo suggests an autoimmune etiology. A number of other autoimmune disorders, including Addison's disease and Hashimoto's thyroiditis, are more common among patients with vitiligo and their relatives.

Figure 792

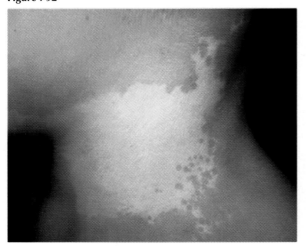

Figure 793

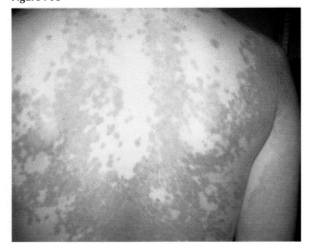

Vitiligo These are more illustrations of fairly extensive cases of vitiligo. The condition tends to progress and may even become universal. A variety of treatment modalities are commonly employed, with varying degrees of success. The patient and family should be made aware of the sophisticated cover-up cosmetics that are now available. The use of broad-spectrum sun-

screen lotions during the summer months minimizes the contrast between normal and involved skin. For some patients, the application of topical corticosteroids early in the course of the disease may induce repigmentation. Finally, varying combinations of topical or oral psoralens and ultraviolet A light (PUVA) are used in the treatment of vitiligo.

Figure 794

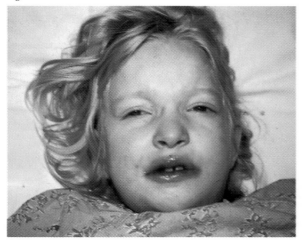

Chédiak-Higashi syndrome   This genetic disorder, recessive in mechanism of transmission, is extremely rare. It is characterized by albinism, photophobia, lymphadenopathy, hepatosplenomegaly, and susceptibility to pyogenic infection. The peripheral blood smear reveals giant granules within lymphocytes. The high incidences of serious infection and lymphoreticular malignancy contribute to a poor prognosis.

Figure 795

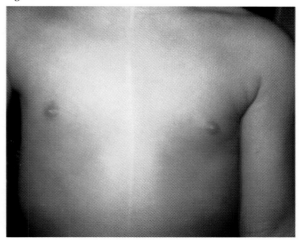

Linea alba   This linear stripe of hypopigmentation in the mid-chest and abdomen is termed *linea alba. Linea nigra* is its hyperpigmented counterpart. This is one of several locations for the extremely common and completely benign pigmentary demarcation lines. Other sites include the upper lateral arms, the mid–posterior legs, and the central back. There may also be two symmetrical lines crossing from the midclavicle to the areolae.

Figure 796

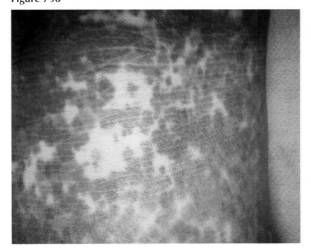

Postinflammatory hypopigmentation   A wide variety of dermatologic diseases may leave either temporary or permanent hypopigmentation. Figure 796 shows loss of pigment in the popliteal fossa of a child who has atopic dermatitis. This process results from the inflammatory disease itself and from chronic scratching. The same phenomenon is shown on the face in Fig. 797. This is probably also the result of atopic dermatitis. Postinflammatory hypopigmentation can usually be easily differenti-

Figure 797

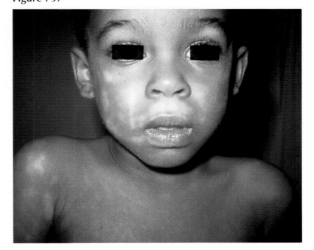

ated from vitiligo. The lesions that follow inflammatory skin disease are less well defined and are more off-white than stark white. The symmetry that may occur in vitiligo is not seen here. For most children, postinflammatory hypopigmentation is temporary. Parents should be reassured that even the most disfiguring patterns of pigmentary alteration will resolve with proper therapy and time.

25

Artifacts

Figure 798

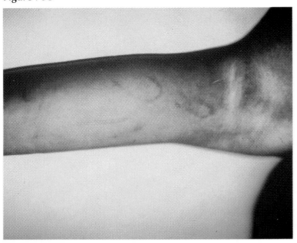

Figure 799

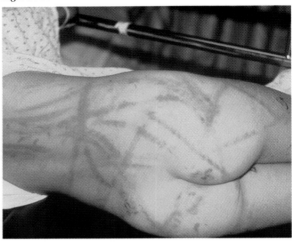

Child abuse The physical abuse of children accounts for many deaths each year in the United States. Physicians who care for children must acquaint themselves with the signs of battering, sexual abuse, and nutritional deprivation. For the protection of children, the laws in all states require the reporting of all cases of suspected child abuse. Illustrated here are typical loop marks in a child who was struck with a doubled-over

rope or electrical cord. The presence of ecchymoses or scars on the lower back or buttocks is almost always the result of physical abuse. Slap marks, human bites, and lash marks each leave bruises of a distinctive shape and distribution. The presence of bruises of this sort is evidence of force used without restraint and is a definite sign of child abuse.

Figure 800

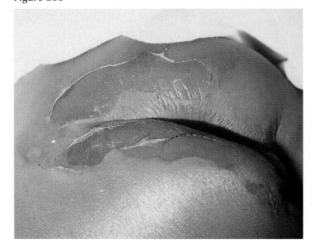

Figure 801

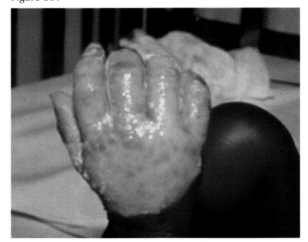

Child abuse Ten percent of the cases of physical abuse in children involve the deliberate infliction of burns as a form of punishment. Cigarette burns, which appear as uniform round erosions, are often located on the palms and soles. Second-degree burns may also occur when a child is held against a radiator or hot plate. Illustrated here are two burns that resulted from forcible immersion in hot water. Symmetrical blistering of

the perineum (Fig. 800) is evidence of a child being lowered into a hot bath. Figure 801 is illustrative of forcible immersion of a hand. In general, the presence of an injury for which the history seems implausible should alert the physician to the possibility of child abuse. A delay in seeking medical assistance for the care of an injury should also cause concern.

Figure 802

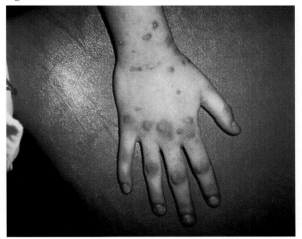

Figure 803

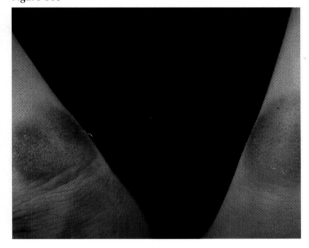

Factitial dermatitis   Injuries to the skin that are induced by the patient or another individual are termed *factitial dermatitis.* This entity, when it occurs in childhood, may be related to a variety of emotional disturbances in either parent or child. The lesions in Fig. 802 are self-inflicted wounds caused by bites. Some are scars and others are inflammatory lesions. The distribution and morphology of lesions of this type are not consistent with any known cutaneous disease, and there is usually no credible history for their development. Other methods of inducing self-injury include scratching, picking, and gouging. The hypertrichosis in Fig. 803 resulted from repeated biting on the skin in a child with severe mental retardation. Self-mutilation of this type is also seen in the Lesch-Nyhan syndrome.

Figure 804

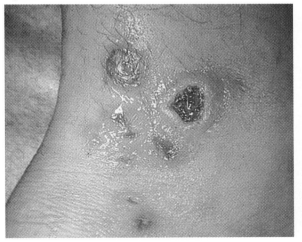

Figure 805

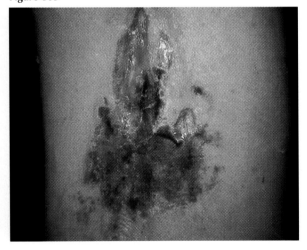

Factitial dermatitis   Figure 804 shows ecthymatous lesions that might have been produced by fingernails. Figure 805 shows the sort of lesions caused by caustic chemicals. Self-induced injury of this sort is associated with a wide range of emotional disturbances or psychiatric disease. Healing of lesions can sometimes be facilitated by occlusion of the area of skin that is being repeatedly injured. Psychiatric referral is often of value.

A particular cause of factitial dermatitis in children is termed *Munchausen syndrome by proxy.* In this condition, a disturbed parent attempts to create the appearance of illness in a child. The presence of this syndrome signals a high level of physical danger for the child, and cases of this sort must be promptly reported to social service agencies as a form of child abuse.

Figure 806

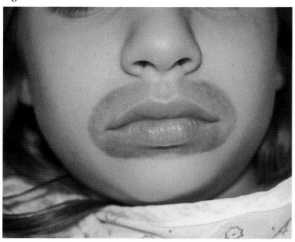

Figure 807

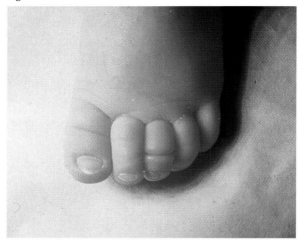

Factitial dermatitis The presence of a localized purpuric eruption in the circumoral area may not indicate a serious disease. This condition is caused by sucking on a glass or cup, creating a negative pressure around the mouth, resulting in the presence of purpura.

Pseudoainhum The word ainhum means "to saw." True ainhum is limited geographically to Africa and usually presents as a groove encircling the small toe. Pseudoainhum refers to a condition that is clinically similar but caused by a wide variety of disease processes. In children, congenital constricting bands may be a cause. More commonly, pseudoainhum occurs as an artifact from the wind of a cord or a long hair buried around a digit. In this illustration, the third toe is affected by a groove whose cause was indeed a buried hair.

Figure 808

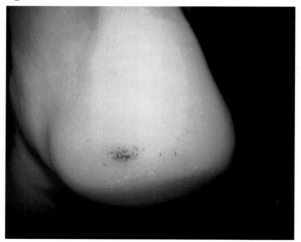

Talon noir (black heel) Stigmata caused by certain operations in occupations and avocations are characteristic. The bump on the radial aspect of the middle finger of a scribe and the callused fingertips of a violinist are examples. The illustration here is of punctate and ecchymotic hemorrhages in a heel of a basketball player. There is something about basketball playing in its jumps, twists, and turns that promotes this type of lesion. Its only significance is that it should not be mistaken for malignant melanoma.

Figure 809

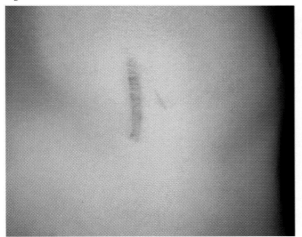

Figure 810

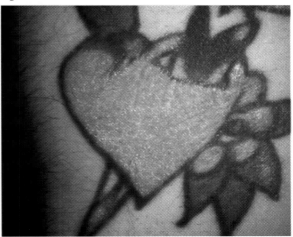

Tattoos The deposition into skin of inert materials that produce colored effects may be accidental or premeditated. The usual material that enters skin accidentally is carbon from mischance, such as fire blast, abrasion on dirty surfaces, and stabs of sharp pencils. Figure 809 shows a stripe of blue color resulting from an incised wound incurred in a fall on a tarred pavement.; Figure 810 is a conventional tattoo placed by a tattoo artist. The pigments used by tattooists to produce colors are carbon for blue and black, cinnabar or cochineal for red, cadmium salts for yellow, and cobalt salts for green. These materials are inert, but on occasion granulomas (Fig. 810) develop, especially from cinnabar. The color produced by carbon is black if placed superficially and progressively dark to light blue the deeper it is placed. The use of lasers for removal can be quite successful.

26

Disorders of Nails and Hair

Figure 811

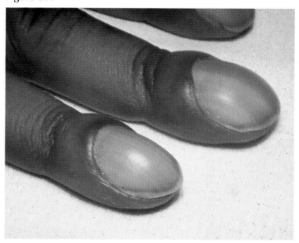

Clubbed nails   Increased curvature of the nail plate may be due to a wide variety of causes. In this patient, the large, convex nails are a hereditary anomaly and were found to be present in both father and brother. Other causes of clubbing of the nails in children include cyanotic congenital heart disease, cystic fibrosis, and chronic inflammatory bowel disease.

Figure 812

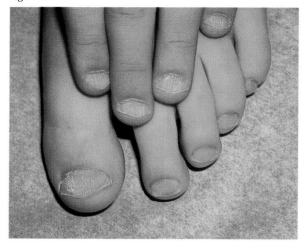

Trachyonychia (twenty nail dystrophy of childhood)   Any skin disease that affects the nail matrix may result in an abnormal nail plate. There are children, though, who only manifest dystrophy of the nail without any other cutaneous lesions, a condition that has been termed *twenty nail dystrophy of childhood.* The nails have a rough, sandpaper-like quality as well as longitudinal ridging and occasional splitting at the distal nail edge. Similar nail changes can be seen in lichen planus and alopecia areata. In many patients the condition spontaneously regresses.

Figure 813

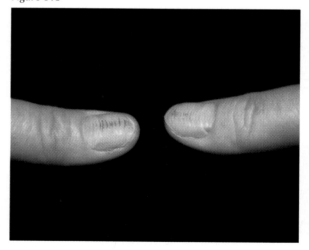

Traumatic onychodystrophy   Trauma to the nail plate or nail folds can produce a wide variety of nail deformities. The one pictured here is the result of a habit tic. This common nail dystrophy is characterized by a longitudinal canal that runs down the center of the entire nail plate. It is caused by manipulation of the proximal nail fold by the index finger of the same hand.

Figure 814

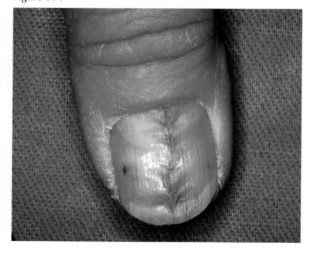

Dystrophia unguis mediana canaliformis   This is a rare condition of unknown etiology that usually involves the thumb. It consists of a canal that runs near the center of the length of the nail plate. Small cracks which that extend laterally from the linear canal give the appearance of an inverted fir tree. This deformity tends to resolve spontaneously over a period of months but often recurs.

Figure 815

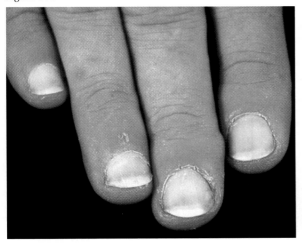

Leukonychia totalis This is a rare nail disorder that is inherited in autosomal dominant fashion. The color of normal nail plates beyond the lunulae is largely pink from the blood in the blood vessels of the nail bed. The whiteness shown here is due to an abnormality in the nail plate. The nails may also be brittle.

Figure 816

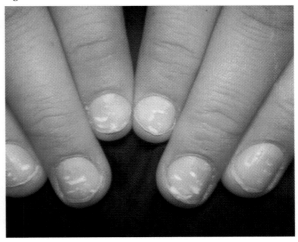

Leukonychia striata The horizontal white streaks pictured here are the result of abnormal keratinization of the nail plate. The tendency toward leukonychia striata is sometimes inherited in an autosomal dominant fashion. In other cases, it can be attributed to vigorous manicuring, to trauma, or to a wide variety of systemic illnesses. In many patients, there is no obvious cause, and the streaks resolve spontaneously.

Figure 817

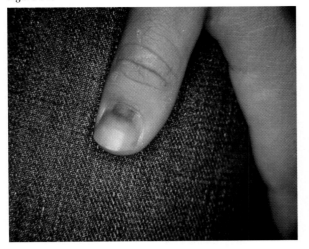

Onycholysis (drug-induced) This word means separation (*-lysis*) of nails (*onycho-*) from nail beds. There are many causes for such a development. The commonest are mechanical. Nails worn long are frequently lifted by being snagged. Excessive soaping and soaking in heavy housework promote separation. The illustration here is of another cause, namely, an idiopathic response by photosensitivity in a patient who had been taking demethylchlortetracycline.

Figure 818

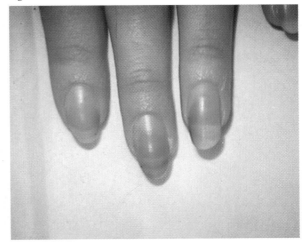

Discoloration of nail plates Many chemicals can discolor nail plates. Solutions of potassium permanganate and silver nitrate stain nail plates brown-purple and jet black, respectively. In the case illustrated here, the stain derived from resorcinol. Such stains are harmless and can be easily removed by superficial scaling with the edge of a glass slide.

Figure 819

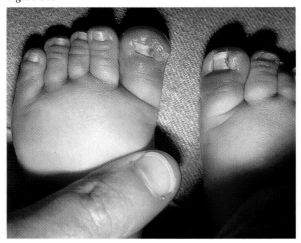

Figure 820

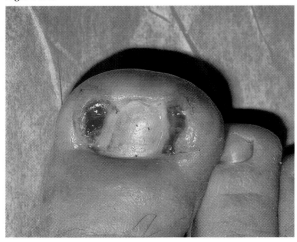

Congenital ingrown toenail   Shortly after birth deformity of the great toe, unilaterally or bilaterally, may occur. Thickening of the lateral nail folds and hyponychium with erythema, edema, and sometimes secondary infection may occur. The growth of the nail may protrude through this thickening at its distal end. This condition is sometimes due to congenital malalignment of the nail plates. Surgical treatment is rarely necessary, as the condition is self-limited with good resolution. Secondary infection should be treated if present.

Ingrown toenail   Improper trimming of nails may lead to the formation of an ingrown toenail. The lateral or medial nail fold becomes erythematous, edematous, and painful with the nail growing into the fleshy portion of the folds. Secondary infection and the formation of granulation tissue typically ensue. Surgical treatment is often necessary when local wound care measures fail to alleviate this condition.

Figure 821

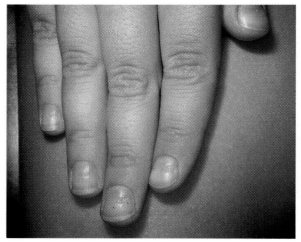

Beau's lines   These transverse lines or furrows begin at the proximal nail fold and grow out with the nail. They represent a brief interference of nail growth secondary to physical stress such as an illness or nutritional deficiency. The lines are not noticed until several weeks after the precipitating event.

Figure 822

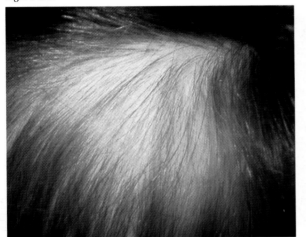

Figure 823

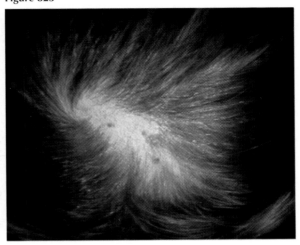

Trichotillomania This is a form of alopecia that is caused by the child's twisting or pulling of his or her own hair. This cause of hair loss is usually easy to recognize. There is often, but not always, a parental awareness of hair-pulling behavior sometimes while the child is studying or watching television or at bedtime. The area of hair loss is usually asymmetric and follows an irregular pattern. Examination of the involved area reveals hairs that are broken off at different lengths. There is never the total hair loss of alopecia areata or the scaling and erythema of tinea capitis. In most cases, trichotillomania is evidence of an innocent and benign habit that is best compared to nail biting. However, trichotillomania may sometimes be evidence of more severe emotional distress. In addition, children who swallow their plucked hairs may develop a gastric trichobezoar. The daily application, by the child if possible, of petrolatum to the affected areas is a useful maneuver. It serves as a reminder to stop pulling or twirling, and it makes the hair slippery and hard to pull out.

Figure 824

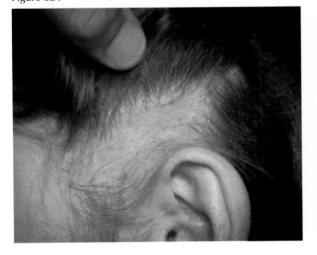

Figure 825

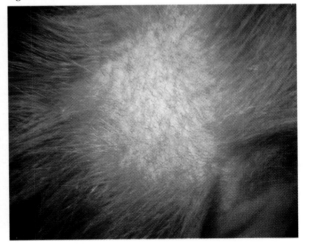

Traumatic alopecia Another traumatic form of alopecia is due to hairstyles that feature braiding with excessive tension. The photograph in Fig. 824 shows hair loss caused by a ponytail. Cornrows or excessively tight braids have a similar effect. The alopecia in this condition is limited to the line of the hair part or to the margins of the scalp. Careful examination reveals broken hairs of varying lengths and sometimes a localized folliculitis. The application of heat or of chemicals to straighten hair will also damage the hair shafts and cause traumatic alopecia. An example of this phenomenon is illustrated in Fig. 825. For most cases of traumatic alopecia, a change in hairstyle is the only treatment that is required.

Figure 826

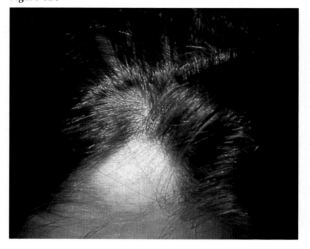

Figure 827

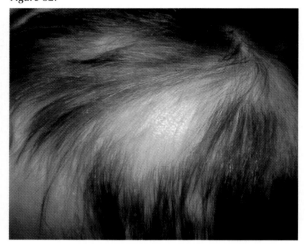

Alopecia areata The children pictured in Figs. 826 and 827 are typical of the most common presentation of alopecia areata. There is usually a history of the abrupt onset of hair loss in one or several circumscribed round or oval patches. There is no history of pruritus or scaling. The occasional association of alopecia areata with diseases such as lymphocytic thyroiditis and vitiligo suggests a possible autoimmune etiology. Fortunately, spontaneous regrowth occurs in most patients over a period of 6 months to 1 year. Prognosis is less favorable in patients with more widespread disease and earlier onset. During the initial onset, parents and children should be counseled with cautious optimism but forewarned that progression of the disorder may occur or that it may recur after a period of complete recovery. The use of topical and intralesional corticosteroids or of topical anthralin ointment seems to hasten the resolution of the process.

Figure 828

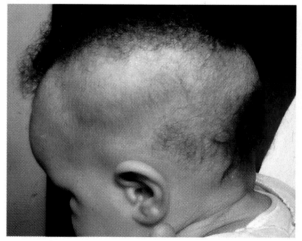

Figure 829

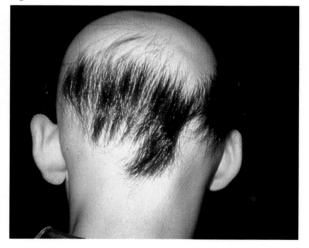

Alopecia areata Illustrated in Fig. 828 is ophiasis, a form of alopecia in which hair loss progresses along the margin of the scalp. Figure 829 is a severe example of alopecia areata that is progressing toward alopecia totalis. Both ophiasis and extensive alopecia areata carry a poor prognosis for regrowth. The use of intralesional steroids in patients with such extensive disease is extremely painful. Topical agents that cause either an irritant or contact dermatitis of the scalp may sometimes stimulate hair growth. However, they do not seem to affect the tendency toward progression and repeated recurrences in patients with severe involvement. Certainly, alopecia areata has enormous implications for the self-image of the affected child or adolescent. Wigs are sometimes helpful. Patients and families should be advised of the availability of support groups related to this disease.

Figure 830

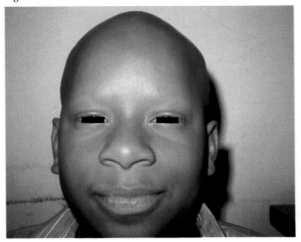

Alopecia universalis   This is the severest expression of the alopecia areata disease process. Complete loss of scalp hair is termed *alopecia totalis*. The patient pictured here has also lost all of his eyebrows, eyelashes, and axillary, body, and pubic hair. Hence, alopecia universalis. The prognosis in this situation is particularly poor, with little chance of responding to therapy or of experiencing spontaneous recovery.

Figure 831

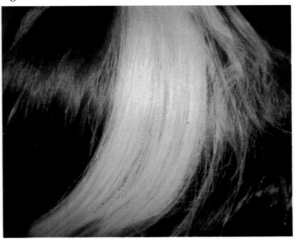

Alopecia areata (recovered)   This illustration is of regrowth of hair in a patch of alopecia areata. The oddity is that the regrowth was with white hair. The phenomenon is not unusual and is temporary. Eventually the regrowth will be in a color that is normal for the patient. It also frequently happens that regrown hair is temporarily of different texture. In time, assuming no relapse, completely normal color and texture supervene.

Figure 832

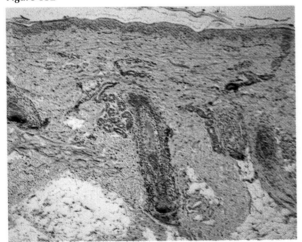

Figure 833

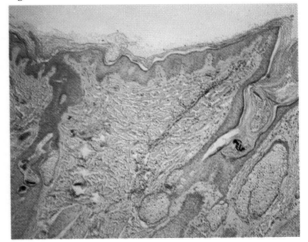

Histopathology of alopecia areata and trichotillomania   Alopecia areata and trichotillomania may at times be difficult to tell apart clinically. Histologically, they are readily distinguished. In alopecia areata (illustrated on the left) hair follicles become diminutive but continue to produce fine hairs. Often there is inflammation, seen here surrounding the centrally situated follicle. At high magnification one can observe mitotic activity in the matrix of the hair bulb, indicating residual viability. In trichotillomania (illustrated on the right) the follicles are not reduced in size, but they no longer produce normal hair shafts. Instead one finds keratinous debris within the pilary canals, which, moreover, are no longer straight, and clumps of dark melanin pigment, seen in both the follicles. In other types of diffuse alopecia, biopsy analysis is of little value. In conditions that terminate in permanent alopecia, scarring can be observed microscopically.

Figure 834

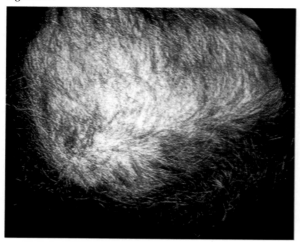

Monilethrix   This word means "beaded hair" and designates a condition in which the hair varies in thickness along its length. Inheritance is autosomal dominant. The result is that the hair remains dry and brittle and fractures easily. Children with this condition may have normal neonatal hairs, but the hair that begins to grow in the second or third month of life will fracture before reaching a normal length. The condition may resolve spontaneously over time or persist into adult life.

Figure 835

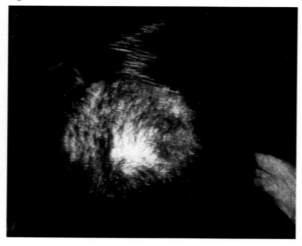

Trichorrhexis nodosa   This is another anomaly of hair growth. It is characterized by dry, fragile hair and results in patches of partial alopecia. The second word in the condition's name derives from the presence of whitish nodes along the hair shaft. These nodes are the site of breakage. This disorder is sometimes, though very rarely, associated with argininosuccinicaciduria and mental retardation. The acquired forms are far more common and seem to be the combined result of trauma to the hair and a genetic predisposition.

Figure 836

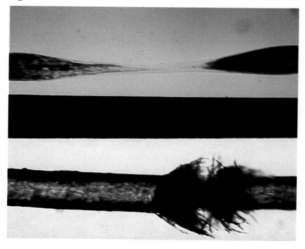

Monilethrix and trichorrhexis nodosa (magnified appearance of hair shafts)   Use of a hand lens or low-power magnification by microscope reveals the anomalies in the hair shafts. The upper part of the figure shows the hair in monilethrix. The nodes are strung on a thin, internodal shaft. The lower part of the picture shows the distinctive appearance of the hair in trichorrhexis nodosa. The nodes look like brushes or brooms. Breakage of hair occurs at the weak internodes of monilethrix and at the brushlike nodes of trichorrhexis nodosa.

Figure 837

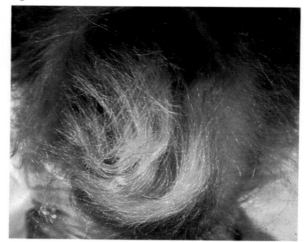

Pili torti   The title means twisted *(torti)* hairs *(pili)*. The gross clinical appearance is of diffuse alopecia and dry, fragile hair. Magnification of hairs in this condition reveals spiral twists at irregular intervals along the long axes of the shafts. Pili torti is seen in association with a number of enzyme deficiencies and hereditary syndromes, including citrullinemia and Bazex syndrome. It may also be associated with sensorineural hearing loss. No effective treatment is available.

Figure 838

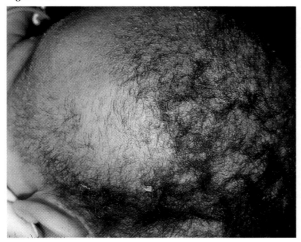

Figure 839

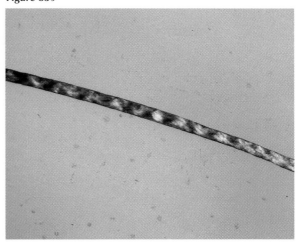

Trichothiodystrophy The term *trichothiodystrophy* describes brittle hair with an abnormally low sulfur content. There are different syndromes that have trichothiodystrophy as a feature along with other findings, including intellectual impairment, decreased fertility, short stature, ichthyosis, and photosensitivity. The hair is short, sparse, and brittle (Fig. 838). Examination of the hair shaft under polarizing light microscopy reveals alternating light and dark bands giving the hair a "tiger-tail" appearance (Fig. 839). The disorder is transmitted in an autosomal recessive fashion. It is unknown whether the different syndromes that have trichothiodystrophy as a feature are distinct entities or represent a single variable syndrome.

Figure 840

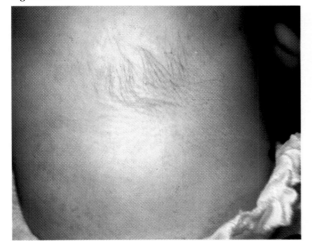

Figure 841

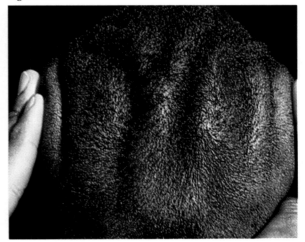

Nevoid hypertrichosis Illustrated here is a hamartoma consisting entirely of hair follicles. A small lesion of this type is completely benign and unimportant. The presence of a patch of hypertrichosis overlying the mid–lower back, however, may be an indication of a significant underlying neurologic abnormality. The so-called faun tail nevus may signal the presence of spina bifida occulta, diastematomyelia, or duplication or tethering of the spinal cord. A thorough neurologic investigation is warranted in such cases.

Cutis verticis gyrata Scalp skin sometimes develops redundantly as a congenital anomaly or in association with a disease such as acromegaly. The consequence is furrowed wrinkling of hyperplastic skin in a pattern that suggests the puzzled pate of a bulldog, in whom the condition is natural. There are cases that are so extreme that hygiene of the scalp is difficult and the cosmetic appearance justifiably disturbing. Plastic surgery is a reasonable treatment.

27

Miscellaneous Anomalies

Figure 842

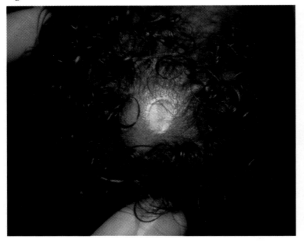

Figure 843

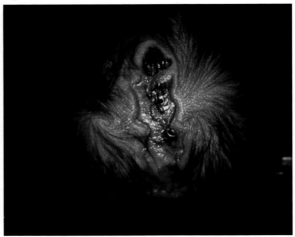

Aplasia cutis congenita　Among the many hazards of intrauterine development and sojourn is failure at times to achieve complete congenital integrity of the integument. It sometimes happens that a child is born with a superficial erosion, as in Fig. 842, or an ulcer, as in Fig. 843. The vertex of the scalp is a common place for the phenomenon to occur; the hands, face, and points over bony prominences are also susceptible. Aplasia cutis congenita is frequently a benign event of only cosmetic importance and in most cases the etiology is not established. However, epidermolysis bullosa, placental infarction, terato-

gens, and some chromosome deletions and trisomies are occasionally implicated as causes. A lesion may be directly adjacent to an epidermal nevus or nevus sebaceus, or it may overlie a defect in the bone. More significant underlying anomalies are meningomyeloceles, spinal dysraphisms, and various cerebral malformations. Hemorrhage and secondary infection may occur, requiring emergency treatment. The combination of aplasia cutis congenita and distal limb reduction is an additional inherited disorder.

Figure 844

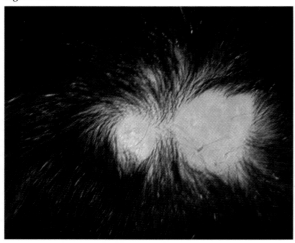

Figure 845

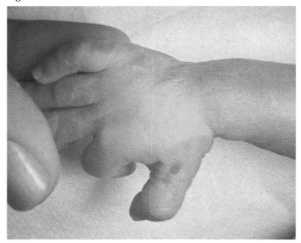

Aplasia cutis congenita　These are examples of cutaneous aplasias that have healed into parchment-like scars. This process may occur in utero or shortly after birth. Figure 844 pictures a lesion that healed postpartum. Note that the defect involved the full thickness of skin and resulted in destruction of the pilar adnexa. In consequence, the scar, healed by secondary intention, is quite bald. In Fig. 845 the same sort of thing is shown on the dorsum of the hand and parts adjacent; it could pass as a scar

consequent to an ordinary thermal burn. Aside from the cosmetic defect, the scars of healed congenital aplasias are good and ordinarily serve normal function well enough. In place like the scalp, alopecic scars of large size that cannot be adequately covered by surrounding hair can be restored to near normal by hair transplants, which fortunately take quite well. In other places, plastic revision could correct undesirable sequelae such as adhesions, if such have occurred.

Figure 846

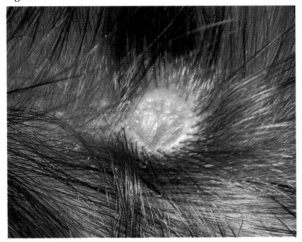

Aplasia cutis congenita Sometimes a thicker, darker growth of hair may be seen around the lesion of aplasia cutis congenita on the scalp. The "hair collar sign" may be a marker for cranial dysraphism such as encephalocele, agenesis of the corpus callosum, and heterotopic brain tissue. This may be a form fruste of a neural tube defect.

Figure 847

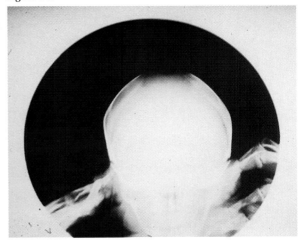

Aplasia cutis congenita This radiograph represents a case of aplasia cutis congenita associated with a significant underlying skull defect. Smaller defects of the skull may occur with smaller cutaneous lesions. These smaller bony defects usually heal in a few months. The larger lesions may require neurosurgical repair.

Figure 848

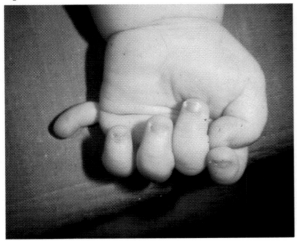

Supernumerary digits Supernumerary digits, like other supernumerary structures, come in all degrees of development, from merest suggestion to nearly full reduplication. This figure shows a fairly well-developed extra digit containing bones, musculature, and nerves and situated in a common site just beyond the last natural finger. More commonly, the vestige consists of a small nubbin of soft tissue in the same location. Treatment is by surgical excision.

Figure 849

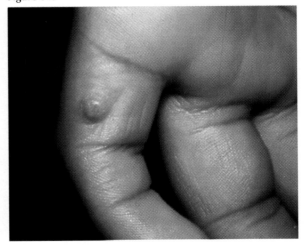

Amputation neuroma Although surgical removal of a supernumerary digit is a technically simple operation, a rare complication is illustrated here. It is an amputation neuroma, a knot of neural tissue formed at the site of the wound of an operation for removal of a structure that had nerves within it. Such a lesion can be tender to touch, spontaneously painful, and possibly productive of phantom symptoms. Reexcision is obviously necessary.

Figure 850

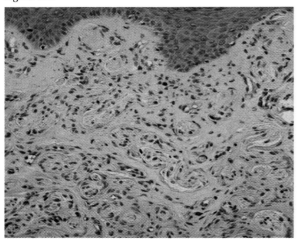

Histopathology of amputation neuroma Small papules found at birth on the ulnar aspect of the fifth finger are remnants of supernumerary digits (pedunculated postminimi). Similar papules may develop after attempted surgical ablation of supernumerary digits. They show the same histopathology as digital traumatic neuromas regardless of cause. In the photomicrograph, one sees marked proliferation of nerves in dense collagenous stroma and Wagner-Meissner corpuscles in the dermal papillae.

Figure 851

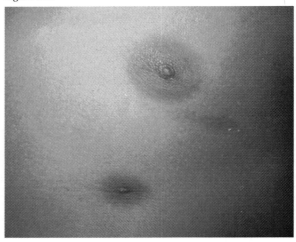

Supernumerary nipple Supernumerary nipples are exceedingly common in both sexes. In women, more than mere nipples, considerable mammary glands may develop along the "milk lines" from axillae to pubes. In males, one or a pair of supernumerary nipples are common enough; two, even three, complete pairs are still not rare. The degree of development may be from vestiges that could be taken for common pigmented moles to well-developed ones like those pictured.

Figure 852

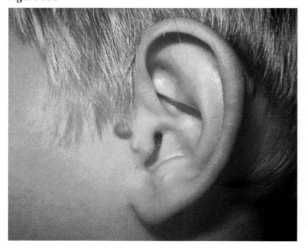

Auricular tags Supernumerary vestiges of the external structures of ears are common. Accessory tragi and auricular tags with or without communication to deeper structures may be deceptively simple. Those in Fig. 852 are probably harmless nubs of tissue that could be sliced off and their bases delicately electrodesiccated. Should that be all there is, the cosmetic result would be fine. Sometimes, however, such structures bear cartilage within them and have communication to uncertain depths

Figure 853

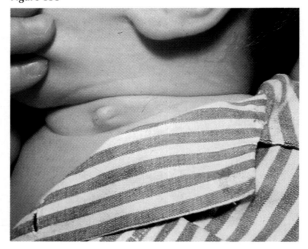

toward the more important structures in the external canal or middle ear. In Fig. 853 there is a bit of reduplicated auricular tissue that had been displaced onto the neck. Again, the anomalous tissue could be easily excised if it had no communication deeper and upward. In the latter event, more thorough dissection of the entire structure would be required. It is not an office procedure.

Figure 854

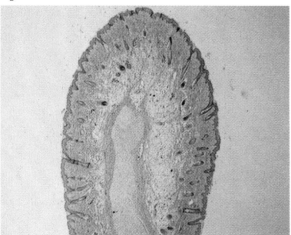

Histopathology of accessory tragi Papules near the normal tragus of the ear are usually rudimentary accessory tragi. In such lesions, one sees epidermis, from which are derived many fine hair–producing follicles. Deep to the dermis, a layer of adipose tissue surrounding a central core of cartilage may often be found. Even if a cartilaginous core is not present, the other features mentioned are sufficient to distinguish an accessory tragus from a soft fibroma.

Figure 855

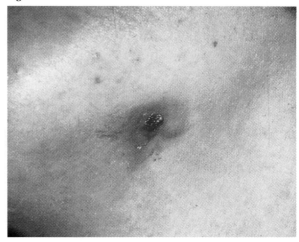

Dental sinus Infection at or around the apex of a tooth may become an abscess that burrows toward exit on the skin. The simplest situation is a channel from a tooth in the lower jaw onto the skin over the mandible, on the underside of the chin or jaw, or on the neck. The presenting lesion may appear, like the one pictured, at the junction of jaw and neck, as a superficial pyoderma or an infected cyst. Simple drainage and topical antisepsis fail to cure. Discovery and extirpation of the internal source are required.

Figure 856

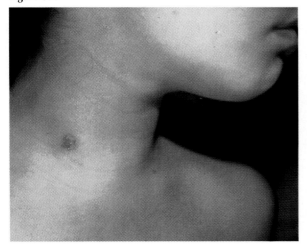

Branchial-cleft cysts The embryogenesis of the head and neck must be a fetus's nightmare. Because so many structures have to come together perfectly from both sides, it is remarkable that they ever do. But they almost always do. An occasional failure of perfect coaptation is to be expected. Cleft palate and cleft lips are well known and easily recognizable. More subtle is failure of perfect development of the branchial arches. The usual clinical lesion is an insignificant-looking

Figure 857

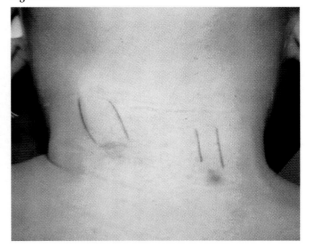

papule or small cystic mass on one side of the neck, anteriorly off center. Figure 856 shows such a lesion. Figure 857 shows a much rarer bilateral anomaly of this nature. Surgical ablation of such embryonic errors is not easy. It takes an operator skilled in head and neck surgery to trace out the unexpected twists and turns of such cysts and sinuses from important structures of the region.

Figure 858

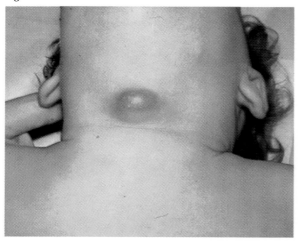

Figure 859

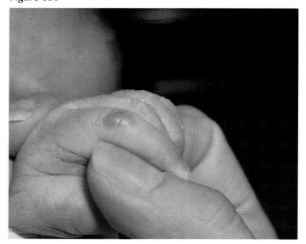

Thyroglossal cyst   This is another example of a dysraphism of midline structures. Thyroglossal cysts and fistulas are similar in appearance to branchial cleft malformations but are usually midline and located near the hyoid bone. These lesions may become complicated by enlargement or secondary infection. Careful excision is recommended.

Sucking blister   The oval blister pictured here was present at birth and is a result of normal sucking behavior in utero. Sucking blisters are fairly common and are usually located on the forearm, wrist, or hand. They most often are solitary and involve only one upper extremity. However, lesions involving both hands, or even involving a foot, are sometimes seen. The sucking blister resolves spontaneously as soon as bottle or breast is offered as a dietary substitute.

Figure 860

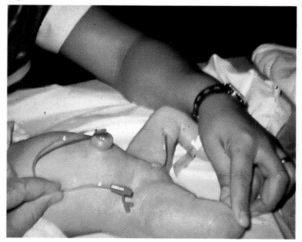

Figure 861

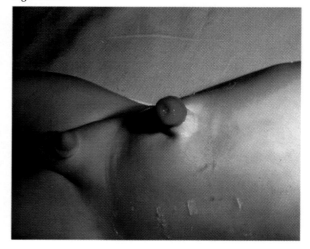

Anomalies of umbilical maldevelopment   A number of developmental abnormalities may accompany an umbilicus with abnormal appearance. Figure 860 shows an umbilicus that gives exit to a patent urachus. The persistent urachus is due to failure of closure of the allantoic duct. This diagnosis is usually suggested by the presence of a clear liquid discharge from the

umbilicus. The bright red polyp in Fig. 861 is a remnant of the distal portion of the omphalomesenteric duct. The mucosal lining of this lesion may represent small intestine, stomach, or colon. Fistulas of the duct, Meckel's diverticulum, and ileal prolapse may accompany this malformation. Treatment in all cases is surgical.

Figure 862

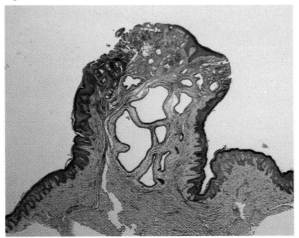

Histopathology of omphalomesenteric duct remnant Of all possible umbilical anomalies, the one related to the gastrointestinal tract is usually missed clinically but is easily diagnosed microscopically. Therefore, persistent abnormalities on and around the umbilicus should be biopsied. Here one sees a sessile lesion covered by stratified squamous epithelium and bearing two foci of enteral epithelium near the summit. There are prominent glands and cystic structures within the lesion.

Figure 863

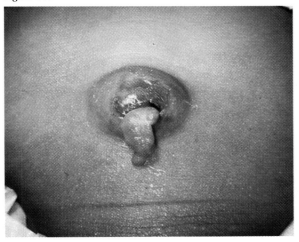

Umbilical granuloma It is normal for the umbilical cord to separate about 6 to 8 days after birth and for the resulting wound to heal within 2 weeks. This process may be slowed by a mild infection at the base of the cord, and it is sometimes complicated by the invasion of true pathogenic organisms. Pictured here is the formation of heaped-up granulation tissue at and in the umbilicus—the so-called umbilical granuloma. Treatment by repeated cauterization with silver nitrate is usually successful.

Figure 864

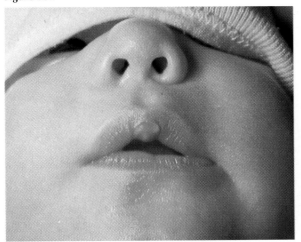

The appearance of the lips of suckling infants The cheeks and lips of neonates are normally well adapted for suckling. The cheeks have fat-padded musculature to produce strong suction, and the lips have surface markings that help to hold a nipple firmly. In this photograph one sees a tubercle in the center of the upper lip and serrations to each side of it and on the entire surface of the lower lip. In feeding, these formations deepen and make grip all the firmer.

Figure 865

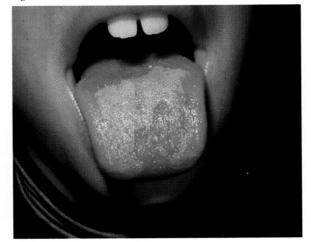

Geographic tongue There is a peculiar condition of the tongue that takes the form of denudations of the lingual surface in patches of redness that shift in position from time to time over hours and days. The cause of the condition is not known; there may be some relationship to psoriasis. No treatment is effective. The condition is largely asymptomatic except for slight tingling when sharp food is taken.

Figure 866

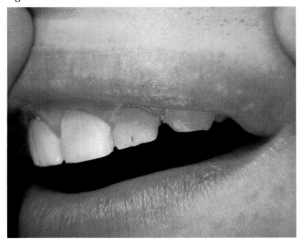

Fordyce's condition   The face abounds in sebaceous glands. Normally their distribution stops sharply at the junction of the skin and vermilion of the lips. Commonly, however, ectopic sebaceous glands are found within the lips under the vermilion and sometimes within the oral mucosa of the lips and even in the buccal mucosa. The condition is harmless and may have been present long before the patient or parents became aware of it. No treatment is required or available.

Figure 867

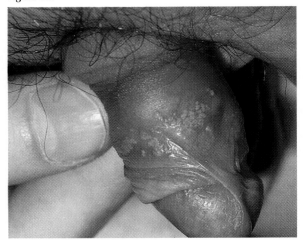

Tyson's glands   The prepuce of the penis has sebaceous glands, known as Tyson's glands, that open directly to the surface of the skin. These glands appear as very small yellow papules and may be prominent in some males, as is seen in this figure.

Figure 868

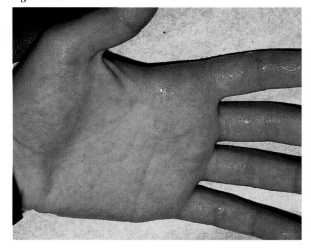

Hyperhidrosis   This disorder entails excessive sweating that may be localized to specific body regions or may be generalized. This figure represents palmar hyperhidrosis. Hyperhidrosis of the palms and soles tends to increase during periods of stress.

Figure 869

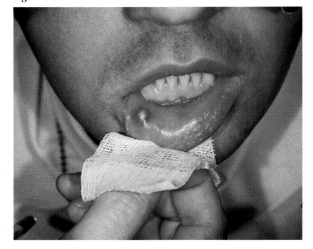

Mucocele   The lower lip is studded with cells that produce mucus. Mucoceles are cysts deriving from such cells. They appear as papules that are visibly and palpably filled with highly viscous fluid. They are harmless and asymptomatic but require extirpation because they make themselves felt when within the mouth and are cosmetically objectionable when on the lips. When reasonably small, like the one pictured here, electrodesiccation and curettage are sufficient; larger lesions may require scalpel surgery.

Index

Note: Reference numbers in this index are the figure numbers.

ISBN 0-07-069249-1

9 780070 692497

90000